THE CANADIAN
ENCYCLOPEDIA
OF
NATURAL
MEDICINE

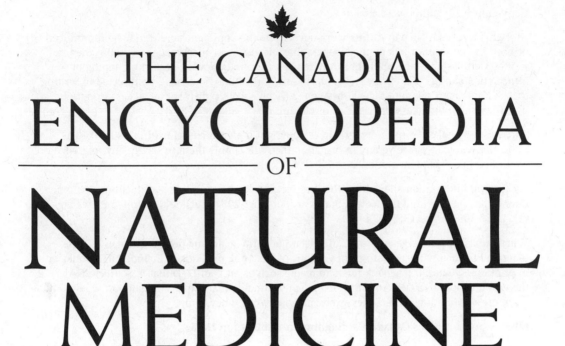

THE CANADIAN ENCYCLOPEDIA
OF
NATURAL MEDICINE

2nd Edition

by Sherry Torkos, BSc Phm

WILEY

John Wiley & Sons Canada, Ltd.

For general information about our other products and services, please contact our Customer Care Department within the United States at (800) 762-2974, outside the United States at (317) 572-3993 or fax (317) 572-4002.

Wiley publishes in a variety of print and electronic formats and by print-on-demand. Some material included with standard print versions of this book may not be included in e-books or in print-on-demand. If this book refers to media such as a CD or DVD that is not included in the version you purchased, you may download this material at http://booksupport.wiley.com. For more information about Wiley products, visit www.wiley.com.

Library and Archives Canada Cataloguing in Publication Data

Torkos, Sherry
      The Canadian encyclopedia of natural medicine / Sherry Torkos. – 2nd ed.

Includes index.
ISBN 978-1-118-37500-6 (pbk); 978-1-118-57152-1 (ebk); 978-1-118-57153-8 (ebk); 978-1-118-57154-5 (ebk)

      1. Naturopathy—Encyclopedias. 2. Self-care, Health—Encyclopedias. 3. Symptoms—Encyclopedias. I. Title.

RZ433.T67 2012   615.5'3503   C2012-902362-0

Production Credits
Cover design: Ian Koo
Interior text design: Adrian So
Author photo: Precious LaPlante
Managing Editor: Alison Maclean
Production Editor: Lindsay Humphreys
Composition: Laserwords
Printer: Friesens Printing

John Wiley & Sons Canada, Ltd.
6045 Freemont Blvd.
Mississauga, Ontario
L5R 4J3

Printed in Canada

1 2 3 4 5 FP 17 16 15 14 13

CONTENTS

ACKNOWLEDGEMENTS

There are many people that I would like to thank for their help and support with this book.

To my husband Rick, my son Phoenix, and my entire family, who have stood by and supported me as I prepared this second edition, I thank you for your patience and understanding of my commitment to this project and all the long hours it required.

To my medical advisory board: Dr. Elvis Ali, Jean-Yves Dionne, Rhonda Dorren, Donnie Edwards, Sam Graci, Dr. George Grant, Karlene Karst, Brad King, Dr. Michael Lyon, Tracy Marsden, Dr. Joey Shulman, Lorna Vanderhaeghe, and Farid Wassef, I appreciate your time and expertise in reviewing sections of my manuscript. To Dr. Bryce Wylde, many thanks for providing the homeopathic recommendations throughout this book and for sharing your knowledge and passion.

To the team at Wiley: Jennifer Smith, Robert Hickey, Lindsay Humphreys, and the design department, thanks for all your help throughout this project.

To my copyeditor, Leanne Rancourt, I appreciate all your hard work in reviewing my manuscript and your fine editorial assistance.

Finally I would like to thank you, the reader, for your interest in health and wellness and for your desire to read this book.

ADVISORY BOARD

Elvis Ali BSc, FIACA, RAc, DHom, ND

Dr. Ali graduated with a Bachelor of Science majoring in Biology in 1979, and received his Doctorate of Naturopathic Medicine in 1987. He has been in private practice for 25 years, specializing in Chinese medicine, sports medicine, and nutrition. He is a staff member at the Canadian College of Naturopathic Medicine, a professor at the Canadian College of Holistic Health, and a director of the Ontario Board of Acupuncture and Chinese Medicine. Dr. Ali is currently involved in seminars, quality control, and research and development of nutritional products at Swiss Natural. He has published papers, serves on *Alive Magazine*'s editorial advisory board, has written and co-authored several books, has conducted lectures internationally, and has appeared on a number of radio and TV shows.

Jean-Yves Dionne BSc Pharm

Jean-Yves Dionne is a pharmacist, speaker, writer, scientific adviser, and natural health products consultant. He is a regular lecturer at Université Laval and Université de Montréal. He has won several prizes for his work, such as the Aventis Pharma award for outstanding contribution to teaching from Université de Montréal, and Pharmacien de coeur et d'action from his peers and Rogers Communications. Jean-Yves is the author of several books on natural health products both in French and English. In 1999 he co-authored *Herbs: Everyday Reference for Health Professionals*. He is a regular contributor to *L'actualité pharmaceutique*, *Drugstore Canada*, *Québec Pharmacie*, *Vitalité Québec*, and *Alive Magazine*.

Rhonda Dorren BSc Pharm

Rhonda Dorren received her Bachelor of Science degree in Pharmacy at the University of Alberta in Edmonton. A licensed pharmacist in Alberta and an author, she is the founder of ChiQue Pharma Clinic, helping clients with their natural medicine and lifestyle needs using multicomponent interventions.

Donnie Edwards RPh, BSc Pharm

Donnie Edwards is co-owner of Boggio & Edwards IDA pharmacy in Ridgeway, Ontario. He specializes in compounding, pain management, women's health, and addiction services. Donnie is a sought-after speaker and media commentator on issues affecting pharmacists, collaborative health care, and government policy. He is a noted expert on addiction, and had a key role in the implementation of a school-based education program on addiction. He has travelled across Canada educating thousands about substance use, abuse, addiction, and dependence. Donnie is a past chair and former CEO of the Ontario Pharmacists' Association.

Sam Graci

Sam Graci is a Canadian lifestyle researcher and the author of four best-selling books in Canada, including most recently *The Bone-Building Solution,* which he co-authored with Carolyn DeMarco, MD, and Leticia Rao, PhD. His books are written on 100 percent recycled paper with biodegradable vegetable ink, and a portion of the proceeds from their sale are donated to Scouts Canada and to non-profit environmental groups.

George Grant MSc, EdD, CChem, RM

Dr. Grant is a multi-talented scientist and lecturer, a prolific author, and Canada's top stress-management and wellness coach. He is the founder of the International Academy of Wellness, and has pioneered research on beta endorphins, HPLC analysis of B-vitamins, and anti-cancer medicines.

Karlene Karst RD

Karlene Karst is a leading expert on nutrition and natural health. Karlene is the author of several books, including her newly released *The Full-Fat Solution.* She is a frequent guest speaker at educational events around North America and appears regularly on *Canada AM.* Visit her at www.karlenekarst.com.

Brad King MSc, MFS

Brad King is one of Canada's most sought-after authorities on nutrition, obesity, and longevity. He is the author of 10 books, including the international bestsellers *Fat Wars* and *Beer Belly Blues,* and is a 2003 inductee into the Canadian Sports Nutrition Hall of Fame. His free monthly newsletter, *Awaken Your Body,* can be found at www.awakenyourbody.com.

Michael R. Lyon BSc, MD

Dr. Lyon is the Medical and Research Director for the Canadian Centre for Functional Medicine in Vancouver, B.C. He heads a team dedicated to biotechnology, nutritional, and natural health product research. He is involved in collaborative clinical research with various Canadian universities and the Imperial College of Medicine in London, England, in the fields of obesity, diabetes, and appetite regulation, and with the University of British Columbia in the areas of childhood learning and behavioural disorders. Dr. Lyon is the author of *Healing the Hyperactive Brain through the New Science of Functional Medicine* and *Is Your Child's Brain Starving?* He is the co-author of *How to Prevent and Treat Diabetes with Natural Medicine, Beat Diabetes Naturally,* and *Hunger Free Forever: The New Science of Appetite Control.*

Tracy Marsden BSc Pharm

Tracy Marsden earned science and pharmacy degrees from the University of Alberta and worked in a community pharmacy setting for over 15 years. Her enthusiasm for wellness prompted her to obtain additional training in herbals and homeopathy. She worked several years as a natural medicine consultant for a pharmacy chain, and has consulted for several natural products manufacturers and contributed to a variety of natural medicine publications, including a regular CAM Review column for *Pharmacy Post* (now *Drugstore Canada*) and articles in *Natural Medicine Review, VitalLink,* and *Integrated Health Retailer.* She is co-author of the bestselling book *You've Hit Menopause, Now What?* and is currently vice-president of Rocky Mountain Analytical, a private Canadian wellness-focused medical laboratory.

Joey Shulman DC, RHN

Dr. Joey's passion for health and nutrition has been the focus of her career for over a decade. Her philosophy of "improve the quality of your food to improve the quality of your life" has enhanced the health of thousands of people across North America. As a two-time national bestselling author and a well-known media personality, Dr. Joey is a highly regarded authority on weight loss, health, and nutrition. She is a sought-after speaker who inspires, entertains, and educates large audiences in Canada and the United States.

Lorna Vanderhaeghe MSc

Lorna Vanderhaeghe is Canada's leading women's natural health expert. With a Master of Science in Nutrition and a degree in Biochemistry, she is the author of 11 books, including most recently *A Smart Woman's Guide to Hormones* and *A Smart Woman's Guide to Weight Loss*. In 2011, Lorna was listed as one of Canada's top 100 female entrepreneurs. She has a free monthly newsletter available at her website, www.hormonehelp.com.

Farid Wassef BSc Pharm, RPh, CCN

Farid Wassef is a community pharmacist who has been in practice in Stouffville, Ontario, since 1989. In 2003, Farid co-authored *Breaking the Age Barrier: Strategies for Optimal Health, Energy, and Longevity*. He has been invited to appear on a number of radio and television programs to discuss health promotion, disease prevention, and the safe and effective use of prescription medicines and natural health products. In 2006, Farid was honoured as Canadian Pharmacist of the Year for his excellence in patient care and innovation in public health.

Bryce Wylde BSc, RNC, DHMHS, HD

Bryce Wylde is a highly knowledgeable and respected natural health care clinician whose specialty is homeopathy, clinical nutrition, supplementation, and botanical medicine. Bryce holds a Bachelor of Science honours degree in Biology and Psychology, and a Diploma in Homeopathic Medicine and Health Sciences. He is a regular expert guest on many shows, including *The Doctor Oz Show*, *The Marilyn Denis Show*, *Canada AM*, *Breakfast Television*, *Steven and Chris*, The Discovery Channel, W Channel, and ABC's *Good Morning America Health*. Bryce is the author of the national best-seller *The Antioxidant Prescription: How to Use the Power of Antioxidants to Prevent Disease and Stay Healthy for Life* and *Wylde on Health: Your Best Choices in the World of Natural Health*.

INTRODUCTION

A PHARMACIST'S PERSPECTIVE
The Power of Natural Medicine in Modern Health

The history of medicine is a fascinating story of the transition from ancient healing techniques to brilliant scientific and technological advances. We have gone from using medicine men and plant-based remedies to creating pharmaceutical drugs and sophisticated surgical procedures. Undoubtedly, medicine today now provides us with the ability to fight off deadly diseases and live longer lives; however, we must not forget that many solutions can still be found in nature. In fact, many of the prescription medications used today are derived from plants. As well, we must be aware that lifestyle factors—diet, activity level, sleep, and environment—play a critical role in health and disease prevention.

In the last 20 years, we've witnessed a growing desire to look to natural remedies first before taking prescription medications that may have drug interactions, side effects, and high costs. According to a 2010 Ipsos Reid survey, 73 percent of Canadians regularly take natural health products (NHPs) such as vitamins and minerals, herbal products, and homeopathic medicines.

There is increasing interest in prevention for both minor and chronic health concerns and a growing awareness of the need to take responsibility for one's health. In the Ipsos Reid survey mentioned above, some of the most common reasons why people take NHPs were to maintain health, to prevent illness, and an overall general concern about one's health. A large proportion of Canadians (71 percent) believe that natural health products are better for them than chemical products or drugs. People are no longer satisfied with the idea of taking a drug to fix their problems. They are starting to question the indiscriminate use of prescription drugs and the motivations behind the industry, and they are becoming better educated about their options.

I have also witnessed a growing awareness among doctors, pharmacists, and other health care professionals in holistic therapies. When I first started practising pharmacy in 1992, the overall knowledge and acceptance of natural medicine was quite low among most health care professionals. This has gradually been improving over the years, driven primarily by the public's interest and use of these therapies, but we still have a long way to go before mainstream medicine and natural medicine are fully integrated. And that's where I come in. As a traditionally trained pharmacist with a complementary background in natural health, nutrition, and fitness, my goal is to bridge the gap between the two worlds and, in doing so, help people along their journey to optimal health.

MY JOURNEY WITH NATURAL MEDICINE

My interest in natural medicine came from a personal experience. As a young teen I suffered from undiagnosed celiac disease, a genetic condition in which the ingestion of gluten, which is a protein found in many grains, triggers an autoimmune reaction in the body. For several years, I experienced abdominal pain, bloating, weight loss, fatigue, visual impairment, hair loss, and skin rashes. Despite seeing several doctors, I did not get a proper diagnosis and was instead given large doses of unnecessary prescription medications.

I was sick almost every day for nearly four years. As my health continued to deteriorate, I developed both physical and emotional symptoms. I suffered with depression, poor concentration, and impaired memory. What I didn't know at the time was that gluten was destroying the absorptive surface of my intestines, causing malnutrition, wasting, and damage to vital organs.

Luckily for me, my parents never gave up. Finally, after much searching, we found a doctor who immediately recognized my symptoms as celiac disease and put me on a strict gluten-free diet. My stomach symptoms gradually improved on the restricted diet. However, my health was far from restored. I was still quite fatigued and forgetful, and suffered with eczema, poor night vision, and lack of hair growth. This is when I turned to holistic therapies. I read, researched, and investigated how to improve my health. I began taking therapeutic dosages of vitamins, minerals, and essential fatty acids to correct the deficiencies that I had experienced for so many years. Slowly, but steadily, I began to return to a state of optimal health.

Coping with a health problem at such a young age was a life-altering experience and filled me with a passion for health and a willingness to look "outside the box" for answers. After high school, I studied science, pharmacy, and nutrition in Philadelphia and went on to build a holistic pharmacy practice in the Niagara area of Ontario. In my practice, I have worked with many people facing serious health challenges, such as heart disease, diabetes, cancer, and depression, and I have seen how remarkably well the body can heal and repair itself when it is given the proper elements.

ABOUT THIS BOOK

My intention with this book is to have people refer to it for both prevention and treatment of health conditions, and then consult with their health care practitioner for proper guidance and monitoring. *I must stress that the information in this book is not intended to diagnose or replace the advice of your doctor or health care provider. Under no circumstances should you stop taking existing medications or combine supplements with existing medications without consulting your doctor first.* I believe that conventional medicine does offer benefits when used appropriately, but I also believe that nutritional therapies, herbs, exercise, meditation, and other holistic measures can provide potential solutions and significant steps toward prevention and as such should be given equal consideration. Knowledge and understanding about natural therapies is imperative before you can integrate it into your life.

In some cases striking the balance between the two modalities is easier said than done. Difficulties arise because many mainstream health practitioners remain cautious or even skeptical about the benefits of natural remedies. By providing comprehensive, science-based information on natural medicine, I hope to provide you with a sound resource that can be taken to your health care provider when discussing a health concern. As such, the information provided in this book reflects the most recent data from scientific studies, in many cases published in respected medical journals. I refer to research throughout the book, and only recommend supplements and therapies that have been studied and found to be beneficial. I also note drug interactions, contraindications, and side effects where relevant.

The first edition of this book was released in 2007, and I am pleased to say that it has met with tremendous success. I had incredibly positive feedback from folks across the country who used this book as a guide for understanding and improving their health. Reception was just as positive from doctors, pharmacists, nurses, dietitians, and many others who are involved in providing recommendations on NHPs.

Because science and our understanding of disease states and health are constantly evolving, I was eager to put together a second edition of this book. This new edition contains many updates and revisions, including the most recent guidelines for micronutrient intake (vitamins and minerals), expanded information on managing various health conditions, new research on supplements and dietary therapies that can play a role in preventing and treating important health conditions such as diabetes, heart disease, arthritis, and cancer, along with vital precautions about side effects, recently discovered drug–supplement interactions, and many other important facts to help guide you in making decisions about your health.

HOW TO USE THIS BOOK

My book is divided into four sections. In Section One, there are six chapters that outline my Prescription for Successful Living.

- Chapter 1 outlines the macronutrients—the proteins, carbohydrates, and fats that are the basic components of our diet.
- Chapter 2 provides details on the micronutrients—the essential vitamins and minerals.
- Chapter 3 highlights the functional foods that provide health benefits beyond nutrition.
- Chapter 4 will give you my top 10 principles for a healthy diet.
- Chapter 5 describes the benefits of physical activity and offers guidelines and tips on incorporating exercise into your lifestyle.

- Chapter 6 discusses the importance of sleep and stress management, two often overlooked elements that are essential for health.

   In Section Two, you will find The Natural Pharmacy.

- Chapter 7 offers a reference guide to 66 of the most common and widely recommended dietary supplements.
- Chapter 8 provides my principles for safe supplementation—guidelines and recommendations on choosing and using natural remedies, complete with medicine cabinet musts and healthy travel kit ideas.

   Section Three covers the 88 most common health conditions from A to Z.

- Each condition is described, including causes, symptoms, and risk factors. Conventional medical approaches are discussed, after which I offer a natural prescription, including dietary strategies, lifestyle recommendations, and supplements. Throughout this section, renowned homeopath Bryce Wylde has contributed information on homeopathic treatments for some of the most common conditions. (For more about homeopathy, see Appendix F, also contributed by Bryce Wylde.)

   If you are coping with a health condition listed in this book, it is not my intention that you follow every recommendation I make. Instead, implement as many of the lifestyle and dietary strategies as possible and discuss my supplement recommendations with your health care provider. Under my "Top Recommended Supplements" section I list those that are supported by scientific research to offer benefits for the particular condition. Next, I list "Complementary Supplements"—those that offer some benefits or play a supportive role; these would be secondary considerations.

   Because many supplements have similar effects on the body, and there are potential interactions between drugs and supplements, it is recommended that you consult with your health care provider before taking a new product. Unlike many drugs, supplements may take weeks to months before the full effect is achieved, so patience is required.

   In addition to your primary health care provider, you may want to look for additional health care providers who offer different perspectives, such as a naturopathic or homeopathic doctor, registered dietitian, massage therapist, acupuncturist, or chiropractor. When looking for alternative health care providers, make sure they are properly trained and always check references. You may also want to find a pharmacist in your area who, like myself, has a broad range of knowledge in natural medicine. Pharmacists are always available, without an appointment, to answer questions and discuss your concerns, especially about medications.

   Section Four contains the appendices—the supplementary charts, tables, and resources that are referred to throughout this book, along with information about homeopathy and its background, philosophy, and scientific basis.

   Over 20 years ago, I discovered the power of natural medicine for myself. That discovery set a course for my future that has taken me around the world from pharmacies and medical clinics, to lecture halls and conferences, through the writing of several health books, and finally to the publication of this encyclopedia. This latest edition reflects hundreds of hours of research, collaboration with my medical advisory team, and feedback from my readers and my publisher. My message to you is this: Don't wait for health problems to arise. Take a proactive approach now. Learn about the power of nutrition, exercise, supplements, stress management, and other lifestyle factors in the prevention of disease and take the necessary steps today. If you are currently struggling with a health problem, realize that there are options and that a plan that incorporates a variety of healing modalities will most likely provide you with the best possible outcome.

I hope I've provided you with a useful resource to achieve optimum health for you and your family. I wish you all the best as you create your own prescription for successful and healthy living!

Sherry Torkos

SECTION I

PRESCRIPTION FOR
SUCCESSFUL LIVING

CHAPTER 1

MACRONUTRIENTS

Macronutrients are essential nutrients—carbohydrates, proteins, and fats—that the body needs for energy and proper growth, metabolism, and function. They are called "macro" because we need these nutrients in large quantities compared to the micronutrients (vitamins and minerals), which are needed in smaller quantities. In this chapter I will explain the various macronutrients, recommended intakes, and the best food sources. In Chapter 4 I will outline principles for a healthy diet—my top recommendations for a nutritional plan for optimal health and disease prevention.

PROTEIN

Protein is a necessary component for building, maintaining, and repairing many body systems and processes, including

- Production of collagen and keratin, which are the structural components of bones, teeth, hair, and the outer layer of skin; they help maintain the structure of blood vessels;
- Manufacture of hormones, such as insulin and thyroid hormone;
- Production of enzymes that control chemical reactions in the body;
- Proper immune function—production of antibodies, white blood cells, and other immune factors;
- Transportation of oxygen, vitamins, and minerals to target cells throughout the body; and
- Source of energy—the liver can use protein to make glucose when there is not enough carbohydrate available, such as when you skip a meal or follow a low-carb diet.

Food Sources

Protein is found in animal products, nuts, and legumes, and to a lesser extent in fruits and vegetables. Protein is made of smaller components called amino acids. Twelve amino acids are manufactured by the human body and are called non-essential; another nine, called essential amino acids, must be obtained from food.

Proteins that provide all the essential amino acids are referred to as *complete* proteins. Your best sources are chicken, turkey, fish, dairy, and eggs. Choose free-range and organic wherever possible to reduce ingesting harmful hormones and chemicals. Certain plants also provide complete proteins, such as amaranth, buckwheat, chia seed, hemp seed, quinoa, and spirulina.

Plant proteins do not contain all the essential amino acids and are considered *incomplete* proteins. It is possible, though, to combine various plant proteins to get all the essential amino acids. For example, eating oats, lentils, and sunflower seeds either together or separately throughout the day provides all the essential amino acids. Combining beans with rice or hummus with pita bread also provides complete proteins. You could also combine whole-wheat pasta with white kidney beans or tofu with brown rice to get all the necessary amino acids. It just requires careful meal planning.

There are certain advantages to eating plant over animal proteins: Plants provide fibre and phytochemicals (antioxidants), do not contain saturated fat, and may play a role in disease prevention. Soy protein, for example, has been shown to significantly lower cholesterol and triglyceride levels, and protect against bone loss. A number of studies have found a lower risk of chronic disease in those who eat a plant-based diet.

CARBOHYDRATES

Carbohydrates have gotten a bad rap over the past few years, and while eating too many carbohydrates and the wrong types of carbohydrates can have detrimental effects on your health, there are still may reasons why we need to include the right carbohydrates in our diet. Carbohydrates are the body's main source of fuel—glucose, which is needed by every cell in our body. They also provide valuable nutrients (vitamins, minerals, and essential fatty acids) and fibre, which is important for intestinal health.

Food Sources

There are two classes of carbohydrates—simple and complex. Simple carbohydrates include naturally occurring sugars in milk and fruit, and refined sugars (granulated sugar). There is a major difference among these simple carbohydrates: fruits offer a range of nutrients and fibre, while refined sugars provide empty calories and lack nutritional value. Excess sugar consumption is linked to dental caries, obesity, insulin resistance, high triglyceride levels, low HDL (good) cholesterol, and compromised immune function. The World Health Organization recommends reducing sugar intake to below 10 percent of total calories. Aside from candy and baked goods, sugar is also found in soft drinks, condiments (ketchup, barbecue sauce), juices, ice cream, and other sweets.

Complex carbohydrates include starches and indigestible dietary fibre. Starches are found in bread, pasta, rice, beans, and some vegetables. Again, there are major differences among complex carbohydrates. Today many of our starches are refined and processed, which strips the food of its fibre and nutrients. For example, white bread, pasta, and rice are much less nutritious and break down into sugar very rapidly, so choose the brown or whole-grain products.

Dietary fibre is found in fruits, vegetables, beans, and the indigestible parts of whole grains such as wheat and oat bran. In addition to supporting intestinal health and proper elimination, fibre also improves blood sugar balance, lowers cholesterol, reduces the risk of colon and breast cancer, and plays a role in weight management.

The Institute of Medicine, which provides recommendations that are adopted by the United States and Canada, recommends the following daily intake for fibre:

Men 19 to 50 years: 38 grams
Men over 50 years: 30 grams
Women 19 to 50 years: 25 grams
Women over 50 years: 21 grams
Pregnant women: 28 grams
Lactating women: 29 grams

To boost fibre intake, incorporate more raw vegetables, fruits, whole grains, and legumes in your diet and consider a fibre supplement.

Glycemic Index

The glycemic index (GI) is a scale that measures how quickly carbohydrates are broken down into sugar. Those that are broken down quickly—such as simple carbohydrates and refined starches—have a high GI. Foods that are broken down slowly—such as most vegetables, fruits, and unprocessed grains—have a low GI.

Numerous studies have linked high-GI diets to obesity, insulin resistance, type 2 diabetes, and increased risk of heart disease. Eating high-GI foods can lead to blood sugar imbalances that may result in fatigue, increased appetite, and food cravings. For these reasons, it is best to minimize high-GI foods and maximize your intake of low-GI foods. See Appendix B for more information on the glycemic index and the rating for common foods.

FATS

"Fat" has become a negative word as it is associated with obesity, yet we do need a certain amount of fat in our diets and on our bodies, and there are health benefits to be obtained by eating certain fats. The point to keep in mind is that there are *good* fats and *bad* fats.

Good Fats

The good fats are the monounsaturated and polyunsaturated fats. Monounsaturated fats are found predominantly in olive, canola, peanut, palm, and safflower oils. The polyunsaturated fats provide us with essential fatty acids (EFAs), which are broken down into two groups:

Omega-6 fatty acids: Linoleic acid (LA), which is converted into gamma-linolenic acid (GLA) and arachidonic acid (AA)
Omega-3 fatty acids: Alpha-linolenic acid (ALA), which is converted into eicosapentaenoic acid (EPA) and docosahexaenoic acid (DHA)

The body cannot make EFAs, so they must be obtained through diet or supplementation. They are essential for many body processes and functions, including the following:

- Growth and development of the brain, nervous system, adrenal glands, sex organs, inner ear, and eyes;
- Energy (fat is the most concentrated source of energy);
- Absorbing fat-soluble vitamins (vitamins A, D, E, K, and carotenoids);
- Maintaining cell membrane integrity;
- Regulation of cell processes such as gene activation and expression, enzyme function, and fat oxidation; and
- Production of hormones and chemical messengers.

Food Sources

Here is a breakdown of the EFAs and their sources:

- **LA:** Found in vegetable oils such as safflower, evening primrose, sunflower, corn, hemp, canola, palm, olive, and soybean oil.
- **GLA:** Found in borage, black currant, and evening primrose oils.
- **AA:** Found in meat and eggs. We get adequate AA through diet; too much of this fat is not good, as it causes inflammation.
- **ALA:** Found in flaxseed, hemp seed, soy, and canola, and to a lesser extent in nuts, green leafy vegetables, wheat germ, and black currant seeds.
- **EPA and DHA:** Found in fatty fish, such as salmon, mackerel, herring, cod, sardines, and tuna.

There is great controversy over what constitutes the optimal dietary intake ratio of omega-6 to omega-3 fatty acids. It is estimated that we currently get around 15:1, whereas leading EFA authorities recommend a ratio closer to 4:1 or even 2:1.

The Institute of Medicine has set an adequate intake level for linoleic acid for adults 19 to 50 years of age at 17 g per day for men and 12 g per day for women; alpha-linolenic acid at 1.6 g per day for men and 1.1 g per day for women. These levels are lower for younger and older individuals.

Rather than trying to calculate the perfect ratio or intake, aim to have more omega-3s (fish, flaxseed, hemp, and fish oils) and GLA (borage, black currant, or primrose oil) from diet or supplements, as these are the beneficial fats that are commonly deficient.

Diets rich in the omega-3 fatty acids offer cardiovascular protection by lowering blood cholesterol and triglyceride levels, reducing blood clotting, and reducing the risk of heart attack and sudden death. These fats also reduce inflammation and are helpful for arthritis and other inflammatory disorders. GLA also reduces inflammation, prevents clotting, dilates blood vessels, improves skin health, and benefits those with diabetes and arthritis.

Bad Fats

The "bad" fats are the saturated fats, trans fats, and cholesterol. Diets high in these fats have been associated with health risks, namely elevated blood cholesterol levels and an increased risk of heart disease. However, in recent years research has revealed that there are some exceptions in this category.

Saturated Fats

Saturated fats are found in animal products such as meat, poultry, milk, cheese, butter, and lard, as well as in tropical oils (such as palm, palm kernel, and coconut oil) and foods made from these oils. These fats are high in cholesterol, and high cholesterol diets have been linked to heart disease, high cholesterol, obesity, and cancers of the breast, colon, and prostate. However, recent research has revealed that not all saturated fats are the same and some surprising health benefits have emerged with some of these oils. In particular, coconut and palm fruit oil, which are also rich in polyunsaturated fatty acids and various antioxidants and nutrients, have been found to have a neutral or beneficial effect on cholesterol levels when they are consumed as an alternate to other fats in the diet. There may be other benefits with these oils. Emerging science suggests that coconut oil can support immune health and weight management (by raising metabolism) and palm oil offers benefits for cognitive function and brain health.

Most people get 38 percent or more of their day's calories from fat while health authorities suggest no more than 20 to 35 percent, of which less than 10 percent should come from saturated fat. To cut your intake of saturated fat, trim fat and skin from meat, choose lean poultry over red meat, and choose low-fat cheese and dairy (cottage cheese, feta, and hard cheeses have less fat). Butter is fine in moderation.

· ·

BUTTER VS. MARGARINE

For years margarine was considered to be a healthier alternative to butter, but some margarines contain hydrogenated oils (trans fats), which are artificially processed fats linked to heart disease and cancer. The exception is non-hydrogenated margarines, such as Becel. You can also find non-hydrogenated margarines fortified with beneficial plant sterols that can help lower cholesterol. While butter contains saturated fats, they are short-chain saturates, which are easily digested and provide a source of usable energy. Butter also contains nutrients: lecithin, vitamins A and E, and selenium. So the bottom line is: Choose butter or a non-hydrogenated margarine and enjoy in moderation.

· ·

Trans Fatty Acids

Trans fatty acids are naturally found in small amounts in animal products; however, the majority of trans fats in our diet come from the artificial form. Trans fats are created when oils undergo a chemical process called hydrogenation, which solidifies them—this is the process that makes vegetable oil into margarine. Trans fat is also found in cookies, crackers, french fries, baked goods, and other snack foods.

When trans fats were first introduced into our food supply, they were thought to be a healthier alternative to saturated fats. Many years later this was found to be false. Trans fats elevate cholesterol levels, increasing the risk for heart disease and heart attack, and are also linked to cancer, particularly breast cancer. The Institute of Medicine has stated that there is no safe limit for trans fats in the diet and that we should reduce consumption of these dangerous fats. Food companies have been making efforts in this area; many manufacturers have reformulated products to be free of trans fats. You will now see many packaged foods labelled "trans fat free."

Cholesterol

Cholesterol is a waxy substance found in the fats (lipids) in our blood. It is manufactured in the liver and also obtained from consuming foods that contain cholesterol, such as organ meats, whole-milk products, and egg yolks. Cholesterol is seen as a bad fat because high blood cholesterol levels are a known risk factor for heart disease. But cholesterol is not all bad—the body requires it to produce sex hormones and maintain cell membranes and a healthy nervous system.

Aside from diet, cholesterol levels can be elevated by family history, lack of activity, stress, and liver disorders. Eating high amounts of saturated and trans fat can also raise cholesterol levels.

As with fats, there is good and bad when it comes to cholesterol. The good cholesterol is HDL (high-density lipoproteins) and the bad is LDL (low-density lipoproteins). LDL cholesterol can build up in the artery walls of the brain and heart, narrowing the passageways for blood flow, a process known as atherosclerosis, the precursor to heart disease and stroke.

HDL cholesterol is called good cholesterol because it picks up the LDL cholesterol deposited in the arteries and transports it to the liver to be broken down and eliminated.

To lower LDL and raise HDL levels, exercise regularly, minimize saturated fats, avoid trans fats, and don't smoke (smoking lowers HDL).

MACRONUTRIENT INTAKE

The Institute of Medicine recommends ranges for macronutrient intake that are associated with a reduced risk of chronic disease while providing adequate intake of essential nutrients. They suggest that adults get 45 to 65 percent of calories from carbohydrates, 20 to 35 percent from fat, and 10 to 35 percent from protein. Ranges for children are similar except that infants and younger children need a slightly higher proportion of fat (25 to 40 percent).

The recommended calorie intake varies depending on height, weight, gender, and activity level. For example, women ages 31 to 50 who are sedentary should consume around 1,800 calories daily. Those who are moderately active should consume 2,000 calories daily, and those who are active should consume 2,200 calories daily.

Macronutrients provide us with calories as follows:

Carbohydrate: 4 calories per gram
Protein: 4 calories per gram
Fat: 9 calories per gram

For example:

If a food product contains 10 g of carbohydrate, 2 g of protein, and 1 g of fat per serving, it would provide $10 \times 4 = 40$ calories from carbohydrate, $2 \times 4 = 8$ calories from protein, and $1 \times 9 = 9$ calories from fat for a total calorie count of 57 calories per serving.

MICRONUTRIENTS

Micronutrients are vitamins and minerals—nutrients that are required by the body in small amounts, yet have powerful effects. They assist in energy-producing reactions, growth, and development; protect against free radical damage; and perform many vital functions. Micronutrients are essential for health, and a deficiency can lead to health problems and disease.

The Institute of Medicine has developed nutrient references called the Dietary Reference Intakes (DRIs); the most recent report was released in 2010. These values are intended to serve as a guide for good nutrition and provide the scientific basis for the development of food guidelines in both the United States and Canada. These nutrient reference values are specified on the basis of age, gender, and life stage and cover more than 40 nutrient substances.

In this chapter I outline the essential vitamins, minerals, and trace elements, their functions in the body, their role in disease prevention and treatment, deficiency symptoms, drugs that deplete these nutrients, and supplement guidelines.

The table at the end of this chapter summarizes food sources, recommended intake levels, and possible side effects and toxicity for the various nutrients.

WHO NEEDS SUPPLEMENTS?

There are many factors that cause nutrient depletion, such as poor diet, stress, exercise, use of prescription drugs, environmental toxicity, and excessive alcohol intake. For many micronutrients, deficiency, inadequate intake, or nutrient depletion is common relative to the Recommended Dietary Allowance (RDA). This is why supplements are so important in making up for shortcomings in the diet and preventing deficiencies.

VITAMINS

There are 13 essential vitamins that our bodies need for proper growth, function, and maintenance of healthy tissues. Vitamins are divided into two categories: water soluble and fat soluble. The B-vitamins and vitamin C are in the water-soluble category.

The body must use water-soluble vitamins right away or they are eliminated in the urine. The exception is vitamin B12, which can be stored in the liver for many years. Adverse reactions, even with high-dose supplements, are rare with these vitamins. Fat-soluble vitamins (A, D, E, and K) are not readily excreted from the body. They are stored in the body's fatty tissue and have the potential to accumulate and cause adverse effects at high doses.

Vitamin A
- Required for vision, gene expression, reproduction, embryonic development, red blood cell production, and immune function.
- Prescription vitamin A derivatives are used to treat skin conditions (acne), retinitis pigmentosa (genetic eye disease), and acute promyelocytic leukemia.
- Deficiency is rare in Canada, but common in developing countries due to malnutrition. It causes night blindness, dry eyes and skin, and impaired growth. Those with zinc deficiency may be at particular risk.
- Vitamin A deficiency may worsen iron-deficiency anemia; vitamin A supplements can benefit those with iron-deficiency anemia by improving iron levels.
- Drugs that deplete vitamin A include cholestyramine, colestipol, mineral oil, and neomycin.
- Supplements should be avoided by those at risk of lung cancer (smokers) or liver toxicity (alcoholics, those with liver disease).
- Doses greater than 10,000 IU daily should be avoided by pregnant women due to the risk of birth defects. Most prenatal vitamins provide 5,000 IU. Vitamin A from beta carotene does not increase the risk of birth defects.
- Doses of preformed vitamin A greater than 5,000 IU may increase the risk of osteoporosis. This is not a concern with beta carotene.
- Supplements of vitamin A beyond what is provided in a multivitamin are not recommended due to risk of toxicity. To avoid this risk, choose a multivitamin that contains beta carotene, which is converted to vitamin A in the liver but is not associated with health risks.

Vitamin B1 (Thiamine)
- Required for energy production, nerve and muscle function, enzyme reactions, and fatty acid production.
- Deficiency causes beriberi, a disease that affects the cardiovascular, nervous, muscular, and gastrointestinal systems.
- Deficiency is common in developing countries; in North America it occurs in alcoholics, those with kidney disease or malabsorption syndromes (celiac disease), and those with poor diets. Conditions that increase thiamine requirement include pregnancy, breastfeeding, fever, strenuous physical exertion, and adolescent growth.
- Drugs that deplete vitamin B1 include furosemide, antibiotics, oral contraceptives, and phenytoin. Consuming large amounts of coffee or tea (even decaffeinated) can deplete thiamine due to the presence of anti-thiamine factors in these beverages.
- Most people get adequate thiamine from diet or a multivitamin.

Vitamin B2 (Riboflavin)
- Required for energy metabolism, enzyme reactions, vision, and skin/hair/nail health; functions as an antioxidant; activates vitamin B6, niacin, and folate.
- May play a role in preventing migraine headaches and cataracts.
- Deficiency occurs in alcoholics, the elderly, and those with poor diets. Deficiency may affect enzyme systems involved in production of other B-vitamins and increase the risk of deficiency of niacin, folic acid, and vitamin B6.
- Symptoms of deficiency include sore throat; redness/swelling of the mouth, throat, tongue, lips, and skin; cracks or sores on the outside of the lips and corners of mouth; scaly, red skin; decreased red blood cell count; and blood vessel growth over the eyes. Deficiency may impair iron absorption and increase risk of pre-eclampsia in pregnant women.
- Drugs that deplete vitamin B2 include antibiotics, chlorpromazine, amitriptyline, adriamycin, and phenobarbital.
- Most people get adequate riboflavin from diet or a multivitamin.

Vitamin B3 (Niacin)
- Required for energy metabolism, enzyme reactions, skin and nerve health, and digestion.
- High doses of nicotinic acid (3 g daily) can lower cholesterol (reduce LDL and triglyceride levels and increase HDL) and reduce the risk of heart attack and stroke; high dosages should be supervised by a physician. Nicotinamide may play a role in the prevention of type 1 diabetes in children. Preliminary research suggests that high dosages (3 g daily) can protect beta-cells and improve beta-cell function.
- Deficiency causes pellagra, the symptoms of which are skin rash, diarrhea, and dementia, and it may lead to death.
- Deficiency may be caused by poor diet, malabsorption diseases, dialysis, and HIV.
- Drugs that deplete vitamin B3 include antibiotics, isoniazid, and 5-Fluorouracil (chemotherapy).
- High-dose niacin, taken along with statin drugs (e.g., lovastatin), may increase the risk of rhabdomyolysis (muscle degeneration and kidney disease).
- Most people get adequate niacin from diet or a multivitamin; supplements may be recommended for those with high cholesterol. Supplements are available as nicotinamide or nicotinic acid. The latter is the form that has been studied for cholesterol-lowering benefits.

Vitamin B5 (Pantothenic Acid)
- Required for carbohydrate metabolism, adrenal function, enzyme reactions, and production of fats, cholesterol, bile acids, hormones, neurotransmitters, and red blood cells.
- Deficiency is rare, except in malnutrition, and causes burning/tingling in the hands and feet, fatigue, and headache.
- Drugs that deplete vitamin B5 include oral contraceptives, amitriptyline, imipramine, and desipramine.
- Most people get adequate niacin from diet or a multivitamin.

Vitamin B6 (Pyridoxine)

- Necessary for protein and fat metabolism, hormone function (estrogen and testosterone), and the production of red blood cells, niacin, and neurotransmitters (serotonin, dopamine, and norepinephrine).
- Used therapeutically for the treatment of PMS, morning sickness, carpal tunnel syndrome, and heart health (lowers homocysteine, an amino acid that, at high levels, can cause arteriosclerosis and build up arterial plaque).
- Deficiency is uncommon, except in alcoholics and the elderly, and causes seizures, irritability, depression, confusion, mouth sores, and impaired immune function.
- Drugs that deplete vitamin B6 include antibiotics, oral contraceptives, isoniazid, penicillamine, and Parkinson's drugs (levodopa).
- Supplements are recommended for the elderly, alcoholics, and those with poor diets.

Vitamin B12 (Cobalamin)

- Required for nerve function, synthesis of DNA and RNA, metabolism of energy, enzyme reactions, and production of red blood cells.
- Used therapeutically for heart health (lowers homocysteine), male infertility, prevention of neural tube defects, asthma, and cancer prevention.
- Deficiency is common among the elderly and those with poor diets, pernicious anemia, depression, those who have undergone abdominal surgery, or those with malabsorption conditions (such as celiac or Crohn's disease).
- Absorption of vitamin B12 from food requires proper functioning of the stomach, pancreas, and small intestine. Stomach acid and enzymes free vitamin B12 from food, allowing it to bind to proteins and get carried to the intestines where pancreatic enzymes free B12 to bind to intrinsic factor and get absorbed. Low stomach acid or inadequate levels of intrinsic factor can impair absorption of vitamin B12 and lead to deficiency.
- Deficiency symptoms include anemia, appetite loss, constipation, numbness and tingling in the extremities, and confusion. Pregnant women with deficiency have increased risk of giving birth to a child with neural tube defects.
- Drugs that deplete vitamin B12 include acid-lowering drugs (omeprazole, lansoprazole, ranitidine), oral contraceptives, antibiotics, cholestyramine, and metformin.
- Supplements are recommended for those over the age of 50, vegetarians, women planning to become pregnant, and those with poor diets.

Biotin

- Part of the B-vitamin family; involved in the synthesis of fat, glycogen, and amino acids and enzyme reactions; required for DNA replication; important for healthy hair and nails.
- Used therapeutically to treat brittle fingernails. Preliminary research suggests benefits for the treatment of diabetes by stimulating insulin secretion and improving blood glucose levels.
- Deficiency is rare except in those with hereditary disorders of biotin metabolism and liver disease. It is also common during pregnancy (due to increased needs) and

it is estimated that one-third of women develop marginal biotin deficiency during pregnancy. It can also occur in those who consume raw egg whites for prolonged periods (weeks to years), because a protein found in egg white (avidin) binds biotin and prevents its absorption, or in those given intravenous feeding without biotin supplementation.

- Deficiency symptoms include hair loss; a scaly red rash around the eyes, nose, mouth, and genital area; depression; lethargy; hallucination; numbness and tingling of the extremities; and impaired glucose utilization and immune system function.
- Drugs that deplete biotin include primidone, carbamazepine, phenobarbital, phenytoin, valproic acid, and antibiotics.
- Most people get adequate biotin from diet or supplements.

Folate (Folic Acid)

- Part of the B-vitamin family; known as folate when it occurs naturally in foods, or as folic acid when present in supplements or added to foods.
- Required for cell division, growth, amino acid metabolism, enzyme reactions, and production of RNA, DNA, and red blood cells.
- Used therapeutically to lower homocysteine levels and for prevention of cancer (colon and cervical) and birth defects (neural tube). There is also some evidence that folate may play a role in the prevention of Alzheimer's disease (through lowering homocysteine levels).
- Deficiency occurs in alcoholics and those with poor diets or malabsorption syndromes like celiac disease. Pregnancy or cancer results in increased rates of cell division and metabolism, increasing the need for folate.
- Symptoms of deficiency include anemia (megaloblastic), fatigue, weakness, headache, hair loss, diarrhea, and poor immune function.
- Drugs that deplete folate include non-steroidal anti-inflammatory drugs (NSAIDs) such as ibuprofen and aspirin, phenytoin, methotrexate, phenobarbital, cholestyramine, colestipol, trimethoprim, and sulfasalazine.
- Supplements are routinely recommended for women who are pregnant or planning to becoming pregnant for the prevention of neural tube defects. Multivitamins typically provide 400 mcg per day; women who are pregnant, planning to become pregnant, or lactating will need to take additional folic acid to meet the recommended levels for these life stages. Although folic acid supplements can reduce homocysteine levels and high homocysteine levels are associated with an increased risk of heart disease, it is unclear whether supplements can lower the risk of heart disease.

Vitamin C (Ascorbic Acid)

- Required for synthesis of collagen (the structural component of blood vessels, tendons, and bone), norepinephrine (a neurotransmitter), and carnitine (an amino acid involved in energy production); promotes wound healing; supports immune function and gum health; and has antioxidant properties.
- Used therapeutically to prevent cataracts, macular degeneration, heart disease, stroke, cancer, and gout. Vitamin C supplements can help prevent colds in those with poor dietary intake and those under stress, and it has also been shown to

reduce the duration and severity of cold symptoms; improve wound healing and response to stress; reduce bronchial spasms in asthmatics; and prevent lead toxicity.

- Severe deficiency causes scurvy (bleeding, bruising, hair and tooth loss, joint pain, and swelling), which is rare today.
- Marginal deficiencies are common among the elderly, alcoholics, and those with cancer, chronic illness, or stress. Symptoms include fatigue, easy bruising, poor wound healing and appetite, anemia, and sore joints.
- Drugs that deplete vitamin C include oral contraceptives, aspirin, corticosteroids, and furosemide. Stress and smoking also deplete vitamin C levels.
- Large doses of vitamin C (greater than 1,000 mg per day) may reduce the effect of warfarin (a blood-thinning drug).
- Recent research suggests that nearly half of Canadians have suboptimal or deficient levels of vitamin C. Supplements are recommended for those with inadequate dietary intake, smokers, and those under stress or with certain chronic diseases. The Linus Pauling Institute recommends 400 mg of vitamin C daily, which is higher than the RDA, yet much lower than the Tolerable Upper Intake Level (UL). Most multivitamin supplements provide 60 mg of vitamin C.
- Natural and synthetic forms are chemically identical and have the same effects on the body.
- Mineral salts of ascorbic acid (e.g., calcium ascorbate) are buffered and therefore less acidic and less likely to cause upset stomach.

Vitamin D

- Regulates calcium and phosphorus levels and promotes absorption of these minerals for growth of bones and teeth; stimulates cell differentiation and controls cellular proliferation (plays a role in cancer prevention); involved in insulin secretion; modulates immune function; regulates blood pressure.
- Vitamin D can be produced in the skin upon exposure to sunlight (UVB rays) or must be obtained from the diet.
- Used therapeutically to prevent and treat osteoporosis, psoriasis, and autoimmune disease, and to reduce the risk of certain types of cancer (breast, colorectal, prostate).
- Deficiency occurs with inadequate dietary intake, limited sun exposure, kidney or liver disease, and alcoholism. Risk factors for vitamin D deficiency include exclusively breastfed infants, age (the elderly are at greater risk), dark-skinned individuals, obesity, and those with inflammatory bowel disease and fat-malabsorption syndromes (celiac disease, cystic fibrosis, and cholestatic liver disease).
- Deficiency causes rickets (weak, deformed bones) in children, osteomalacia (soft bones) and osteoporosis in adults, dental problems, muscle weakness and pain, and tooth decay.
- Drugs that deplete vitamin D include carbamazepine, phenytoin, phenobarbital, cimetidine, ranitidine, cholestyramine, colestipol, orlistat, and mineral oil.
- Since vitamin D is found in few foods and at low amounts, a supplement is recommended for most people, particularly those discussed above who are at increased risk of deficiency. Most multivitamins provide 400 IU (10 mcg), so additional vitamin D supplements are often required to meet the current recommendations.

Vitamin E

- A family of eight antioxidants: four tocopherols (alpha, beta, gamma, and delta) and four tocotrienols (alpha, beta, gamma, and delta). Alpha-tocopherol is the form that is actively maintained in the body and found in the largest quantities in blood and tissues.
- An antioxidant that protects cell membranes against free radical damage (oxidative damage); prevents LDL oxidation; supports immune function; prevents blood clotting; and dilates blood vessels.
- Used therapeutically to prevent and treat heart disease (although evidence is conflicting) and cancer, to prevent macular degeneration and cataracts, enhance immune response, reduce oxidative stress, and improve cognitive function.
- Deficiency is rare, except in those who are malnourished or who have fat-malabsorption conditions (celiac disease, cystic fibrosis, and cholestatic liver disease); however, suboptimal intake is common and may be associated with increased health risks.
- Symptoms of deficiency include impaired balance and coordination, damage to sensory nerves (peripheral neuropathy), muscle weakness (myopathy), and damage to the retina of the eye (pigmented retinopathy).
- Drugs that deplete vitamin E include cholestyramine, colestipol, isoniazid, mineral oil, orlistat, sucralfate, phenobarbital, phenytoin, and carbamazepine.
- Use of vitamin E supplements along with drugs that have a blood-thinning effect may increase the risk of bleeding. Examples include warfarin, antiplatelet drugs (clopidogrel, dipyridamole), and NSAIDS (aspirin, ibuprofen).
- It is difficult to achieve the RDA from diet alone; most multivitamins provide the RDA. Supplements are particularly necessary to achieve amounts needed for disease prevention.
- Look for natural vitamin E (alpha-tocopherol); the synthetic form (*dl*-alpha-tocopherol) is less bioavailable (i.e., less absorbable) and only half as potent.

Vitamin K

- Essential for blood clotting (coagulation); required for bone formation and cell growth; required for many enzyme reactions in the body.
- Used therapeutically for the prevention of osteoporosis and osteoporotic fractures.
- Deficiency is rare in adults and causes impaired blood clotting. It is more common in newborns because it is not easily transported across the placental barrier and a newborn's intestines are not yet colonized with bacteria that produce vitamin K. Injections of vitamin K1 are typically given to newborns to prevent bleeding disorders. Babies who are exclusively breastfed are at increased risk of vitamin K deficiency because breast milk is relatively low in vitamin K compared to formula.
- Symptoms of deficiency include easy bruising and bleeding (nosebleeds, bleeding gums, blood in the urine or stool, or heavy menstrual bleeding).
- Drugs that deplete vitamin K include antibiotics, aspirin, phenytoin, phenobarbital, cholestyramine, colestipol, orlistat, and mineral oil.

- Large doses of vitamins A or E can reduce levels of vitamin K.
- High intake of vitamin K from foods or supplements can potentially reduce the efficacy of blood-thinning drugs (warfarin). Individuals taking warfarin do not need to avoid eating vitamin K rich foods, such as leafy greens but are advised to maintain a consistent amount in their diet.
- Most people get adequate vitamin K from diet or a multivitamin.

MINERALS, TRACE MINERALS, AND ELECTROLYTES

Minerals are elements that originate in the earth. The body cannot make minerals so they must be obtained through diet or supplements. Both plant and animal foods provide minerals. Plants obtain minerals from the soil they are grown in. Animals get minerals from the plants they eat, and then we get these minerals indirectly by eating the animal products. There are also some minerals present in drinking water, but this varies with geographic location, as does the mineral content of plants.

Minerals are categorized according to our daily requirements. Calcium, magnesium, and phosphorus are considered major minerals since we require a substantial amount of these for health and wellness. The trace minerals, which are required in smaller amounts, are chromium, copper, fluoride, iodine, iron, manganese, molybdenum, selenium, and zinc. The minerals potassium and sodium are known as electrolytes, substances that dissociate into ions (charged particles) in solution, making them capable of conducting electricity.

Minerals
Calcium
- The most abundant mineral in the body; essential for building and maintaining bones and teeth; required for muscle contractions and nerve function; regulates blood pressure, blood vessel contractions, and clotting; involved in enzyme reactions.
- Used therapeutically for the prevention of osteoporosis, pre-eclampsia, and lead toxicity and for the treatment of premenstrual syndrome and high blood pressure. Increased calcium intake has also been associated with a lower risk of colorectal cancer, although more research is needed.
- Deficiency can occur with poor diet, abnormal parathyroid function (the gland that regulates blood calcium levels), kidney failure, and vitamin D or magnesium deficiency.
- Symptoms of deficiency include bone loss and weakening, muscle cramps, heart palpitations, tooth decay, back and leg pain, insomnia, nervous disorders, and rickets (bone deformities in children).
- Drugs that deplete calcium include cimetidine, ranitidine, omeprazole, aluminum antacids, corticosteroids, cholestyramine, mineral oil, phenytoin, and furosemide.
- A high intake of sodium (salt), protein, phosphorus (soft drinks and food additives), or caffeine (more than 3 cups of coffee or 400 mg of caffeine per day) can promote calcium losses.

- Calcium supplements may reduce the efficacy of calcium channel blockers (drugs used to lower blood pressure); use with thiazide diuretics increases the risk of hypercalcemia (high blood calcium levels); calcium supplements may reduce absorption of antibiotics (tetracycline, quinolones), bisphosphonates (osteoporosis drugs), and levothyroxine (thyroid hormone).
- It is difficult to meet the RDA through diet alone unless dairy intake is high. Most multivitamin/mineral supplements provide a small amount of calcium because it is quite bulky. Therefore, a separate calcium supplement may be necessary, especially for those at risk of osteoporosis and those with high blood pressure. Dosages higher than the RDA are not generally recommended and may cause potential health risks.
- There are several forms of calcium: Carbonate provides the highest amount of calcium (40 percent) and is inexpensive; citrate provides 21 percent calcium, but may be better absorbed in the elderly and those taking acid-lowering drugs.
- To maximize absorption, take no more than 500 mg of elemental calcium at one time, take with meals, and ensure adequate vitamin D intake (as this is required for calcium absorption).
- Separate calcium-rich foods and supplements by two hours from iron supplements (calcium reduces iron absorption); avoid drinking tea with meals, as the tannins in tea reduce calcium absorption.
- Some vegetables contain chemicals that inhibit the absorption of calcium, such as oxalic acid, which is found in raw spinach, rhubarb, sweet potato, and dried beans. Cooking these foods releases calcium that is bound to oxalic acid, thus improving the amount you can absorb. Phytic acid, which is found in wheat bran or dried beans, also reduces calcium absorption.

Magnesium

- Required for nerve and muscle function, formation of bones and teeth, synthesis of the antioxidant glutathione, health of cell membranes, and body temperature regulation; involved in energy production, numerous enzyme reactions, and synthesis of DNA and RNA.
- Used therapeutically to prevent heart disease and in the treatment of high blood pressure, pre-eclampsia, heart disease, diabetes, osteoporosis, migraine headaches, and asthma.
- Deficiency is uncommon, but may occur in those with poor diets, malabsorption syndromes (celiac disease), Crohn's disease, intestinal surgery or inflammation, kidney disease, diabetes, and alcoholism, and in the elderly due to lower dietary intake and reduced absorption.
- Marginal deficiency (consuming less than the RDA) is common and is estimated to affect 75 percent of people, particularly the elderly.
- Symptoms of deficiency include muscle cramps and spasms, weakness, insomnia, poor appetite, kidney stones, osteoporosis, nervousness, irritability, anxiety, depression, and high blood pressure.
- Drugs that deplete magnesium include furosemide, hydrochlorothiazide, cholestyramine, and oral contraceptives.

- Other interactions: Magnesium reduces absorption of digoxin, nitrofurantoin, antimalarial drugs, quinolone antibiotics, tetracycline, chlorpromazine, alendronate, and etidronate, so separate intake of magnesium from these drugs by two hours.
- High doses of zinc (greater than 140 mg per day) reduce magnesium absorption.
- Low blood magnesium levels can cause low blood calcium levels, resistance to parathyroid hormone action, and resistance to some of the effects of vitamin D.
- It is difficult to meet the RDA through diet alone; therefore, a multivitamin/mineral supplement is recommended. Those with certain medical conditions or health risks may require an additional magnesium supplement.

Phosphorus
- Required for maintaining the structure of bones, teeth, soft tissue, and cell membranes (phospholipids); energy production and storage; enzyme reactions; hormones; formation of DNA and RNA; and maintaining acid–base balance.
- Deficiency is rare except among alcoholics and those with kidney disease, malabsorption syndromes (celiac or Crohn's disease), or poor diets.
- Symptoms of deficiency include poor appetite, anemia, muscle weakness, bone pain, rickets in children, osteomalacia in adults, increased risk of infection, and numbness and tingling of the extremities.
- Drugs that deplete phosphorus include aluminum and magnesium (antacids and supplements), cholestyramine, and digoxin.
- Most people get adequate phosphorus through diet; supplements are rarely necessary.

Trace Minerals
Chromium
- Involved in glucose metabolism (enhances the effect of insulin) and enzyme reactions.
- Used therapeutically for the treatment of diabetes and for those with impaired glucose tolerance. There is conflicting evidence as to whether chromium supplements can lower cholesterol and triglyceride levels and support weight loss.
- Severe deficiency is rare, but marginal deficiency is common; it is estimated that 90 percent of adults consume less than the RDA.
- The main cause of deficiency is poor dietary intake (high-sugar diets increase urinary excretion of chromium).
- Deficiency results in impaired glucose utilization and may be a contributing factor to the development of type 2 diabetes; symptoms include elevated blood sugar, numbness, tingling in the extremities, and nerve problems.
- Drugs that deplete chromium include corticosteroids (prednisone).
- Other interactions: Chromium may enhance the blood sugar–lowering effects of insulin and oral diabetic drugs (glyburide and metformin), thus requiring a dosage adjustment.
- Since marginal deficiencies are common, a multivitamin/mineral complex containing chromium is recommended. Chromium is available in several forms. Most studies involving chromium were done with the picolinate form, which is readily absorbed and used by the body. Certain individuals (diabetics and those at risk for diabetes) may require an additional supplement.

Copper

- A component of enzymes, which are required for energy production, connective tissue formation, iron metabolism, brain and nervous system, synthesis of neurotransmitters, melanin, myelin, hemoglobin, and the antioxidant superoxide dismutase; involved in regulating gene expression.
- Severe deficiency is rare, but marginal deficiencies are common. The typical diet provides about 50 percent of the RDA. Those at risk of deficiency include premature and low birth-weight infants with diarrhea; infants fed only cow's milk formula, which is low in copper; those with malnutrition, malabsorption syndromes (celiac disease), or cystic fibrosis; those receiving intravenous feeding; and those taking prolonged high doses of zinc (50 mg or more daily).
- Deficiency leads to iron deficiency and anemia, low white blood cell count (neutropenia), and increased risk of infection, osteoporosis, loss of skin pigment, and impaired growth in children.
- Drugs that deplete copper include penicillamine, ethambutol, and zidovudine.
- A varied diet provides adequate copper for most individuals. Taking a multivitamin/mineral complex will provide the RDA.

Fluoride

- Essential for formation and maintenance of healthy bones and teeth.
- Used to prevent cavities and harden tooth enamel. Fluoride has been shown to increase bone mineral density in those with osteoporosis; however, most studies have not found that supplements can reduce fracture risk and its use is associated with several side effects (upset stomach, joint pain, stress fractures, calcium deficiency, and dental fluorosis).
- Deficiency causes tooth decay and dental caries (cavities).
- Drugs that deplete fluoride include calcium supplements and calcium- and aluminum-containing antacids, which reduce fluoride absorption (separate intake of fluoride from these supplements by two hours). Calcium and magnesium present in foods can also reduce fluoride absorption.
- Most Canadians get adequate fluoride through the small amount present in food, municipal drinking water, and use of fluoride toothpastes and rinses. Supplements are available by prescription and are recommended only for children living in areas with low water fluoride concentrations who are at risk of tooth decay; they are rarely required for adults. Excessive fluoride intake can result in fluorosis (mottling of tooth enamel).
- People who consume well water should have the fluoride content of their water tested.

Iodine

- Required to make thyroid hormones, which regulate metabolism, energy production, and body temperature, and are essential for growth and reproduction.
- Used for prevention of radiation-induced thyroid cancer in those with iodine deficiency and to treat fibrocystic breast disease.

- Deficiency may occur in those who do not consume salt, fish, or sea vegetables. It is estimated that over 30 percent of the world's population is deficient in iodine. Iodine deficiency has been rare in Canada since the introduction of iodized salt, but it is becoming more common in the general population due to restrictions on salt intake for blood pressure.
- Deficiency reduces thyroid hormone production, causing hypothyroidism, fatigue, weight gain, goiter, miscarriage, birth defects, mental retardation, and stunted growth. It is also the most common cause of brain damage worldwide.
- Drugs that deplete iodine include lithium, possibly resulting in hypothyroidism.
- Other interactions: Amiodarone (a heart drug) contains high levels of iodine and may affect thyroid function; potassium iodide may decrease the anticoagulant effect of warfarin.
- A deficiency of selenium, vitamin A, or iron can worsen iodine deficiency.
- Foods containing goitrogens—such as cabbage, broccoli, cauliflower, Brussels sprouts, and soybeans—inhibit the synthesis of thyroid hormone. These foods are a concern only for those who are iodine deficient and consume high amounts of them. Cooking deactivates the goitrogens.
- Most multivitamins contain potassium iodide and provide the RDA for iodine. Additional supplements are rarely necessary, but should be considered for pregnant and lactating women if dietary iodine is insufficient to meet the RDA, and in those who avoid salt, fish, and sea vegetables.
- A daily prenatal supplement providing 150 mcg of iodine will help to ensure that pregnant and breastfeeding women consume sufficient iodine during these critical periods.

Iron

- Required to produce hemoglobin and myoglobin (proteins involved in the transport and storage of oxygen) and amino acids (carnitine); required for cellular energy production; produces enzymes that have antioxidant effects; supports DNA synthesis and immune function.
- Used therapeutically for prevention of anemia in pregnancy and in others at risk, and in the treatment of restless leg syndrome.
- Deficiency is common, especially in women with heavy menstrual bleeding and during pregnancy (due to increased needs for the developing baby); vegetarians, those with malabsorption syndromes (celiac disease), bleeding ulcers, copper deficiency; and those who have undergone surgery.
- Deficiency leads to depleted iron stores, impaired red blood cell formation, and anemia. Symptoms include fatigue, paleness, headache, hair loss, brittle nails, rapid heart rate, increased risk of infections, and rapid breathing on exertion.
- Drugs that deplete iron include antacids, cimetidine, ranitidine, omeprazole, lansoprazole, aspirin, anti-inflammatory drugs, and cholestyramine.
- Iron supplements can bind to and reduce absorption and efficacy of levodopa, levothyroxine, methyldopa, quinolones, tetracyclines, bisphosphonates, and zinc and calcium supplements. To avoid this, separate intake of iron supplements from these products by two hours.

- Vitamin C–rich foods and supplements enhance the absorption of non-heme iron (the form of iron found primarily in plants).
- A multivitamin/mineral complex providing the RDA is recommended for most pre-menopausal and pregnant women and those at risk of deficiency.
- Men and post-menopausal women should choose iron-free multivitamin/mineral supplements to avoid iron excess.

Manganese

- Required for the production and activation of enzymes that are involved in energy metabolism; bone, cartilage, and collagen formation (wound healing); and the production of antioxidants.
- Deficiency is uncommon, but may occur in those with epilepsy, hypoglycemia, diabetes, schizophrenia, and osteoporosis.
- Deficiency symptoms include impaired growth and reproductive function, skeletal abnormalities, impaired glucose tolerance, and altered carbohydrate and fat metabolism.
- Drugs that deplete manganese include magnesium-containing antacids and laxatives and tetracycline.
- Absorption is reduced by calcium, phosphate, and iron.
- Supplements beyond the amount provided by diet or a multivitamin and mineral complex are not necessary and can cause neurotoxicity.

Molybdenum

- Required for the production of enzymes that are cofactors in amino acid metabolism, formation of uric acid, and the metabolism of drugs and toxins.
- Deficiency is extremely rare and may occur in those with a rare genetic condition; deficiency causes seizures, developmental delays in neonates, tachycardia, brain damage, and coma.
- Drugs that deplete molybdenum include high intakes of copper or sulphate.
- Supplements beyond the amount provided by diet or a multivitamin and mineral complex are not necessary.

Selenium

- Component of enzymes that function as antioxidants; involved in detoxification; converts thyroid hormone to its active form; supports immune function; enhances the antioxidant activity of vitamin E.
- Used therapeutically to strengthen immune function, prevent infection, and to prevent oxidative stress and support immune system function in those with HIV/AIDS.
- Deficiency is uncommon, but may occur in those with poor diets, those who live in areas where the soil is depleted in selenium, and those with Crohn's disease and malabsorption syndromes (celiac disease).
- Symptoms of deficiency include muscular weakness and wasting, degeneration of cartilage, cardiomyopathy (inflammation of the heart), pancreatic damage, and impaired immune function. There is some evidence that selenium deficiency can

heighten cancer risk (liver, lung colon, and prostate) and supplements may offer benefits, although the research is conflicting.
- Drugs that deplete selenium include valproic acid and corticosteroids (prednisone).
- Supplements beyond the amount provided by diet or a multivitamin and mineral complex may be necessary for some individuals.

Zinc

- Involved in numerous enzyme reactions; required for growth and development, immune and neurological function, and reproduction and regulation of gene expression; stabilizes the structure of proteins and cell membranes.
- Used therapeutically to support immune function, reduce severity and duration of the common cold, and delay the progression of macular degeneration.
- Severe deficiency is rare, except in those with a genetic disorder (acrodermatitis enteropathica) that reduces zinc uptake, and in those with severe malnutrition or malabsorption, severe burns, or chronic diarrhea.
- Marginal deficiencies are common, especially among malnourished individuals, alcoholics, vegetarians, pregnant women, the elderly, and those with celiac disease, Crohn's disease, colitis, and sickle cell anemia.
- Symptoms of deficiency include impaired growth and development, skin rashes, severe diarrhea, immune system deficiencies, impaired wound healing, poor appetite, impaired taste sensation, night blindness, clouding of the corneas, and behavioural disturbances.
- Drugs that deplete zinc include diuretics, anticonvulsants, iron supplements, penicillamine, ACE-inhibitor drugs, acid-reducing drugs, and oral contraceptives.
- Zinc supplements can reduce copper levels, so look for a multivitamin that contains copper as well as zinc.
- Zinc supplements can reduce absorption of antibiotics (tetracycline and quinolones), so separate intake of zinc supplements from these products by two hours.
- Since the average zinc intake is below the RDA and many conditions and drugs deplete zinc levels, a supplement should be considered. Most multivitamin and mineral complexes provide at least the RDA for zinc. Additional zinc supplements may be necessary for some individuals.

Electrolytes
Potassium

- Required to maintain fluid balance; required for nerve conduction and muscle function; cofactor for enzymes involved in energy production and carbohydrate metabolism.
- Used therapeutically for prevention of stroke, osteoporosis, and kidney stones, and in the treatment of high blood pressure.
- Deficiency (hypokalemia) is common, particularly among those with prolonged diarrhea or vomiting, alcoholism, kidney or heart failure, laxative abuse, anorexia, or magnesium deficiency.

- Deficiency symptoms include fatigue, muscle weakness and cramps, bloating, constipation, and abdominal pain. Severe hypokalemia may result in muscular paralysis or abnormal heart rhythms.
- Drugs that deplete potassium include furosemide, hydrochlorothiazide, corticosteroids, pseudoephedrine, caffeine, and high-dose penicillin.
- Drugs that enhance potassium (may cause hyperkalemia) include spironolactone, triamterene, amiloride, ACE-inhibitors, anti-inflammatory drugs (ibuprofen), heparin, digoxin, and beta-blockers.
- The average dietary potassium intake is about 2,300 mg per day for women and 3,100 mg per day for men. Evidence suggests that diets supplying at least 4,700 mg per day are associated with a decreased risk of stroke, hypertension, osteoporosis, and kidney stones, and this is the Adequate Intake (AI) level set by the Institute of Medicine.
- Multivitamin/mineral complexes typically provide 99 mg of potassium per serving. Depending on dietary intake and personal risk factors for chronic disease, additional potassium supplements may be necessary for some people.
- Take supplements with meals or choose a microencapsulated form to reduce the risk of upset stomach.

Sodium

- Regulates fluid balance along with potassium; required for nerve conduction and muscle function; assists absorption of chloride, amino acids, glucose, and water; regulates blood volume and blood pressure.
- Excess sodium intake is linked to gastric cancer, osteoporosis, high blood pressure, heart disease, and kidney stones. Reducing sodium intake may help to reduce the risk of these conditions.
- Deficiency is rare even among those on low-sodium diets. Low blood levels of sodium (hyponatremia) may be caused by fluid retention or excess sodium loss (excessive sweating, prolonged exercise, severe and prolonged vomiting and diarrhea, and kidney disease).
- Symptoms of hyponatremia include headache, nausea, muscle cramps, fatigue, confusion, and fainting. Severe cases may lead to swelling of the brain, seizures, coma, and brain damage.
- Drugs that deplete sodium include diuretics, anti-inflammatory drugs, carbamazepine, codeine, morphine, and some antidepressants.
- Supplements are rarely necessary, except in the above-mentioned conditions.
- The Adequate Intake (AI) level for sodium and sodium chloride (salt) is based on the amount needed to replace losses through sweat in moderately active people and to achieve a diet that provides sufficient amounts of other essential nutrients. Most adults consume an amount much greater than the AI.

NUTRIENT RECOMMENDATIONS

The table below contains nutrient recommendation for individuals 19 years and older, and women 19 years and older who are pregnant or lactating. To access guidelines for infants, children, and teenagers, refer to the Institute of Medicine's website at www .iom.edu. In this table I have outlined the following:

• Best food sources to obtain the particular nutrient.
• *Recommended Dietary Allowance (RDA):* The average daily dietary nutrient intake level sufficient to meet the nutrient requirement of nearly all (97 to 98 percent) healthy individuals in a particular life stage and gender group.
• *Adequate Intake (AI):* The recommended average daily intake level based on observed or experimentally determined estimates of nutrient intake of apparently healthy people that are assumed to be adequate. The AI is given when an RDA cannot be determined.
• *Tolerable Upper Intake Level (UL):* The highest average daily nutrient intake level that is likely to pose no risk of adverse health effects for almost all individuals in the general population. As intake increases above the UL, the potential risk of adverse effects may increase.
• Side effects and toxicity.

For some nutrients an RDA has not been established, but an AI is provided (indicated by an asterisk). It is important to note that the RDA is mainly based on information on short-term effects. The optimum nutrient intake for health and disease prevention may be higher than the RDA and varies with age, state of health, diet, and other factors.

Vitamins	Food Sources	RDA or AI*	UL	Side Effects/ Toxicity
Vitamin A	Liver, dairy products, and oily fish (Beta carotene is found in orange and green vegetables and fruit)	(mcg/day) Men = 900 Women = 700 Pregnancy = 770 Lactation = 1,300	(mcg/day) Men = 3,000 Women = 3,000 Pregnancy = 3,000 Lactation = 3,000 *Note:* 1 mcg = 3.33 IU	Liver toxicity and birth defects (associated with vitamin A, not beta carotene). Toxicity is associated with long-term consumption of high-intake vitamin A (8,000– 10,000 mcg/day or 25,000–33,000 IU/day)
Vitamin B1 (thiamine)	Brewer's yeast, organ meats, enriched whole grains and bread products, legumes, and nuts	(mg/day) Men = 1.2 Women = 1.1 Pregnancy = 1.4 Lactation = 1.4	Not determined	No adverse effects known with food or supplements
Vitamin B2 (riboflavin)	Dairy, whole grains, organ meats, eggs, dark green vegetables, and fortified cereals	(mg/day) Men = 1.3 Women = 1.1 Pregnancy = 1.4 Lactation = 1.6	Not determined	No adverse effects known with food or supplements

(continued)

Vitamins	Food Sources	RDA or AI*	UL	Side Effects/ Toxicity
Vitamin B3 (nicotinic acid, nicotinamide)	Fish, meat, poultry, eggs, nuts, seeds, legumes, avocado, whole grains, and fortified cereals	(mg/day) Men = 16 Women = 14 Pregnancy = 18 Lactation = 17	35 mg/day	No adverse effects from niacin in foods; supplements may cause flushing and upset stomach; higher doses (500 mg/ day) may cause liver problems, particularly with time-release products
Vitamin B5 (pantothenic acid)	Liver, kidney, egg yolk, brewer's yeast, broccoli, chicken, beef, whole grains, and legumes	(mg/day)* Men = 5 Women = 5 Pregnancy = 6 Lactation = 7	Not determined	No adverse effects known from foods or supplements
Vitamin B6 (pyridoxine)	Fortified cereals, bananas, spinach, avocado, chicken, soy, legumes, salmon, and organ meats	(mg/day) Men and women 19–50 = 1.3 Men > 50 = 1.7 Women > 50 = 1.5 Pregnancy = 1.9 Lactation = 2.0	(mg/day) Men = 100 Women = 100 Pregnancy = 100 Lactation = 100	No adverse effects from food; high-dose supplements may cause neuropathy (pain and numbness in the extremities)
Vitamin B12 (cobalamin)	Meat, poultry, fish, milk, and fortified cereals	(mcg/day) Men = 2.4 Women = 2.4 Pregnancy = 2.6 Lactation = 2.8	Not determined	No adverse effects known from foods or supplements
Biotin	Egg yolk, liver, wheat bran, yeast, oatmeal, soybeans, cauliflower, mushrooms, and nuts	(mcg/day)* Men = 30 Women = 30 Pregnancy = 30 Lactation = 35	Not determined	No adverse effects known from foods or supplements
Folate (folic acid)	Dark leafy vegetables, fortified cereals, citrus fruits, and legumes (beans, lentils, and peanuts)	(mcg/day) Men = 400 Women = 400 Pregnancy = 600 Lactation = 500	(mcg/day) Men = 1,000 Women = 1,000 Pregnancy = 1,000 Lactation = 1,000	No adverse effects known from foods or supplements
Vitamin C (ascorbic acid)	Citrus fruit, tomatoes, red peppers, broccoli, spinach, cabbage, strawberries, and potatoes	(mg/day) Men = 90 Women = 75 Pregnancy = 85 Lactation = 120	(mg/day) Men = 2,000 Women = 2,000 Pregnancy = 2,000 Lactation = 2,000	Upset stomach, diarrhea, kidney stones (in those at risk), excess iron absorption

Vitamin D	Fatty fish (mackerel, salmon, sardines), fish liver oils, eggs from hens fed vitamin D, milk, and fortified cereals	(mcg/day)* Men and women 19–70 = 15 > 70 = 20 Pregnancy = 115 Lactation = 15	(mcg/day) Men = 100 Women = 100 Pregnancy = 100 Lactation = 100 *Note:* 1 mcg = 40 IU	Hypercalcemia (calcium deposits in kidneys, arteries, heart, ears, and lungs, and bone loss); symptoms include headache, weakness, nausea, vomiting, constipation
Vitamin E	Vegetable oils (olive, sunflower, safflower oils), nuts, whole grains, meat, and green leafy vegetables	(mg/day) Men = 15 Women = 15 Pregnancy = 15 Lactation = 19	(mg/day) Men = 1,000 Women = 1,000 Pregnancy = 1,000 Lactation = 1,000 *Note:* 1 mg alpha-tocopherol = 1.5 IU	No adverse effects from vitamin E–containing foods; supplements may increase the risk of bleeding in some individuals, particularly those taking blood-thinning drugs
Vitamin K	Green leafy vegetables, cabbage, Brussels sprouts, vegetable oils (canola, soybean, cottonseed, and olive)	(mcg/day)* Men = 120 Women = 90 Pregnancy = 90 Lactation = 90	Not determined	No adverse effects known from foods or supplements; those taking anticoagulant drugs should monitor their intake of vitamin K

Minerals	Food Sources	RDA or AI*	UL	Side Effects/ Toxicity
Calcium	Dairy, calcium-set tofu, cabbage, kale, broccoli, bok choy, and legumes	(mg/day)* Men and women 19–70 = 1,000 > 70 = 1,200 Pregnancy = 1,000 Lactation = 1,000	(mg/day) Men 19–50 = 2,500 Men > 50 = 2,000 Women 19–50 = 2,500 Women > 50 = 2,000 Pregnancy = 2,500 Lactation = 2,500	May cause kidney stones, hypercalcemia (high blood calcium), soft tissue calcification, and kidney problems in those at risk; high doses may cause constipation and gas
Magnesium	Leafy green vegetables, unrefined grains, nuts, seeds, meat, milk, soybeans, tofu, legumes, and figs	(mg/day) Men 19–30 = 400 Men > 30 = 420 Women 19–30 = 310 Women > 30 = 320 Pregnancy 19–30 = 350 Pregnancy > 30 = 360 Lactation 19–30 = 310 Lactation > 30 = 320	(mg/day) Men = 350 Women = 350 Pregnancy = 350 Lactation = 350	No adverse effects from magnesium in food; high-dose supplements may cause diarrhea

(continued)

Minerals	Food Sources	RDA or AI*	UL	Side Effects/ Toxicity
Phosphorus	Dairy products, meat, fish, eggs, nuts, lentils, cereals, and bread	(mg/day) Men = 700 Women = 700 Pregnancy = 700 Lactation = 700	(mg/day) Men 19–70 = 4,000 Men > 70 = 3,000 Women 19–70 = 4,000 Women > 70 = 3,000 Pregnancy = 3,500 Lactation = 4,000	High doses may cause calcification of soft tissues (kidneys), reduced calcium absorption and bone mass; those with kidney disease are at greatest risk of toxicity

Trace Minerals	Food Sources	RDA or AI*	UL	Side Effects/ Toxicity
Chromium	Wheat germ, brewer's yeast, some cereals, green beans, apples, bananas, spinach, meat, liver, eggs, poultry, oysters, and fish	(mcg/day)* Men 19–50 = 35 Men > 50 = 30 Women 19–50 = 25 Women > 50 = 20 Pregnancy = 30 Lactation = 45	Not determined	Reports of kidney failure and impaired liver function with high doses (greater than 1,200 mcg/day) over long periods of time
Copper	Organ meats, shellfish, nuts, seeds, whole grains, prunes, cocoa products, and dark green vegetables	(mcg/day) Men = 900 Women = 900 Pregnancy = 1,000 Lactation = 1,300	(mcg/day) Men = 10,000 Women = 10,000 Pregnancy =10,000 Lactation = 10,000	Toxicity is rare and causes abdominal pain, vomiting, liver and kidney damage, and coma; doses up to 10,000 mcg/ day are not associated with toxicity, except in those with Wilson's disease, Indian childhood cirrhosis, or idiopathic copper toxicosis
Fluoride	Fluoridated drinking water, marine fish with bones, and tea	(mg/day)* Men = 4 Women = 3 Pregnancy = 3 Lactation = 3	(mg/day) Men = 10 Women = 10 Pregnancy = 10 Lactation = 10	Dental and skeletal fluorosis may occur at doses greater than two times the AI; acute toxicity seen at doses of 5 mg/kg body weight causes nausea, abdominal pain, and diarrhea

Iodine	Salt, seafood, sea vegetables (kelp), and vegetables grown in iodine-rich soil	(mg/day) Men = 150 Women = 150 Pregnancy = 220 Lactation = 290	(mg/day) Men = 1,100 Women = 1,100 Pregnancy = 1,100 Lactation = 1,100	High intakes may cause hypothyroidism and goiter; toxicity is rare and occurs only with very high doses; symptoms include burning of the mouth, throat, and stomach; fever, nausea, and vomiting; those with iodine deficiency, goiter, cystic fibrosis, or thyroid disease may be more susceptible to adverse effects
Iron	Fruits, vegetables, fortified bread and cereals, meat, poultry, and fish	(mg/day) Men = 8 Women 19–50 = 18 Women > 50 = 8 Pregnancy = 27 Lactation = 9	(mg/day) Men = 45 Women = 45 Pregnancy = 45 Lactation = 45	Iron supplements (regular doses) may cause nausea, vomiting, and constipation; overdose can be fatal; individuals with genetic disorders of iron overload (hemochromatosis), alcoholic cirrhosis, and liver disease may experience adverse effects with intakes below the UL
Manganese	Whole grains, nuts, legumes, leafy green vegetables, avocados, egg yolks, and teas	(mg/day)* Men = 2.3 Women = 1.8 Pregnancy = 2.0 Lactation = 2.6	(mg/day) Men = 11 Women = 11 Pregnancy = 11 Lactation = 11	Elevated blood levels can cause tremors; inhaled manganese dust and high levels in drinking water can be toxic to the brain; those with liver disease may be at increased risk of adverse effects from manganese, such as tremors and psychosis
Molybdenum	Legumes, nuts, whole grains, liver, and hard drinking water	(mcg/day) Men = 45 Women = 45 Pregnancy = 50 Lactation = 50	(mcg/day) Men = 2,000 Women = 2,000 Pregnancy = 2,000 Lactation = 2,000	Toxicity is rare and may cause gout-like symptoms and neurological problems; those with copper deficiency are at increased risk of molybdenum toxicity

(continued)

Trace Minerals	Food Sources	RDA or AI*	UL	Side Effects/ Toxicity
Selenium	Organ meats, seafood, and plants and grains grown in selenium-rich soil	(mcg/day) Men = 55 Women = 55 Pregnancy = 60 Lactation = 70	(mcg/day) Men = 400 Women = 400 Pregnancy = 400 Lactation = 400	Toxicity may occur at doses greater than 400 mcg/day and causes hair and nail brittleness and loss, upset stomach, skin rash, fatigue, and irritability
Zinc	Red meat, shellfish, eggs, whole grains, and fortified cereals	(mg/day) Men = 11 Women = 8 Pregnancy = 11 Lactation = 12	(mg/day) Men = 40 Women = 40 Pregnancy = 40 Lactation = 40	Zinc toxicity causes abdominal pain, diarrhea, nausea, and vomiting; high dosages of supplements may reduce copper levels

Electrolytes	Food Sources	RDA or AI*	UL	Side Effects/ Toxicity
Potassium	Bananas, baked potatoes, oranges and orange juice, raisins, artichokes, avocados, spinach, nuts, seeds, lima beans, meat, cod, chicken, and salmon	(mg/day)* Men = 4,700 Women = 4,700 Pregnancy = 4,700 Lactation = 5,100	Not determined	Potassium supplements can cause nausea, vomiting, abdominal pain, and diarrhea; symptoms of toxicity include tingling in the extremities, muscle weakness, temporary paralysis, and abnormal heart rhythm
Sodium	Salt, processed foods (deli meats), soy sauce, pickles, snack foods (chips, pretzels, salted nuts), and canned tomato juice	(g/day)* [Salt] Men and women: 19–50 = 1.5 [3.8] 51–70 = 1.3 [3.3] > 70 = 1.2 [3.0] Pregnancy = 1.5 [3.8] Lactation = 1.5 [3.8]	For all adults: 2.3 g/day of sodium 5.8 g/day of salt Note: 2 g of sodium = 5 g of salt (sodium chloride)	Ingestion of a high amount may cause edema, elevated blood pressure, increased risk of cardiovascular disease and stroke, nausea, vomiting, diarrhea, and abdominal cramps

*Adequate Intake (AI) recommendation

CHAPTER 3

FUNCTIONAL FOODS

Hippocrates wisely stated back in 400 BC, "Let food be your medicine and medicine be your food." Modern research has validated this doctrine. Today we know that what we eat is a major determinant of health, and that food provides both nutritive and healing properties.

According to the Bureau of Nutritional Sciences of the Food Directorate of Health Canada, "a functional food is similar in appearance to, or may be, a conventional food, is consumed as part of a usual diet, and is demonstrated to have physiological benefits and/or reduce the risk of chronic disease beyond basic nutritional functions." In other words, these foods provide more than just vitamins and minerals; they contain compounds that have beneficial actions in the body and can reduce the risk of chronic disease. These are foods that you want to include more of in your daily diet. Look for organic products to reduce your exposure to harmful pesticides.

Many compounds found in functional foods are available in supplement form. Supplements often provide a standardized amount of the active compounds, are easy to take, and are a great way to complement the diet.

In this chapter I will provide examples of functional foods and their associated health benefits.

A FUNCTIONAL FOOD PANTRY

Apples provide both soluble and insoluble fibre (one medium apple with skin provides about 3 g of fibre). Apple skins are a major food source of a type of flavonoid called quercetin, which is a potent antioxidant that helps protect against heart disease and cancer. These flavonoids, along with vitamin C, give apples immune-bolstering properties. Phenolic compounds found in apple skins provide protection against many chronic diseases and have recently been found to provide UVB sun protection. So there is a lot of truth to the saying "An apple a day keeps the doctor away." Fuji apples have the highest concentration of phenolic and flavonoid compounds, but Red Delicious apples are also quite high.

Berries, cherries, and red grapes contain plant pigments called anthocyanidins, which give these fruits their radiant red and purple colour. Anthocyanidins have antioxidant properties, preventing free radical damage and reducing the risk of chronic disease. These compounds are also important for proper brain and blood vessel function.

Broccoli contains sulphoraphane and indole-3-carbinol, antioxidants that neutralize free radicals, enhance detoxification, and may reduce the risk of certain types of cancer, particularly breast cancer. These compounds are found in other cruciferous vegetables, such as kale, cauliflower, and cabbage. Try to have a serving of these foods every day.

Carrots are an excellent source of many antioxidant compounds, particularly beta carotene, which is part of the carotenoid family. Carotenoids help protect against cardiovascular disease, cancer, macular degeneration, and cataracts, and they also promote good night vision. New research is looking at the effects of another phytonutrient in carrots called falcarinol and its ability to reduce the risk of colon cancer. To get the maximum amount of nutrients from carrots, eat them raw or lightly steamed.

Chocolate and cocoa provide various flavonoids that provide antioxidant benefits for the heart and other organs. Dark chocolate contains more antioxidants and less fat than milk chocolate. Look for products that contain 70 percent or more cocoa.

Citrus fruits contain flavanones (a type of flavonoid), antioxidants that reduce free radicals, prevent cellular damage, reduce cancer risk, and boost defences against viral infections. Oranges, grapefruit, lemons, and limes offer a wide range of nutrients (vitamin C, folate, and fibre).

Collard greens and kale contain plant pigments called lutein and zeaxanthin, which are important for eye health and can reduce the risk of macular degeneration (age-related blindness). Supplements of lutein have been shown to improve vision in those with macular degeneration and prevent disease progression. One to two servings of kale or collard greens per week provide the recommended amount of lutein and zeaxanthin. Other food sources of lutein and zeaxanthin include spinach, broccoli, and leeks, but they contain a lesser amount.

Cranberries contain proanthocyanidins, which have been shown to reduce the risk of urinary tract infections. Preliminary research also shows that these compounds may help lower cholesterol, improve gum health, prevent ulcers, and prevent brain damage after a stroke. The bladder benefits are seen with one to two glasses of juice daily. Look for pure cranberry juice or low-sugar juice cocktail.

Fish and fish oils contain omega-3 fatty acids (EPA and DHA), which have been found to reduce the risk of coronary heart disease. Specifically, they reduce triglyceride levels, increase HDL (good cholesterol), reduce inflammation, prevent clotting, and reduce blood pressure. They are also known to be beneficial for vision and brain health. Choose wild (not farmed) fish.

GET YOUR OMEGA-3s

The recommended intake of fish oils for heart health is 1 g to 3 g daily from supplements or one to two servings of fish per week. Sadly, our fish supply is contaminated with PCBs, dioxins, and pesticides, which increase the risk of cancer. Farmed fish, especially salmon, contains the highest amount of toxins. Health authorities recommend consuming no more than six meals per year of farmed salmon. Wild Pacific salmon has fewer toxins and can be eaten once or twice a month. You can also get your omega-3s through a fish oil supplement. Look for a quality product that is tested for purity and provides a 3 to 2 ratio of EPA to DHA.

Flaxseed provides lignans, plant compounds with antioxidant activity that may protect against heart disease and some cancers. It lowers LDL cholesterol, total cholesterol, and triglyceride levels. Flaxseed is a good source of dietary fibre (14 g of fibre per 50 g serving) and is thus used to relieve constipation and to treat ulcerative colitis and irritable bowel syndrome. Flaxseed also contains beneficial omega-3 fatty acids. To obtain all the benefits, eat the milled flaxseed or get whole seeds and crush them in a food processor or coffee grinder. Take 15 mL (1 tbsp) once or twice daily. Store milled seeds in the refrigerator or freezer in an opaque, airtight container; they will be stable for 90 days.

Garlic contains sulphur compounds, which offer a number of health benefits. Studies have shown that garlic mildly reduces cholesterol, reduces LDL oxidation (atherosclerosis), prevents blood clotting, and fights cancer. It also possesses anti-inflammatory, antibacterial, and antiviral effects. Studies have found benefits with as little as 900 mg of garlic per day, which is approximately equivalent to one clove.

Ginger has a long history of use for relieving stomach problems. Clinical studies have validated its benefits for preventing the symptoms of motion sickness (especially sea sickness) and in the treatment of nausea and vomiting associated with pregnancy and migraine. The active compounds in ginger, called gingerols, have potent anti-inflammatory effects, making it helpful in the treatment of arthritis and other inflammatory conditions. New research suggests that ginger may also help fight cancer. Choose fresh ginger over the dry (powder) form to maximize intake of the active compounds.

Green tea is rich in catechins (a type of flavonoid) called epigallocatechin gallate (EGCG). This compound has been found to reduce the risk of certain cancers, reduce the size of existing tumours, and inhibit tumour growth. It also supports heart function by lowering blood pressure and reducing the risk of fatal heart attacks. EGCG also supports nerve function and may benefit those with Parkinson's and Alzheimer's disease. Recently EGCG has been found to reduce body fat and improve metabolism. Most studies evaluating the health benefits of green tea involved drinking 750 mL to 2,500 mL daily. Black tea, white tea, oolong tea, and other teas derived from the plant *Camellia sinensis* may offer similar health benefits but are not as widely researched.

Oat bran contains a soluble fibre called beta-glucan, which has been shown to lower cholesterol and reduce the risk of heart disease. Studies have found that 3 g of beta-glucan daily can reduce total cholesterol by an average of 5 percent. This amount can be found in approximately 60 g of oatmeal or 40 g of oat bran. Other good forms of soluble fibre are chia seed, psyllium, apples, and beans.

Onions contain a variety of nutrients, such as vitamin C and chromium. Powerful sulphur compounds in onions are responsible for their pungent odour and for many of their health benefits. They can help reduce blood sugar, cholesterol, and blood pressure. Onions provide a concentrated source of the flavonoid quercetin, which helps reduce inflammation and may halt the growth of cancer. Cooking meats with onions may help reduce the amount of carcinogens produced when meat is cooked at high heat. There are many varieties of onions. In general, the more pungent an onion, the more active compounds and health benefits it has.

Soybeans contain isoflavones (daidzein and genistein), which help reduce cholesterol levels, fight cancer, increase bone density, and reduce menopausal symptoms. Research suggests that consuming 25 g of soy protein daily can provide a significant cholesterol-lowering effect. Aside from soybeans and tofu, you can get the benefits of soy protein by eating soy nuts, soy milk, soy yogurt, and bars and shakes containing soy protein.

Tomatoes contain an antioxidant called lycopene, which has been found to reduce the risk of prostate and colon cancer, support prostate health, reduce blood clotting and inflammation, and reduce heart attack risk. Most studies found health benefits with an intake of 8 mg to 10 mg daily. Lycopene is also present in tomato sauce, tomato paste, and ketchup, which contain a higher amount of lycopene than fresh tomatoes. To obtain 10 mg of lycopene, you would have to eat about 10 to 15 raw tomatoes, 60 mL (2 ounces) of ketchup, or 20 mL (4 tsp) of tomato paste. Lycopene is also found in papaya, strawberries, watermelon, guava, and pink grapefruit.

Yogurt contains active bacteria cultures known as probiotics or friendly bacteria, which improve gastrointestinal health (digestion and elimination) and immune function. These active cultures also help digest the naturally occurring sugar (lactose) in dairy products that causes bloating and diarrhea in some people. Avoid the "diet" or "light" yogurts, since they are sweetened with aspartame, a chemical whose safety in food is questionable. The amount of probiotics in yogurt varies with brand and storage. For this reason those looking for the consistent benefits of probiotics often opt for supplements.

TEN PRINCIPLES OF A HEALTHY DIET

With so many important vitamins and minerals to include in the diet and good and bad fats to keep straight, it's easy to see how people can feel overwhelmed when making food choices. Eating a healthy diet, however, is actually quite simple.

In this chapter I will share with you my 10 principles for a healthy diet, elements that I recommend based on current science for optimal health, energy, and disease prevention.

1. MAKE QUALITY FOOD CHOICES

Fresh, natural, unprocessed foods should form the basis of your diet. Look for organic produce to reduce ingestion of toxic pesticides. If organic is not available, look for locally grown fruits and vegetables. Items from foreign countries may contain higher levels of pesticides and bacteria. To preserve the nutrients in your food, minimize storage time and cooking or reheating.

Choose unprocessed whole grains (brown rice, multigrain breads) over the refined and processed products. Refined grains (white bread) have most of the vitamins, minerals, and fibre removed.

Quality protein sources include free-range and organic meat and poultry, legumes, nuts, seeds, eggs, and tofu. If you are following a vegetarian diet, be sure to incorporate a variety of plant-based proteins to ensure that all essential amino acids are consumed.

Consume health-promoting fats from fish, nuts, seeds, and quality oils (hemp, chia seed, flaxseed, canola, olive, sunflower, and safflower).

Avoid or minimize eating fast/processed foods, as they are typically high in calories, poor in nutritional value, and laden with potentially dangerous chemicals and preservatives. Read your labels carefully.

• •

FORGET THE FADS

Avoid fad diets, which can be hard to follow, have few nutrients, and can even be dangerous. Whether your goal is weight loss or better health, stay away from the latest fad and make healthier food choices.

• •

2. ENJOY VARIETY

To get a broad range of nutrients in your diet, enjoy a variety of foods rather than sticking to your favourites. This is particularly important with vegetables and fruits, as their nutrient profiles vary greatly. To obtain the many antioxidants, vitamins, minerals, and phytonutrients, eat a variety of plant foods every day. Experiment with new foods and recipes, and try to reintroduce previously disliked foods.

3. MODERATION: KNOW YOUR CALORIE REQUIREMENTS AND PORTION SIZES

Your caloric requirements depend on your age, gender, height, weight, and activity level. To discover your recommended calorie intake, consult Health Canada's website www.hc-sc.gc.ca. Note that those engaged in vigorous physical activity or who are pregnant or lactating have increased calorie requirements.

To figure out how many calories you should consume from carbohydrates, fat, and protein, consider the ranges set out by the Institute of Medicine (IOM). They recommend that adults get 45 to 65 percent of their calories from carbohydrates, 20 to 35 percent from fat, and 10 to 35 percent from protein.

According to the most recent national survey among Canadian adults, 7 in 10 men and 5 in 10 women had energy intakes that exceed their energy expenditure. Consuming excess calories, whether from fat, protein, or carbohydrates, can lead to weight gain and associated health risks.

••

AVOIDING PORTION DISTORTION

Overeating can lead to obesity, high triglyceride levels, insulin resistance, free radical damage, and shortened life expectancy. To prevent overeating, control your portion sizes and eat slowly. A serving equals 1 piece of fruit, 1 cup of raw or ½ cup of cooked vegetables, 1 slice of bread, ½ cup of cooked rice or pasta, or 2 to 3 ounces of meat. Eating slowly allows your stomach to send a message to your brain that you are full. Chew your food thoroughly and drink water to allow for proper digestion. It should take you 20 to 30 minutes to eat a meal.

••

4. EAT SMALL AND FREQUENT MEALS

Try to eat every three hours—three small meals and two snacks daily. This will improve metabolism (calorie burning) and blood sugar balance, which improves energy and mood.

Breakfast is essential to fuel your body. If you aren't very hungry in the morning, then have a light meal such as yogurt and berries or a protein shake. Try not to eat too late in the evening (after 8 p.m.), as this could impact sleep. Don't skip meals, even if you are trying to lose weight, since this causes fatigue, poor concentration, and sluggish metabolism, and triggers food cravings.

5. DRINK PLENTY OF WATER

Water is essential to health—it helps regulate body temperature, removes wastes, and transports nutrients throughout the body. A lack of water causes dehydration, which can be deadly. To keep your body well hydrated, drink water throughout the day. The Institute of Medicine recommends that men consume 3.0 L (13 cups) and women consume 2.2 L (9 cups) of water daily. Water purified by reverse osmosis is best because tap water may contain high amounts of chlorine and other chemicals, which can be harmful to the stomach and bladder. Keep in mind that intense physical activity and heat exposure increases water loss and the need for more fluids.

6. BOOST FIBRE INTAKE

Most Canadians are getting only a fraction of the recommended amount of fibre, which is 21 g to 38 g daily depending on age and gender. Health Canada recommends 38 g per day for men between the ages of 19 and 50, 30 g per day for men 51 and older, 25 g per day for women between the ages of 19 and 50, and 21 g per day for women 51 and older.

Fibre is critical because it can reduce your risk of chronic diseases, such as diabetes, heart disease, and certain cancers, plus it keeps your bowels regular, improves blood sugar control, and plays a role in weight management. Dietary fibre is found in fruits, vegetables, beans, nuts, seeds, and whole grains such as wheat and oat bran. If your diet is lacking in fibre, look for a supplement.

7. REDUCE THE SALT AND INCREASE THE POTASSIUM

Salt (sodium) is necessary for health, as it helps maintain fluid balance and aids muscle and nerve function; however, according to Health Canada the majority of Canadians consume sodium in quantities that exceed the upper limit, the amount associated with an increased risk of adverse health effects. In particular, excessive sodium intake can contribute to high blood pressure, especially in older individuals, Black Canadians, and those with diabetes and kidney disease.

The IOM recommends adults consume 3.8 g of salt daily to replace the amount lost through sweat. The Tolerable Upper Intake Level (maximum recommended amount) is 5.8 g per day, and most adults regularly consume more than this amount; we need to cut back.

There is naturally occurring salt in dairy, seafood, vegetables, breads, and grains; however, the majority of our salt intake comes from processed and prepared foods, such as deli meats, condiments (ketchup), dressings and sauces (soy), and snack foods (chips, pretzels), so cut back on these foods and season food with herbs or flavoured oils and vinegars rather than using the salt shaker.

Potassium is another important nutrient for regulating fluid balance. It is also important for nerve and muscle function and supports cell structure and integrity. The IOM recommends that adults consume at least 4.7 g of potassium per day to lower blood pressure, blunt the effects of salt, and reduce the risk of kidney stones and bone loss. Most Canadians consume much less than this recommended amount. To boost potassium intake, eat more bananas, oranges and orange juice, avocado, peaches, and tomatoes.

8. MINIMIZE SUGAR

The typical adult consumes about 72.5 kg of sugar each year, which is clearly too much. Sugar is naturally present in foods like fruits and it is added to numerous foods such as sauces (ketchup), dressings, baked goods (breads, cookies, muffins), and snack foods. Excessive sugar intake has been linked to diabetes, obesity, elevated triglycerides, tooth decay, emotional swings, weakened immune function, and other health problems. Refined (white) sugar contains propyl alcohol, which cannot be broken down in the body. Accumulation of this chemical in the intestines can disrupt digestion and be toxic to the body.

The World Health Organization recommends restricting consumption of added sugar—including sugar from honey, syrups, and sweetened drinks/juices—to less than 10 percent of calories.

To satisfy a craving for sweets, have fruit (fresh or dried). Fruit contains natural sugar (fructose), but it also provides vitamins, minerals, and fibre. Mashed bananas or apple sauce are great substitutions for sugar in baked goods. Artificial sweeteners such as aspartame and saccharin should be minimized or avoided because they have been linked to headaches, mental illness, brain damage, and cancer. Stevia, a natural sweetener obtained from a plant, is a good substitute. It can provide up to 300 times the sweetening power of sugar without the calories.

9. CONTROL CAFFEINE

Caffeine is naturally present in coffee, tea, and to a small degree chocolate. It is also added to energy drinks and soft drinks. An excessively high intake of caffeine is associated with various health problems including calcium loss from bones, increased blood pressure, reduced fertility in men and women, sleep disturbances (insomnia), irritability, anxiety, and tremors. It is also highly addictive—abrupt withdrawal, even if you drink only one cup of coffee daily, can cause headaches, irritability, and fatigue within hours of missing your usual drink.

The news is not all bad with respect to caffeine, though. Moderate consumption of coffee, tea, and chocolate is associated with various health benefits because of the presence of antioxidants. To reap the benefits of these foods while minimizing risk, it is generally recommended to cap caffeine intake at 300 mg per day, which is equivalent to about three (regular size) cups of coffee. Drip coffee has the highest caffeine content at 100 mg to 200 mg. Black tea and green tea contain approximately 35 mg to 45 mg, but the effects of caffeine are blunted by an amino acid (theanine), which has a calming effect. Cola contains about 35 mg per can, and chocolate contains 6 mg to 20 mg per 30 g piece.

10. LIMIT ALCOHOL

Heavy and chronic drinking (more than three drinks per day) is linked to liver and cardiovascular disease, pancreatitis, immune system depression, increased risk of cancer (esophagus, mouth, liver, breast, and colon), brain shrinkage, sexual dysfunction (impotence), infertility, and malnutrition. Alcohol and what it is mixed with floods the body with excess calories, which can contribute to weight gain.

There are some benefits with moderate alcohol consumption. Research has found that moderate consumption and reduces the risk of heart disease, likely due to its ability to increase HDL (good) cholesterol and reduce blood clotting, and due to the increased antioxidant activity, as seen with red wine and dark beer. The Heart and Stroke Foundation of Canada recommends that if you drink alcohol, limit yourself to no more than 2 drinks a day (to a weekly maximum of 10 drinks) for women and 3 drinks a day (weekly maximum of 15 drinks) for men. A drink means 341 mL (12 ounces or 1 bottle) of regular-strength beer (5% alcohol), 142 mL (5 ounces) wine (12% alcohol), or 43 mL (1 and 1/2 ounces) spirits (40% alcohol).

PUTTING IT ALL TOGETHER

As you read through this chapter, you probably identified some areas where you need to make changes. This is the first step—realization. Next, work on slowly making healthier food choices, such as cutting out fast food, eating more vegetables, drinking more water, or limiting your sugar or caffeine intake. By gradually making changes, you will be more likely to stick with your nutritional plan.

Take time to plan your meals so that you are not reaching for fast food or unhealthy snacks.

Don't get discouraged by an occasional overindulgence. If you have a bad diet day, don't let it perpetuate. Get back on track the next day—consistency counts.

By following a healthy diet you will notice that you have more energy, a better mood, and an overall improved sense of well-being.

EXERCISE FOR BETTER HEALTH

There is no getting around it—regular exercise and physical activity are essential for good health and must be part of your daily life. You will notice recommendations throughout this book for exercise, as virtually every parameter of health can be improved with exercise. Numerous studies have shown that regular exercise cuts your risk of chronic, debilitating diseases such as heart disease (by reducing cholesterol and blood pressure), osteoporosis, cancer, and diabetes, and it also prevents premature death! Exercise is essential to develop and maintain both a healthy body weight and muscular strength. Plus it offers emotional benefits, as exercise reduces stress and anxiety, and improves sleep and overall emotional well-being.

With today's busy, fast-paced lifestyle, exercise usually falls to the bottom of the priority list while it should be at the top. There are plenty of reasons why people don't exercise. Lack of time is the most common excuse, so in this chapter I show you ways to boost the activity in your life. Many people find they don't have the energy to exercise, yet they don't realize that exercise actually gives them more energy. Some people have a misconception that exercise is expensive, but that is only true if you join a fancy health club. There are plenty of activities you can do with little or no cost. Some are concerned about health problems (arthritis and back problems), yet exercise can actually benefit and improve these problems. Regardless of your health status, age, or current fitness level, there are activities that you can do to improve your health. So now that we have put aside the common obstacles, let's take a look at the various types of exercise and how to build them into our lifestyle.

CARDIOVASCULAR (AEROBIC) EXERCISE

Cardiovascular activities involve large muscle groups and increase heart rate for more than a few minutes. Examples include brisk walking, swimming, biking, aerobics, dancing, and rollerblading. These exercises help burn calories and also improve cardiovascular and respiratory (lung) function by conditioning the lungs to use more oxygen while increasing your heart's efficiency (decreasing heart rate).

Aim for 30 minutes to an hour five times per week. If you are currently not exercising, then start slowly—five minutes on your first day and then increase gradually. With time, endurance improves.

Pick activities that you enjoy and do them in the morning or right after work, preferably on an empty stomach. Morning is best because you will have more energy and will continue to burn calories for several hours afterward.

To determine the intensity level for optimal cardiovascular (and fat-burning) benefits, check your heart rate. The activity should increase your heart rate to 60 to 80 percent of your maximum rate for 30 minutes or longer. To find your maximum rate, subtract your age from 220. Then calculate 60 to 80 percent of that figure. Beginners should aim for 60 percent, while more advanced exercisers can aim for 80 percent.

For example, if you are 40 years old:

220 − 40 = 180
60–80 percent of 180 = 108–144

So you should keep your heart rate between 108 and 144 beats per minute for 30 minutes.

Other ways to gauge your intensity level are as follows:

Breath sound check: Your breathing should be heavier and audible.
Talk test: You should be capable of talking, but not with great ease.

To increase intensity, add resistance or power to the movements. For example, when a brisk 30-minute walk becomes easy, add hand weights or walk on hills. Moving your arms above your heart will also increase your heart rate.

RESISTANCE TRAINING

Activities that challenge your muscles against resistance increase strength, endurance, and muscle mass, and strengthen bones. This can be achieved with weightlifting, exercise machines, bands/tubes, using your own body weight, or lifting heavy objects. These activities are particularly important for older adults because they help prevent and slow the muscle and bone loss that occurs with aging.

Try to spend 20 to 30 minutes three to four times a week doing resistance activities. Choose two body parts per workout. For example, do chest and triceps on Monday, back and biceps on Wednesday, and legs and shoulders on Friday. Pick two exercises per body part and do two or three sets of 8 to 12 repetitions of that exercise. Vary your activities and routine to continually challenge your muscles.

One effective form of resistance training that has gained popularity over the past decade is Pilates. Pilates incorporates controlled resistance activities and breathing to build strength and improve flexibility, balance, and endurance.

STRETCHING

Stretching after a workout is a great way to improve flexibility and joint health and prevent next-day soreness. Spend about five to ten minutes stretching all your muscles. Stretch slowly and gently, breathe deeply, and hold each position for at least 10 seconds. Yoga, which involves breathing techniques along with controlled poses and stretches, is a great way to reduce stress and improve flexibility and posture.

HOW MUCH EXERCISE DO YOU NEED?

The Canadian Society for Exercise Physiology has created the Canadian Physical Activity Guidelines, which provide recommendations based on age. These guidelines recommend that adults should accumulate a minimum of 150 minutes of moderate- to vigorous-intensity aerobic physical activity per week, in bouts of 10 minutes or more. They also suggest adding muscle- and bone-strengthening activities, using major muscle groups, at least twice a week.

BUILDING ACTIVITY INTO YOUR DAY

If you don't have time to dedicate to exercise, work on incorporating more activity into your daily routine. Every little bit helps. Studies have actually shown that the benefits of exercise are cumulative (i.e., performing a few minutes of exercise at a time is as effective as performing all the exercise at once). Here are some suggestions:

• Do housework or gardening with vim and vigour.
• Take the stairs instead of the elevator.
• Use your break at work to go for a brisk walk.
• Ride your bike to the store.
• Park your car farther away and walk to your destination.
• Wash your car by hand instead of using the car wash.

Of course, if you can set aside the recommended 150 minutes each week for exercise, that is great.

EXERCISE FOR WEIGHT LOSS

Regular exercise is essential for losing body fat and maintaining muscle mass. In fact, it has been found that those who work out five times a week lose three times as much fat as those who exercise only two or three times weekly. Exercise supports fat loss by

• Burning calories and stored fat;
• Raising the metabolic rate (the rate at which you burn calories) for 4 to 24 hours afterward;
• Slowing the movement of food through your digestive tract, so you feel full longer; and
• Balancing blood sugar—exercise pulls stored calories (energy) in the forms of glucose and fat out of tissues, which helps balance blood glucose levels, making you less likely to feel hungry

MORE MUSCLE BURNS MORE CALORIES

It is a common misconception that aerobic exercise is the most effective way to lose body fat. Aerobic activities do burn calories, but resistance training plays a stronger role because it builds lean muscle mass, which boosts your metabolism, burns calories, and encourages the body to use fat more efficiently as fuel. The bottom line is the more muscle you have, the more calories you burn. In fact, 1 pound (0.5 kg) of muscle burns roughly 50 calories per day, compared to 1 pound (0.5 kg) of fat, which burns only 2 to 3 calories per day.

CREATING YOUR FITNESS PROGRAM

If you have been sedentary all your life, the prospect of getting active may be intimidating, so take it slowly. If you do too much too soon, you may injure yourself or become too discouraged to continue. Here are some important points to keep in mind:

- Before you start an exercise program, consult with your doctor, especially if you have any health conditions or are taking medication.
- For guidance on proper exercise technique and help in designing a workout tailored to your needs, see a certified personal trainer.
- To keep your motivation high, get a workout partner, vary your activities, and most importantly have fun.
- Don't expect overnight results. Set reasonable goals, be consistent with your exercises, and you will see both the physical and emotional rewards.
- Be sure to drink lots of water during and after your workout, and make time to stretch your muscles.
- Ensure adequate protein intake to maintain and repair muscles. Research shows that by consuming a high-quality protein shake (especially whey protein isolate) immediately after performing resistance exercise, you can greatly increase your body's ability to recuperate. This is largely due to a very powerful amino acid in protein— essential to early muscle repair—called leucine.

CHAPTER 6

THE IMPORTANCE OF SLEEP AND STRESS MANAGEMENT

Right along with proper nutrition and regular exercise are two other essential elements for healthy living: adequate sleep and stress management. These essential but often overlooked factors are paramount for physical and emotional well-being and disease prevention. In this chapter we take a closer look at the value of sleep, how to get a better night's rest, and how to deal with stress more effectively.

SLEEP

Sleep is one of the body's most basic needs for health and well-being, yet with today's busy lifestyles sleep deprivation has become all too common. In fact, nearly half of all adults report having difficulty sleeping.

While we think of sleep as a relaxing and passive state, there is actually quite a lot going on in the body during sleep. During sleep our body's major organs and regulatory systems are busy repairing, restoring, and regenerating. Sleep is required for the rejuvenation of our immune, nervous, skeletal, and muscular systems, and various hormones are secreted during sleep.

There are five stages of sleep defined by brain wave activity, muscle tone, and eye movement. Stage one is referred to as drowsy sleep and represents the onset of sleep. During stage two, conscious awareness of the external environment disappears. During stages three and four, the body goes into a deeper sleep, and the brain produces what are called delta waves. Delta sleep is our deepest sleep, the point when our brain waves are least like what they are when we are awake. It is during this time that the body's major organs and regulatory systems are busy working on repair and regeneration, and certain hormones, such as growth hormone, are secreted. Stage five, known as REM (rapid eye movement) sleep, is the stage during which we dream.

The exact amount of sleep needed varies among individuals, but is thought to be between seven and nine hours for adults. Infants and children require more sleep.

An occasional sleepless night is not a concern, but persistent difficulty in falling asleep, waking up too early, awakening frequently during the night, or waking up feeling tired and not refreshed could indicate insomnia. Getting less than six hours of sleep is associated with numerous health problems. Lack of sleep, particularly deep (delta) sleep, not only makes us feel tired, but it has serious consequences such as memory loss, poor concentration, depression, headache, irritability, increased response to stress, high blood pressure, depressed immune function, and low libido. Worse yet, studies have found that lack of sleep increases the risk of heart disease, stroke, and certain types of cancer, including breast and colon cancer. More recently sleep deprivation has been linked to obesity due to hormonal changes that reduce metabolism and increase appetite.

Causes of Insomnia

There are many factors that can affect the quality of sleep, such as stress, medical problems (depression, anxiety), side effects of medications, alcohol, poor nutrition, noise/light, the need to go to the bathroom during the night, and poor sleep hygiene (going to bed at different times). Insomnia and its causes and treatments are covered in greater detail in Section 3 of this book.

Tips for a Better Night's Rest

For a good night's sleep, consider the following:

- Establish a regular bedtime and wake time.
- Do relaxing activities before bed—read a book, have a warm bath, or meditate.
- Reserve your bedroom for intimacy and sleep only. Don't watch TV or do computer work in your bedroom.
- Make your bedroom dark, quiet, and comfortable.
- Avoid caffeine (coffee, tea, soft drinks, chocolate) and smoking within four hours of bedtime, as this can affect your ability to fall asleep.
- Choose your bedtime snacks wisely. Sugary foods such as cookies, ice cream, and candy bars can cause a "sugar rush" and affect your ability to fall asleep. Avoid these foods within four hours of bedtime. Also avoid heavy and spicy foods before bed as they can trigger heartburn and reflux and affect your ability to stay asleep. If you want a bedtime snack, choose a food that contains tryptophan, an amino acid that stimulates the release of serotonin, a brain chemical that facilitates sleep. Examples include whole-grain crackers and cheese or turkey, a banana, or a small bowl of cereal.
- Be aware that some medications can contribute to sleep problems, such as decongestants, beta-blockers, thyroid medications, antidepressants, and pain medications (some of which contain caffeine).
- Avoid alcohol; it may help you fall asleep, but drinking alcohol causes nighttime wakening and reduces sleep quality.
- Exercise regularly early in the day. Do not exercise in the evening, as this can be stimulating and affect your ability to fall asleep.
- If you work shifts or travel to different time zones, try a supplement of melatonin (a hormone naturally secreted in response to darkness), as it helps promote good sleep. Other remedies for promoting better sleep are discussed in the insomnia section of this book.

STRESS

Stress has become a common complaint of life in the fast lane. We don't have enough time, take on too much, worry about health and wealth, and feel overwhelmed and stressed out on a regular basis. Sound familiar? According to recent reports, 43 percent of all adults suffer the adverse health effects of stress, and stress-related ailments account for 75 to 90 percent of all visits to physicians. These numbers have been steadily climbing over the past few decades.

Understanding Stress

Stress, as defined by Hans Selye, an Austrian-born Canadian physician who studied the physiological and biochemical results of stress and anxiety, is "the non-specific response of the body to any demand placed upon it." He claimed that it isn't stress that harms us but distress, a phenomenon that occurs when we have prolonged emotional stress and don't deal with it in a positive manner. In other words, stress is not an external force but rather how we react internally to external stimuli—how we feel and respond to traffic, deadlines at work, or any event that we perceive as stressful.

To understand why stress can be harmful to your health it is important to look at what happens in your body when you are stressed. Your body undergoes a series of changes called the stress response. There are three stages to this response: *alarm, resistance,* and *exhaustion.*

Alarm is the start-up stage, which defines the first reaction to the stressor. Stress hormones called catecholamines (adrenaline and noradrenaline) and glucocorticoids (cortisol) are released. These hormones, which are secreted by the adrenal glands, prepare the body to either fight or flee—hence the term "fight-or-flight" for this response. When this occurs, our body enters a catabolic state, where our fuels (glucose, fats, and amino acids) are broken down to provide energy. Heart rate, blood pressure, blood volume, and pulmonary (lung) tone increase to enhance the function of the heart and lungs. Muscle tone increases to improve strength and performance.

The second stage is known as *resistance.* If the stressor persists (and in this case it does), it becomes necessary to attempt some means of coping with the stress. Although the body begins to try to adapt to the strains or demands of the environment, the body cannot keep this up indefinitely, so its resources are gradually depleted.

The third and final stage is *exhaustion.* The body's resources are depleted and the body is unable to maintain normal function.

This stress response, an innate mechanism, was designed to help us cope with short bursts of stress, such as running away from a predator. The problem is that our bodies have not adapted to handle a continuous onslaught of stress and the continuous release of stress hormones.

Stress and Disease

Our emotional state can affect our physical or biological state. Many studies have found that people who are positive, optimistic, and don't worry excessively (i.e., don't sweat the small stuff) have less chronic disease and live longer.

Stress has the very opposite effect on health. It literally wreaks havoc on almost every system in our body. The most commonly experienced consequences are headaches, insomnia, anxiety, muscle tension, and upset stomach. Stress also hampers immune function, memory, and concentration; impairs fertility; reduces sex drive; and can accelerate the aging process. Stress is also associated with depression, anxiety, and obesity, and is linked to some of our most serious and debilitating diseases, namely heart disease, diabetes, and cancer.

Stress Management

Stress can certainly take a toll on your body and mind, so it is absolutely crucial to find ways to cope effectively. Start by identifying your stressors and then look for ways to change your reaction to those situations. It may be a matter of analyzing and rethinking your natural reaction, avoiding certain situations, or using one of the following stress-reducing strategies. Seeking help from a counsellor or psychologist can be very helpful to learn coping techniques and strategies.

Meditation

Meditation is the practice of focusing the mind and consciously relaxing the body for a sustained period. It is common among Eastern cultures and is gaining popularity in North America. Focusing on a single object or your breath or a sound occupies your mind and diverts it from the problems that are causing you stress. Many studies have found meditation to be an effective and practical way to manage stress. All you need is a quiet, comfortable area. Sit down and close your eyes. Relax all your muscles starting with your feet and working up. Focus your attention on your breathing or a calming sight or sound. Breathe in slowly and deeply and then out. Do this for 10 or 20 minutes. You can do this when feeling stressed, or make a habit of meditating once or twice a day for better health and relaxation.

Breathing Techniques

Taking slow, controlled breaths is a great way to promote calming when feeling stressed or anxious. Sit down comfortably and close your eyes. Place the tip of your tongue against the roof of your mouth just behind your front teeth. Begin by exhaling through your mouth around your tongue, then close your mouth and inhale deeply through your nose for four seconds. Hold your breath for five seconds and then completely exhale through your mouth, making a *whoosh* sound. Repeat this cycle four or five times. This technique can be done anytime, anywhere.

Exercise

Getting regular exercise is a great way to reduce stress, promote calming, and improve both physical and emotional well-being. Exercise can help elevate your mood, lessen anxiety and anger, and increase blood flow to the muscles, which tend to be tense from stress. Walking, cycling, swimming, and dancing are just a few examples of stress-busting activities. Keep in mind, though, that you also need to find ways to change your reaction to stress (counselling). Yoga and tai chi are excellent forms of exercise to promote relaxation, as they incorporate breathing and visualization.

Visualization

This technique involves concentrating on images in your mind that make you feel calm and relaxed. Close your eyes, take a few deep breaths, and visualize a picture or event that make you feel calm and centred. Focus on the details—the sounds, images, and smells.

Other Considerations

- Massage, acupuncture, and acupressure promote relaxation of the body and mind.
- Supplements that help relieve stress include theanine, B-vitamins, and magnesium. This is discussed further in Section Three of this book.
- Learn to say no. Taking on too much leads to feeling overwhelmed and pressed for time. Being able to say no (no excuse needed) when asked to take on a new task will make you feel empowered and relieved.
- Avoid negativity, as negative people, places, and events can create stress.
- Channel stress in positive ways—exercise, paint, or clean your house.
- Talk about it—share your feelings and concerns and get support from friends, family, or a therapist.

FINAL THOUGHTS

Improving the quality of your sleep and dealing more effectively with stress will bring many health rewards—fewer physical and emotional ailments and overall improved well-being. Identify the areas where you are struggling, seek help, and work on adopting positive changes.

SECTION II

THE NATURAL PHARMACY

CHAPTER 7

REFERENCE GUIDE TO DIETARY SUPPLEMENTS, HERBAL REMEDIES, AND BRANDED INGREDIENTS

In this chapter you will find concise information on various nutritional supplements. This list is not all-inclusive—there are thousands of supplements on the market, but I chose to include those with the most research and proven health benefits. In cases where clinical research has been done on a specific branded product or ingredient, I have included that name. As well, I have noted important drug interactions, side effects, and precautions.

You will find other nutritional supplements that have specific uses listed under the individual ailments in Section Three. For example, supplements used specifically for weight loss are included in the discussion on obesity.

It is always a good idea to check with your health care provider before taking any new product, particularly if you are taking medications or have a health condition. Dosages are not included here, as they vary with the intended use, age of the person, existing medical problems, and other factors.

AGED GARLIC EXTRACT (KYOLIC)

Garlic is well known for its myriad health benefits and its strong odour. Aged garlic extract is unique in that it is odourless, processed from organically grown garlic, standardized to potent sulphur compounds, and the most widely researched garlic product available. Studies have shown that the unique antioxidant compounds in aged garlic extract provide benefits for heart health by lowering blood pressure and cholesterol, slowing the progression of atherosclerosis, reducing homocysteine levels and inflammation, and improving circulation. It also supports liver detoxification and immune function, and may play a role in cancer protection.

ALOE VERA

Aloe vera is a plant that has a long history of use to promote skin healing. It contains amino acids, vitamins C and E, zinc, and essential fatty acids. Research supports the use of topical aloe for genital herpes (to improve healing of lesions), seborrhea, and psoriasis; preliminary research shows benefits with oral aloe to improve blood sugar in type 2 diabetes and for treatment of ulcerative colitis.

ALPHA-LIPOIC ACID

Alpha-lipoic acid, an antioxidant found inside every cell of the body, helps the body convert glucose into energy to meet the body's needs, and is found naturally in liver, yeast, potatoes, spinach, and red meat. Levels may be depleted in those with diabetes, liver cirrhosis, and atherosclerosis. It is used to improve glucose levels in diabetics, to treat diabetic neuropathy, and for burning mouth syndrome. Side effects are rare and may include skin rash and upset stomach.

ARGININE

An amino acid found in many foods, such as dairy, meat, poultry, and fish, arginine is involved in cell division, wound healing, removal of ammonia from the body, immunity to illness, the secretion of hormones, and the production of nitrous oxide, a substance that dilates blood vessels. Research supports its use for congestive heart failure, intermittent claudication, angina, impotence, and sexual dysfunction in women; preliminary evidence shows benefits for diabetes and improving recovery from surgery. High dosages (greater than 20 g per day) are not recommended for those with kidney and liver disease.

BETA-GLUCAN

A type of soluble fibre found naturally in plants such as oats, wheat, and barley, beta-glucan is also available in supplements. Studies have shown that beta-glucan can modestly improve cholesterol levels; it may also reduce blood pressure and improve blood sugar levels in diabetics. There are no known side effects or drug interactions.

BLACK COHOSH

Black cohosh is an herb used for the treatment of menopausal symptoms; several studies show that it can reduce hot flashes and improve mood. It may also help reduce vaginal thinning and protect the bones. Research involving black cohosh plus St. John's wort has shown benefits for both hot flashes and depression in menopause. Do not use during pregnancy or breastfeeding, and use cautiously if you have liver disease. High doses may cause upset stomach, nausea, and headache.

BOSWELLIA

An herb with a long history of use in Ayurvedic medicine, boswellia is used for arthritis, respiratory diseases, and diarrhea. Its anti-inflammatory properties have been studied and found beneficial for the treatment of rheumatoid and osteoarthritis, asthma, and inflammatory bowel disease. It is generally well tolerated; there are no known drug interactions.

BREWER'S YEAST

A product derived from dried, pulverized cells of the fungus *Saccharomyces cerevisiae*, brewer's yeast is a rich source of B-vitamins, protein, and minerals like chromium. Supplements are used to treat acute diarrhea and to lower cholesterol and improve blood sugar balance in diabetics. Recent research suggests that a form of brewer's yeast

(EpiCor) may also help prevent the common cold and influenza. Brewer's yeast is available in powders, flakes, tablets, and liquid forms; some forms of brewer's yeast require refrigeration. Side effects are rare, but some people are allergic to brewer's yeast.

BROMELAIN
Bromelain is a combination of protein-digesting enzymes (called proteolytic enzymes) found in pineapple juice and in the stem of pineapple plants. It is used to reduce inflammation, treat sinusitis, improve healing from injuries, and support immune function. Side effects are rare, but allergic reactions are possible. It may thin the blood, so use cautiously with blood-thinning drugs like warfarin as dosage adjustments may be necessary.

BUTCHER'S BROOM
Butcher's broom is an herb with a long history of use as a diuretic and for urinary problems. Research has demonstrated benefits for reducing the pain, swelling, and fatigue associated with chronic venous insufficiency; it may also be helpful for hemorrhoids, varicose veins, and lymphedema. It is generally well tolerated; there are no known drug interactions.

CARNITINE
Carnitine is an amino acid that the body uses to turn fat into energy. Levels may be depleted in those with kidney, liver, or brain disease, and in those taking antiseizure drugs such as phenytoin and valproic acid. Research supports benefits for angina, intermittent claudication, congestive heart failure, heart attack recovery, diabetic neuropathy, chronic obstructive pulmonary disease, and male sexual function and infertility. Carnitine is very safe and well tolerated, but should be used cautiously by those with low thyroid hormone.

CAYENNE
Cayenne is a pepper that is part of the capsicum family. Creams containing cayenne are used to reduce pain (arthritis, strains, sprains, fibromyalgia, back pain, headache, and shingles); it helps reduce the itching caused by psoriasis and the symptoms of neuropathy; it may reduce the stomach irritation caused by non-steroidal anti-inflammatory drugs (NSAIDs). Wash your hands after applying this cream because it can cause burning and stinging if you rub your eyes. Oral cayenne may increase the absorption of theophylline, a drug used for asthma and lung disease.

CELADRIN
Celadrin is a patented blend of cetylated fatty acids derived from beef tallow. Studies show benefits for reducing the pain and inflammation associated with osteoarthritis; it may also benefit other inflammatory conditions such as rheumatoid arthritis, eczema, psoriasis, and gout. There are no known drug interactions or side effects. It is available in cream and oral supplements.

CHAMOMILE
An herb popular for its calming properties, chamomile is found in teas, oral supplements, and creams. It is used orally (tea and supplements) to reduce anxiety and promote

relaxation. Topical products are used to promote healing. Compounds in chamomile have blood-thinning properties, so it should be used cautiously by those taking warfarin or other blood thinners, as dosage adjustments may be necessary.

CHONDROITIN SULPHATE
Chondroitin sulphate is a naturally occurring substance in the body that is a major constituent of cartilage, the connective tissue found in joints. Oral supplements are used to reduce the symptoms of osteoarthritis (improve mobility and reduce pain); it may also reduce the progression of the disease. Topically it is used to improve wound healing. It is usually well tolerated, although high doses may cause upset stomach.

COENZYME Q10
Coenzyme Q10, an antioxidant naturally found in our bodies, is involved in energy production in every cell. Strong evidence supports supplement use for congestive heart failure; it is also used for high blood pressure, heart attack recovery, mitral valve prolapse, cardiomyopathy, gum disease, diabetes, Parkinson's disease, and migraine headache. Q10 levels may be depleted by statin drugs, beta-blockers, and antidepressants. Deficiency causes fatigue, gum disease, heart problems, and increased risk of infections. Supplements are well tolerated even at high dosages.

COLOSTRUM
Colostrum, a component of breast milk, is produced during the first day or two after birth. It provides newborns with a rich mixture of antibodies and growth factors. Supplements are derived from cow colostrums and are used for immune support, for treatment of infectious diarrhea, and in sports products.

CRANBERRY
Cranberry contains antioxidants called proanthocyanidins (condensed tannins), which prevent bacterial adhesion to the bladder wall. Cranberry juice and supplements may also help lower cholesterol and protect against gum disease and *H. pylori* infection (the cause of ulcers). Cran-Max is a proprietary cranberry supplement that has been found in numerous studies to prevent urinary tract infections. It is unique from other cranberry products in that it is made with all of the parts of the cranberry (skin, seeds, pulp and juice) with a patented technology called Bio-Shield, which protects the bioactives from destruction in the stomach.

CREATINE
Creatine is a naturally occurring substance that plays an important role in the production of energy in the body. Several studies have shown that creatine can increase athletic performance in sports that involve intense but short bursts of activity. It may also offer benefits for weight training and to prevent muscle loss in seniors. Side effects include diarrhea and muscle cramping. It should be avoided by those with kidney disease.

D-CHIRO-INOSITOL

D-Chiro-Inositol is a natural ingredient derived from carob juice that is sold commercially as Chirositol. Numerous clinical studies have found that D-Chiro-Inositol can stimulate insulin function with a positive effect on blood sugar and lipid levels, reduce androgens, and modulate serotonin. It is used for the treatment of diabetes, metabolic syndrome, skin tags, polycystic ovarian syndrome, infertility, and conditions of excess androgens, and to assist in weight management. Chirositol is well tolerated.

D-GLUCARATE

A supplemental form of glucaric acid, which is a phytonutrient found in fruits and vegetables (apples, Brussels sprouts, broccoli, and cabbage), D-glucarate helps the liver detoxify and eliminate excess hormones (particularly estrogen). It is used for the treatment of PMS, fibrocystic breast disease, uterine fibroids, and other conditions of estrogen excess; it is also used for prevention of hormone-dependent cancers of the breast and prostate. There are no known side effects or drug interactions. However, many drugs are metabolized in the liver and D-glucarate may enhance the elimination of certain drugs, requiring dosage adjustments.

DIGESTIVE ENZYMES

Digestive enzymes are protein compounds that aid in the breakdown and digestion of food. They are found naturally in raw foods and are also produced by the body. There are three classes: proteolytic enzymes digest protein, lipases digest fat, and amylases digest carbohydrates. Supplements are used to aid digestion and may be particularly helpful in those with digestive problems such as irritable bowel syndrome, celiac disease, and food intolerances. Proteolytic enzymes may also help reduce pain and inflammation from injuries, osteoarthritis, and surgery. Side effects and allergic reactions are rare.

DIOSMIN

Diosmin is a flavonoid that improves the tone and strength of the blood vessels, reduces swelling, fights free radical damage, and stimulates lymphatic flow. Over 30 clinical studies have found it effective for improving vein disorders, including varicose veins, chronic venous insufficiency, nighttime leg cramps, and hemorrhoids. It has a quick onset of action (one to two weeks) and is not associated with any side effects or drug interactions. Look for a product standardized to 95 percent diosmin and 5 percent hesperidin.

ECHINACEA

Echinacea is an herb that supports immune function. Most studies have found that it shortens the duration of colds and flus and may halt a cold if it is taken at the first sign of symptoms, but most research suggests that it is not effective as a preventative. Side effects are rare; it is not recommended for those with autoimmune disorders like lupus. Allergic reactions may occur, especially in those with sensitivity to ragweed, mums, or daisies.

EVENING PRIMROSE OIL

Obtained from the seeds of the primrose plant, evening primrose oil provides a rich source of gamma-linolenic acid (GLA), which is an omega-6 fatty acid. It has anti-inflammatory properties and is important for brain function. Research supports benefits for the treatment of arthritis, diabetic neuropathy, eczema and dry skin, cyclic mastalgia (breast pain with menstrual cycle), fibrocystic breast disease, and Raynaud's disease. Side effects (upset stomach) are rare.

FENUGREEK

Fenugreek, an herb used as a medicine and spice for thousands of years in India and Egypt, aids in lactation, wound treatment, bronchitis, digestive problems, arthritis, and kidney problems. Studies show that it can reduce blood sugar and cholesterol levels in diabetics; it may also relieve constipation. It is usually well tolerated, although high doses may cause upset stomach. It is not recommended during pregnancy. Diabetics may require adjustment in therapy, as fenugreek can lower blood sugar levels.

FEVERFEW

Feverfew is a plant extract that is used for headache prevention. The main active component, parthenolide, prevents platelet clumping and inhibits the release of serotonin and inflammatory chemicals. Several studies have shown that it can reduce the severity, duration, and frequency of migraine headaches. Recent research on a combination of feverfew and ginger in an olive oil emulsion (called LipiGesic M) found it effective in the acute treatment of migraine. This product is taken sublingually (under the tongue) and has been found in studies to significantly reduce pain and prevent a migraine from becoming severe. Feverfew is well tolerated; there are no known drug interactions.

FISH OIL

Fish oil is a rich source of the omega-3 fatty acids DHA (docosahexaenoic acid) and EPA (eicosapentaenoic acid), which have anti-inflammatory effects. DHA is important for brain function, vision, and joint health. EPA supports immune function, blood clotting, and circulation. Numerous studies have shown that fish oil can reduce the risk of heart attack and stroke; it lowers triglyceride levels, raises HDL (good) cholesterol, reduces clotting, lowers homocysteine, and may reduce blood pressure. Some research suggests benefits for rheumatoid arthritis, menstrual pain, depression, bipolar disorder, attention deficit disorder, and Raynaud's disease. Side effects are rare; some supplements cause fishy burps.

5-HYDROXYTRYPTOPHAN (5-HTP)

5-HTP is an amino acid that the body uses to make serotonin, a brain chemical that regulates mood, sleep, appetite, pain sensation, and sexual behaviour. Research shows benefits for depression, migraine headaches, weight loss, insomnia, and fibromyalgia. Side effects are rare or minor (upset stomach). Use cautiously with Parkinson's drugs, antidepressants, and drugs or supplements that affect serotonin.

FLAXSEED

Flaxseed is a tiny seed that provides fibre, omega-3 (alpha-linolenic acid) and omega-6 fatty acids, and lignans, which are a type of phytoestrogen. Flaxseed oil is used to reduce inflammation, improve circulation, and treat dry skin; however, there is less research to support its proposed health benefits compared to fish oils. Whole flaxseeds are taken for their laxative benefits. Milled (ground) flaxseed provides the beneficial oils, fibre, and lignans that may help in cancer prevention. Flaxseed is generally well tolerated.

FRUCTOOLIGOSACCHARIDES (FOS)

These are short chains of fructose molecules that occur naturally in foods and are also put into supplements. The body cannot digest these substances, but they serve as a food for probiotics (friendly bacteria) in the digestive tract, so are known as prebiotics. Some research shows that FOS lowers triglyceride levels and cholesterol, and preliminary evidence shows benefits for digestion and intestinal health. FOS may cause bloating, flatulence, and upset stomach at doses of 15 g or higher.

GINGER

Ginger is a plant that is used as a spice and therapeutically as an herbal medicine. Research shows benefits for nausea associated with pregnancy, motion sickness, upset stomach, and migraine headache. There are no significant side effects. Ginger has blood-thinning properties. Studies on ginger supplements in normal amounts have not found any significant effect on coagulation, but it should be used cautiously by those taking anticoagulant drugs like warfarin.

GINKGO BILOBA

Ginkgo biloba, a plant, has a long history of use. Ginkgo has undergone extensive research for a variety of health conditions. It is an antioxidant, improves blood circulation by dilating blood vessels, and reduces the stickiness of blood platelets. Research supports benefits for Alzheimer's disease, improving memory and cognitive function, and treatment of intermittent claudication and anxiety. Preliminary research shows benefits for macular degeneration, PMS, Raynaud's disease, and vertigo. Side effects are rare and minor (upset stomach, headaches, and skin reactions); it may enhance the blood-thinning effect of anticoagulants, so dosage adjustments may be necessary.

GINSENG, AMERICAN AND ASIAN

American and Asian (Panax) ginseng are very similar in composition and properties. Ginseng has adaptogen properties (helps the body deal with stress, whether physical or emotional) and enhances immune function. One particular extract of North American ginseng called COLD-FX has been extensively studied and found to help reduce the frequency, severity, and duration of cold and flu symptoms by boosting the immune system. Both Asian and American ginseng may help to improve blood sugar control. Asian ginseng has been found to enhance mental/cognitive function, sports performance, and overall well-being. Preliminary research shows benefits for improving erectile function, enhancing fertility, and treating attention-deficit/hyperactivity disorder

(ADHD). Ginseng may enhance the blood sugar–lowering effects of insulin or diabetic medications and may decrease the effect of blood-thinning drugs. It is generally well tolerated, but there are some reports of nervousness, insomnia, and upset stomach. Use cautiously with uncontrolled high blood pressure. It is not recommended during pregnancy or breastfeeding, or for those with breast cancer.

GINSENG, SIBERIAN

Also known as *Eleuthero*, Siberian ginseng is not a true ginseng, but has some similar properties as an adaptogen. It is commonly used to support immune function, mental acuity, and athletic performance and to help reduce the effects of stress. Side effects may include upset stomach, insomnia, and increased blood pressure. It is not recommended for those with uncontrolled high blood pressure.

GLUCOSAMINE

Glucosamine occurs naturally in the body and is a building block used to manufacture components of cartilage, the material that cushions joints. Numerous studies have found that it can improve osteoarthritis symptoms (joint pain, mobility); it may also prevent the progression of the disease. Preliminary research suggests possible benefits for irritable bowel syndrome. It is well tolerated, but may cause mild upset stomach.

GRAPE SEED EXTRACT

Grape seed extract provides a source of a potent group of antioxidant compounds called oligomeric proanthocyanidin complexes (OPCs). Research supports benefits for the treatment of chronic venous insufficiency and varicose veins and the prevention of blood clots while flying, and reducing postsurgical edema. Preliminary research suggests benefits for ADHD, PMS, erectile dysfunction, asthma, allergies, hemorrhoids, improving blood sugar control in diabetics, and prevention of atherosclerosis. A patented form of grape seed extract sold as MegaNatural BP has been shown in clinical studies to reduce blood pressure and improve blood vessel flexibility. Grape seed extract is very well tolerated, but may cause minor upset stomach. High dosages may enhance the effect of blood-thinning drugs.

GREEN TEA

Green tea is derived from the plant *Camellia sinensis*. Unlike black and oolong tea, it is not fermented, which preserves the active constituents. It provides a high level of antioxidants called polyphenols, particularly the catechin called epigallocatechin gallate (EGCG). Numerous studies have found green tea to be beneficial for heart health, cancer prevention, cervical dysplasia, weight loss, liver disease, and gum health. Green tea contains some caffeine, but much less so than coffee. Side effects are rare; large amounts may cause insomnia and nervousness.

HAWTHORNE

Hawthorne is an herb with a long history of use for heart ailments. Research has demonstrated that it can improve the heart's pumping action and is helpful in the treatment of congestive heart failure. It may also lower blood pressure and reduce palpitations and angina. It is generally well tolerated; side effects are minor and may include dizziness, upset stomach, headache, and skin rash.

INDOLE-3-CARBINOL

Indole-3-carbinol is a nutrient found in cruciferous vegetables such as broccoli, Brussels sprouts, cabbage, cauliflower, and kale. It has anticancer properties, aids in detoxification of estrogen, reduces the levels of free radicals, and protects liver function. It has been shown in preliminary research to reduce estrogen-promoted cancers (cervical and breast) and to reverse cervical dysplasia. Recent research on a formula containing indole-3-carbinol, D-glucarate, milk thistle, and other nutrients (femMED Breast Health) found that it had a positive effect on the estrogen metabolism ratio, increasing urinary levels of 2-hydroxyestrone (2-OHE) and decreasing levels of 16-alpha-hydroxyestrone (16α-OHE). This effect is associated with a decreased risk of breast cancer. There are no known side effects.

IPRIFLAVONE

Ipriflavone, a synthetic flavonoid derived from soy, is widely used for osteoporosis (available as a supplement in Canada, yet sold as a prescription drug in many other countries). Many studies have shown that when combined with calcium, it can slow and even reverse bone breakdown; it also helps reduce the pain of fractures caused by osteoporosis. It is generally well tolerated; one study found that long-term use (three years) reduced levels of lymphocytes (white blood cells). Use under doctor's supervision if you have immune deficiency (HIV) or kidney disease, or are taking immune-suppressant drugs.

LECITHIN

Lecithin is a source of phosphatidylcholine, a phospholipid (a fat-soluble component of all cell membranes). Supplements of lecithin are broken down in the body into choline, which promotes methylation and is used to make acetylcholine, a nerve chemical essential for proper brain function. Some research supports benefits for liver disease, lowering homocysteine, and the treatment of bipolar, Alzheimer's, and other neurological disorders. It is generally well tolerated.

LICORICE

Licorice is an herb with a long history of use for digestion and immune support. It contains glycyrrhizin, which causes fluid retention and can raise blood pressure; supplements of deglycyrrhizinated licorice (DGL) do not cause these effects. DGL has been studied for ulcer prevention and treatment, and is generally well tolerated. Licorice is used for cough and asthma; topical products may help relieve eczema. It may raise blood pressure, lower testosterone in men, and have estrogenic effects; it is not recommended during pregnancy or breastfeeding, or for use by those with cancer.

L-THEANINE

L-theanine is an amino acid naturally present in green tea that promotes a relaxation effect. Suntheanine is a patented and clinically studied pure form of L-theanine. Research has shown that it promotes an alert state of relaxation without drowsiness. There is also evidence that it can improve the quality of sleep, improve learning performance, reduce the symptoms of premenstrual syndrome, heighten mental acuity, promote concentration, reduce the negative side effects of stress and caffeine, and support immune function. Suntheanine is well tolerated; there are no known drug interactions.

LUTEIN

Lutein, an antioxidant pigment in the carotenoid family, is found in dark green and yellow vegetables. It is highly concentrated in the macula of the eye (behind the retina) and plays a role in protecting the retina from oxidative damage and UV light. Research supports benefits for prevention of cataracts and macular degeneration. It is very well tolerated; there are no known drug interactions.

LYCOPENE

Lycopene is a potent antioxidant (carotenoid) naturally present in red vegetables and fruits (tomatoes, pink grapefruit, and watermelon). Research supports benefits for prevention of prostate cancer and pre-eclampsia, and treatment of asthma; it may also help prevent macular degeneration, cataracts, and heart disease. Lyc-O-Mato is a patented lycopene complex that contains lycopene along with other antioxidants naturally present in tomatoes (beta carotene, phytofluene, tocopherols, and phytosterols). Research suggests that Lyc-O-Mato helps support prostate and heart health and protect the skin from the oxidative stress caused by free radicals produced from sun exposure. Lycopene is very well tolerated; there are no known drug interactions.

LYSINE

Lysine is an amino acid naturally present in meat, poultry, dairy products, eggs, and beans. Regular supplement use has been shown to prevent cold sores; it may also prevent genital herpes flare-ups. It is generally well tolerated.

MELATONIN

Melatonin, a hormone that is produced in the brain and released in response to darkness, regulates our biological clock (sleep–wake cycle). Supplements have been shown to help shorten the time needed to fall asleep, improve sleep quality, and help with disrupted sleep cycles (such as with travellers and shift workers). It may also help in the treatment of depression, seasonal affective disorder, anxiety, schizophrenia, and cluster headaches, and to improve quality of life in cancer patients. Supplements are taken half an hour to one hour before bed to promote better rest. It is well tolerated and does not cause next-day drowsiness; it is not recommended during pregnancy or breastfeeding.

METHYLSULFONYLMETHANE (MSM)

MSM is a naturally occurring sulphur compound in the body; it is also present in certain foods (vegetables). It may be helpful for osteoarthritis, recovery from sports injuries, and growth of nails and hair, although more research is needed. It is very well tolerated; there are no known drug interactions.

MILK THISTLE

Milk thistle, an herb with a long history of use for liver and spleen disorders, contains a flavonoid complex called silymarin, which is responsible for its antioxidant, detoxifying, and liver health benefits. Research supports its use for the treatment of viral and alcoholic hepatitis and liver cirrhosis. Preliminary research suggests that it might protect the liver against drug-induced toxicity caused by acetaminophen (Tylenol) and phenytoin (Dilantin). It is generally well tolerated; there are no known drug interactions.

MODUCARE

Moducare, a patented blend of plant sterols and sterolins (plant fats), helps to restore, strengthen, and balance the immune system. Several studies have demonstrated its immune-modulating effects. It is not recommended for use by those with organ transplants or those taking immune-suppressant drugs; use only under doctor's supervision if pregnant, lactating, or diabetic, or if you have an immune disorder.

NATURAL EGGSHELL MEMBRANE (NEM)

NEM is a supplement made from the membranes of eggshells through a patented process. It contains naturally occurring glycosaminoglycans, including chondroitin and hyaluronic acid, along with collagen and other beneficial proteins. Preliminary research suggests that it can reduce joint pain and stiffness and improve flexibility in those with osteoarthritis. Unlike most joint health products, the benefits of using NEM are often noticed within 10 days.

NETTLE

Nettle is an herb widely used for the treatment of benign prostatic hyperplasia; many studies show benefits for reducing symptoms. Preliminary research suggests benefits for allergies; topical products are used to relieve the pain of osteoarthritis. It may be more beneficial when combined with pygeum and/or saw palmetto, and is generally well tolerated.

PHOSPHATIDYLSERINE

Phosphatidylserine, a phospholipid (a fat-soluble component of all cell membranes) made by the body, performs vital functions such as moving nutrients into cells and pumping waste products out of them. Research shows that supplements can help improve memory, mental function, and depression in the elderly, and it is useful in the treatment of Alzheimer's. It is well tolerated, but may cause mild upset stomach; it may enhance the effect of blood-thinning drugs and supplements, requiring dosage adjustments.

PHYTOSTEROLS/PHYTOSTANOLS

Phytosterols (also known just as sterols) and phytostanols (stanols) are naturally occurring compounds (fats) found in almost all plants. There is significant evidence that stanols/sterols and their ester forms can lower LDL and total cholesterol, similarly to some drugs. Several studies have found benefits with beta-sitosterol (a phytosterol) for reducing symptoms of prostate enlargement. Sterols and stanols are added to foods (such as CoroWise plant sterols, which are added to margarine spreads and orange juice) and sold as supplements. They are very well tolerated.

POLICOSANOL

Policosanol is a waxy substance obtained from sugar cane. Several studies have shown that it can substantially lower cholesterol, similarly to prescription drugs, although the quality of this research has been questioned. Policosanol may enhance the effects of blood-thinning drugs and supplements, so dosage adjustments may be necessary; it is not recommended during pregnancy or breastfeeding.

PROBIOTICS

Also known as friendly or beneficial bacteria, probiotics are microorganisms normally present in the mouth, digestive and urinary tracts, and vaginal area. There are numerous strains (types) of probiotics. Some of the most common strains include *Lactobacillus* (L) *acidophilus*, *L. reuteri*, *L. casei*, *Bifidobacterium bifidum*, and the yeast *Saccharomyces boulardii*.

Probiotics provide many health benefits by protecting against infection by harmful bacteria (yeast and bacteria), aiding in detoxification, producing vitamins, aiding digestion, and supporting immune function. Research supports benefits for travellers' diarrhea, constipation, irritable bowel, ulcerative colitis, eczema, infantile colic, allergies, and tooth decay. They also improve immune function, reduce cholesterol, prevent and treat yeast infections, and enhance ulcer treatment. Probiotic supplements vary greatly in potency (the number of bacteria), therapeutic use (some have been researched for a specific aspect of health), and form (capsules, tablets, powders, liquids). Choose products that are backed by research, tested for potency and stability, and made from human strains. Some require refrigeration. Beneficial bacteria are also present in some fermented dairy foods (live culture yogurt and kefir), although potency and stability is questionable. Probiotics are generally well tolerated.

PYGEUM

Pygeum is a tree whose bark contains phytosterols and compounds that reduce inflammation and modulate testosterone activity in the prostate. Studies have found it beneficial for improving symptoms of an enlarged prostate (benign prostatic hyperplasia); it may also be beneficial for prostatitis (prostate infection). It is often combined with saw palmetto or nettle root, which are also beneficial for reducing prostate symptoms, and is very well tolerated.

RED CLOVER

Red clover is a plant with a history of use for skin disorders and cough, and as a diuretic. Recent research has focused on its isoflavones, which work as phytoestrogens, with possible benefits for menopause. Several (but not all) studies found red clover helpful for reducing hot flashes. It may help reduce blood pressure and cholesterol levels and protect against osteoporosis by reducing bone loss. It is not recommended during pregnancy or breastfeeding, or for use by those with breast or uterine cancer. It may enhance the effect of blood-thinning drugs, so dosage adjustments may be necessary.

RELORA

Relora, a proprietary blend of extracts of magnolia and phellodendron, has been studied for its stress-relieving properties. It promotes relaxation without sedation, normalizes stress hormones, and reduces stress-related eating. It is generally well tolerated, but may cause mild upset stomach.

RHODIOLA

Rhodiola, an herb classified as an adaptogen, was used historically to combat stress and fatigue and to speed recovery from illness. Studies have demonstrated benefits for reducing fatigue and enhancing mental function. Preliminary research suggests that it may help with altitude sickness and may aid cancer chemotherapy by protecting the liver against drug-induced damage. There are no known side effects or drug interactions.

RIBOSE

Ribose is a carbohydrate that is critical for the manufacture of ATP (adenosine triphosphate), which is the major source of energy used by all cells in the body. Studies suggest supplements may help increase exercise tolerance and endurance, particularly in those with heart disease, and aid recovery from heart attack. It may also offer benefits for enhancing athletic performance, although the research is mixed.

S-ADENOSYLMETHIONINE (SAMe)

SAMe is a naturally occurring nutrient in the body that is involved in hormone and neurotransmitter production, detoxification, joint health, and many other vital bodily processes. Research shows that supplements can benefit those with depression, osteoarthritis, liver disease, and fibromyalgia. It may also reduce depression associated with Parkinson's disease. It is generally well tolerated, but may cause mild upset stomach. It is not recommended for those with bipolar disorder; use cautiously with other products that affect serotonin levels.

SAW PALMETTO

Saw palmetto is an herb that has been widely studied for its benefits for prostate health. Studies show that it can help reduce an enlarged prostate and improve urinary symptoms in those with benign prostatic hyperplasia, similarly to prescription drugs, but it is better tolerated. It may also be helpful for the treatment of prostatitis and is generally well tolerated.

SOY

Soy contains a range of beneficial compounds including isoflavones (a type of phytoestrogen), protein, fibre, and sterols. Numerous studies have shown that soy foods can lower LDL cholesterol levels and improve the ratio of LDL to HDL (usual dosage is 47 g per day). However, studies on soy isoflavones alone (rather than whole soy or soy protein) have not yielded the same benefits for cholesterol reduction. Soy and soy isoflavones may help reduce menopausal symptoms (hot flashes); preliminary research suggests they may reduce the risk of breast, uterine, and colon cancer, and benefit those with osteoporosis and osteoarthritis. Soy can reduce absorption of thyroid hormone and inhibit the function of the thyroid gland, particularly in those who are deficient in iodine, so it should be used cautiously in those with impaired thyroid function. High supplemental intake is not recommended during pregnancy.

ST. JOHN'S WORT

St. John's wort is an herb with a long history of use for treating emotional disorders. Research supports its use for mild to moderate depression and seasonal affective disorder with effects comparable to those of prescription antidepressant drugs. Side effects are rare and include skin rash and mild upset stomach. It may cause increased sensitivity to the sun. Use cautiously with other antidepressant products. St. John's wort may reduce the efficacy of many drugs, including oral contraceptives, organ transplant medications, digoxin, statins, warfarin, proton-pump inhibitors (ulcer drugs), and anaesthetics; consult with your pharmacist before taking this herb.

SYTRINOL

Sytrinol is a patented formula derived from natural citrus and palm fruit extracts that contains various antioxidant compounds (polymethoxylated flavones, and delta, gamma, and alpha tocotrienols) with benefits for heart health. Clinical trials have shown that this supplement can significantly improve total cholesterol by lowering LDL cholesterol and triglyceride levels while increasing HDL levels. There is also some evidence that it can reduce arterial plaque, improve glycemic control, and reduce blood platelet aggregation.

TEA TREE

Oil from this tree is widely used for its antiseptic properties; it kills bacteria, viruses, and fungi upon contact. Topical products have been found effective for improving acne and athlete's foot. It may also help in the treatment of gum disease and dandruff. When used topically tea tree may cause skin irritation in some individuals; orally it can be toxic in high amounts.

TONGKAT ALI

Tongkat ali has traditionally been used to increase energy, enhance sexual potency, strengthen erection, boost metabolism, and improve fertility. Modern research has confirmed these effects. Tonkat ali works by increasing testosterone and cGMP production. Physta is a standardized and clinically studied extract of the Malaysian plant Tongkat ali (*Eurycoma longifolia*) made through a patented technology. This extract contains numerous phenolic components, tannins, polysaccharides, and other beneficial compounds. It is well tolerated.

TURMERIC

An herb that is part of the ginger family, turmeric contains a compound called curcumin, which has anti-inflammatory and antioxidant properties. Numerous studies have been conducted on curcumin showing that it can help in the treatment of arthritis, digestive problems such as dyspepsia, and ulcerative colitis. There is also preliminary research suggesting benefits for preventing Alzheimer's disease, cataracts, and multiple sclerosis, and reducing cholesterol. Turmeric and curcumin supplements are very safe and well tolerated.

VALERIAN

Valerian is an herb that is used for its calming and sedating properties. Some (but not all) studies show that it is useful for insomnia and chronic sleep disorders; it may take a few weeks to get the optimal effect. Some studies have found benefits with valerian when it is combined with hops and/or lemon balm. It is generally well tolerated, and does not cause next-day drowsiness when taken at bedtime. It is not recommended for use in conjunction with prescription sleep aids.

WILLOW

Willow is an herb with a long history of use for pain and fever. It contains salicin, a compound that can be purified to salicylic acid (similar to the active ingredient in aspirin). Research supports benefits for back pain and osteoarthritis. It may also help with dysmenorrhea, tension and migraine headaches, rheumatoid arthritis, tendonitis, and bursitis. It is generally well tolerated, but may cause upset stomach, although not to the same extent as aspirin, which causes stomach irritation and bleeding. Willow doesn't impair blood coagulation to the same extent as aspirin; however, it should still be used cautiously by those taking blood thinners.

CHAPTER 8

PRINCIPLES OF SAFE SUPPLEMENTING

Mounting clinical research is demonstrating that nutritional supplements can play an important role in health·and disease prevention. Every day we are learning of new products, new uses, and new benefits. While these advances in science are exciting and offer great hope, how do we take this information and put it into practical use in our own lives? Choosing an appropriate supplement and creating a supplement program requires careful thought and consideration. In this chapter I outline the role of nutritional supplements, my recommended "foundation" supplements, tips on creating a supplement program, and suggestions for your medicine cabinet and travel essentials.

WHY TAKE SUPPLEMENTS?

You may have heard the phrase, "If you eat a healthy diet, then you don't need to take supplements." If you eat a whole foods diet, with plenty of nutrient-dense fruits and vegetables, whole grains, lean protein, and healthy fats every day, then it may be possible to get what your body needs from diet alone. However, the reality is that most people don't eat healthily on a daily basis. Fast foods and processed foods are prevalent in our diet, and these foods are typically devoid of nutrients. Furthermore, there are a number of factors that actually deplete nutrients from our bodies, such as stress, environmental toxins, and the use of prescription medications.

Nutritional supplements are often necessary not only to make up for dietary deficiencies and depletion but to achieve optimum health and help prevent chronic disease. Throughout this book you will see recommendations for supplements that can help manage or prevent various health conditions. But keep in mind that supplements are intended to complement, not replace, a healthy lifestyle.

CREATING YOUR SUPPLEMENT PROGRAM

There are so many different supplements available, and if you took everything that sounds beneficial you could end up popping pills all day long, which is not necessary to achieve good health. It is important to first look at your diet, lifestyle, and health needs when determining what supplements to take. There are a few supplements that I consider "foundation supplements." These supplements, which include multivitamins and minerals, green foods, probiotics, and essential fatty acids, should be considered by most people as they offer broad health benefits.

Multivitamins and Minerals

It is my professional opinion that almost everyone can benefit from taking a daily multivitamin and mineral complex. As noted above, even if you eat a healthy diet, you could be lacking in certain nutrients. Aside from diet, there are many factors that increase your need for vitamins and minerals, such as smoking, exposure to pollution, use of prescription medication, intense exercise, stress, and certain medical conditions such as osteoporosis, heart disease, alcoholism, and malabsorption diseases (celiac and Crohn's diseases). Those on a strict vegetarian diet may also have difficulty in getting enough essential nutrients from diet alone. Taking a daily multivitamin ensures that your body gets all the essential nutrients it needs to function optimally. Think of a multivitamin as a form of "health insurance."

Since our nutritional needs vary with age and lifestyle factors, it is important to look for products designed for your particular needs. For example:

- Children who are picky eaters could be lacking in various nutrients, such as vitamin C and iron. Those with developmental issues may benefit from essential fatty acid supplements.
- Teenagers who don't eat a healthy diet (too much fast food) may be lacking in vitamins. Growing teens also require extra calcium to build strong bones.
- Women of childbearing age may need extra calcium and iron, especially if they have heavy menstrual cycles.
- Higher amounts of folic acid—to reduce the risk of birth defects—are recommended for women who plan to get pregnant.
- Women who are pregnant or lactating should take a prenatal supplement, which contains higher amounts of nutrients needed to support a growing baby and the increased demands of breastfeeding. These supplements also contain lower amounts of vitamin A since it can lead to birth defects in high amounts (greater than 5,000 IU daily).
- Athletes require extra antioxidants to compensate for free radicals generated during intense activity.
- Seniors require extra calcium and vitamin D to protect the bones. Vitamin B12 and other B-vitamins may be deficient in older individuals depending on diet, medical conditions, and prescription drug use.
- Seniors should not take products containing iron unless advised by their doctor.

Chapter 2 provides extensive information on vitamins and minerals, including dosage ranges based on age and gender, as well as nutrients that may be depleted by prescription drugs or certain health conditions.

Green Foods

Most people find it difficult to consume the recommended seven to ten servings of fruits and vegetables per day that provide our primary dietary source of vitamins, minerals, and fibre. To complement your diet, you may want to consider taking a green foods supplement. Green foods such as chlorella, spirulina, barley grass, and wheat grass provide vital nutrients such as antioxidants, minerals, and fibre, which can help boost energy levels, support detoxification, and enhance well-being. There are many green food supplements on the market, which vary in composition. Greens+ is one of my top recommended brands as it contains the highest quality ingredients and has been clinically studied. You can add your Greens+ to your morning protein shake, or mix with juice or water. For best results, it is important to take this product daily.

Probiotics

Also known as friendly or beneficial bacteria, probiotics are microorganisms normally present in the mouth, digestive and urinary tracts, and vaginal area. There are numerous strains (types) of probiotics. Some of the most common strains include *Lactobacillus (L) acidophilus, L. reuteri, L. casei, Bifidobacterium bifidum,* and the yeast *Saccharomyces boulardii.*

Probiotics provide many health benefits by protecting against infection by harmful bacteria (yeast and bacteria), aiding in detoxification, producing vitamins, aiding digestion, and supporting immune function. Research supports benefits for travellers' diarrhea, constipation, irritable bowel, ulcerative colitis, eczema, infantile colic, allergies, and tooth decay. They also improve immune function, reduce cholesterol, prevent and treat yeast infections, and enhance ulcer treatment. Probiotic supplements vary greatly in potency (the number of bacteria), therapeutic use (some have been researched for a specific aspect of health), and form (capsules, tablets, powders, liquids). Choose products that are backed by research, tested for potency and stability, and made from human strains. Some require refrigeration. Beneficial bacteria are also present in some fermented dairy foods (live culture yogurt and kefir), although potency and stability is questionable. Probiotics are generally well tolerated.

Essential Fatty Acids (EFAs)

EFAs are good fats that are *essential* for health throughout life. They are required for growth and development of the brain, nervous system, adrenal glands, sex organs, and eyes. They maintain the health of cell membranes, produce hormones and brain chemicals, and regulate various cell processes.

The body cannot make EFAs, so they must be obtained through diet or supplementation. As discussed in Chapter 1, the two main classes of EFAs are the omega-3s and omega-6s. Most people get adequate omega-6s as they are found abundantly in vegetable oils. Omega-3s are present in fish and, to a lesser extent, in some plants (flaxseed and leafy green vegetables). Omega-3 deficiency is thought to be quite common, and supplementing with omega-3s offers a number of health benefits, such as reducing the risk of heart attack and improving brain function and skin health. Omega-3 supplements are also recommended for women who are trying to get pregnant or who are pregnant as these good fats are essential to the growing brain, eyes, and nervous system of the baby.

Fish oil provides the highest amount of omega-3s. Look for a pharmaceutical-grade, cold-pressed fish oil from a reputable manufacturer. Those who cannot tolerate fish oils can take flaxseed oil or chia seed. The usual dosage for omega-3s is 1 g to 3 g daily. There are specific formulas for children with improved taste.

BEYOND THE FOUNDATION

Beyond these foundation supplements I would suggest that you look at your particular health needs and any underlying medical problems in determining what other supplements to take. For example, if you have osteoporosis you may require extra minerals, vitamin D, and other nutrients. If you have heart disease, it would be wise to take coenzyme Q10 along with extra antioxidants. Focus on one concern at a time, exploring different nutritional supplements that may offer help. If you invest the time in creating a supplements program that's right for your individual needs, your reward should be improved quality of life.

In Section Three I provide concise guidelines on supplement recommendations for various health conditions. Keep in mind that it is always wise to consult with a professional for advice on which supplements to take, the appropriate dosage, and any precautions.

TIPS ON SELECTING SUPPLEMENTS

There are many factors to consider when choosing a supplement. Before choosing a product, consider my list of do's and don'ts below.

Do's

- Research your options—consult with your pharmacist or health care provider and find out as much as you can about the products you are considering. In particular ask if there are any possible interactions with medications or side effects.
- When buying a multivitamin, look for one that contains a complete array of essential vitamins, minerals, and antioxidants in one formula. This will keep the amount of pills you take to a minimum and will also be easier on your budget. Depending on your diet and needs, you may still need to take additional vitamin C, E, and calcium as it is difficult to fit all of these nutrients into one tablet.
- Buy from a reputable manufacturer. Ask your pharmacist or health food store adviser for a recommendation.
- Remember it may take four to six weeks or longer to notice benefits, and some supplements that are taken for prevention may not offer benefits that you can feel.
- If you are pregnant, breastfeeding, or have a chronic medical condition, be sure to consult a nutrition specialist before purchasing or taking any supplements.
- Read the labels carefully. Look for an expiration date and make sure the product is not past its expiration. If there is no expiration date on the label, don't buy it.
- If you have questions about a certain brand, call the manufacturer and ask your questions.

Don'ts

- Don't take supplements with sugar, starch, corn, wheat, iron, dairy, salt, artificial flavourings and colourings (dyes), and preservatives. These are unnecessary ingredients that can cause allergic reactions in some people.
- Don't choose a supplement based on price. Some vitamins are more expensive because of company marketing and advertising costs and are not necessarily made with better ingredients. On the other hand, some products are very cheap because they contain less active ingredients and more fillers.
- Don't continue to take a supplement if you have a bad reaction, such as prolonged upset stomach or rash.
- Don't stop taking a prescribed drug or substitute a supplement for a prescribed drug unless under the advice and supervision of your health care provider.
- Don't take a higher dosage of a product than is recommended on the label unless advised to do so by your health care provider.

NATURAL MEDICINE CABINET

Below is a list of certain products that you may want to have on hand to deal with minor ailments.

- Activated charcoal for stomach upset, food poisoning, and drug overdose
- Aloe vera gel for minor sunburn
- Arnica gel for bruises
- Boswellia or curcumin for minor injuries and inflammation
- Calendula cream for skin rashes, minor wounds, and irritation
- Ginger for nausea and upset stomach
- Lavender oil for relaxation and headache relief
- Magnesium liquid or tablets as a natural laxative for constipation
- Melatonin as a natural sleep aid
- North American ginseng (COLD-FX) for prevention of colds
- Probiotics for diarrhea. *Lactobacillus (L.) acidophilus* and *L. reuteri* (BioGaia) are among the strains that have been studied and found beneficial. Apple pectin, carob powder, and chamomile are also helpful for treating diarrhea. Note: Severe cases of diarrhea, especially in children, need to be seen by a physician.
- Tea tree oil as an antiseptic for treatment of minor skin irritations, insect bites, and stings
- Zinc lozenges for sore throat and colds

NATURAL TRAVEL ESSENTIALS

Depending on whether you are travelling north or south, here are some suggestions for remedies to pack for your trip:

- Activated charcoal for stomach upset, food poisoning, and drug overdose
- Aloe vera to soothe sunburn
- Ginger tea or supplements for motion sickness and sea sickness

- Natural insect repellant—look for products that contain eucalyptus oil, catnip oil, garlic, and/or citronella
- Probiotics to take during your trip, especially when travelling overseas, to prevent travellers' diarrhea and upset stomach. Keep in mind that some types/brands of probiotics require refrigeration. For ease of use when travelling, look for a product that is stable at room temperature.
- Tea tree oil to relieve insect bites and clean wounds
- Zinc oxide for sun protection

SECTION III

COMMON HEALTH CONCERNS AND CONDITIONS

ACID REFLUX (GERD)

Acid reflux, known medically as gastroesophageal reflux disease (GERD), is a disease in which stomach acid flows back (refluxes) into your esophagus (food pipe). This causes burning and pain, which is commonly known as heartburn. Many people experience an occasional episode of heartburn, which is usually not a cause for concern, but when it occurs continually, it could indicate GERD.

GERD is a common disorder, affecting up to 60 percent of people at some point during the course of a year, and 20 to 30 percent of people at least weekly.

Normally when you swallow, the lower esophageal sphincter, which is a circular band of muscle around the bottom of the esophagus, relaxes to allow food and liquid to flow down into your stomach. Then it closes again. If this valve becomes weakened or relaxes when it shouldn't, stomach acids can flow up into the esophagus, causing heartburn.

When stomach acids continually reflux upward, they can cause irritation and inflammation of the lining of the esophagus, which is known as esophagitis. This can cause chest pain after eating, difficulty swallowing, and breathing problems.

Although GERD is uncomfortable, there are a number of dietary and lifestyle modifications that can help relieve symptoms.

SIGNS & SYMPTOMS

- Chest pain that may be worse when lying down

- Coughing, wheezing, asthma, and sore throat

- Difficulty swallowing

- Heartburn, a burning in the chest that may go up into the throat

- Regurgitating food and liquid

- Sour taste in mouth

If left untreated, GERD can lead to other conditions such as esophageal narrowing (due to formation of scar tissue) and an esophageal ulcer.

RISK FACTORS

- Asthma: Coughing and laboured breathing put pressure on the stomach; asthma medications may relax the esophageal sphincter.

- Connective tissue disorders (scleroderma) and diseases that affect the muscles.

- Diabetes: Gastroparesis (delayed stomach emptying) is a complication of diabetes.

- Hiatal hernia: The stomach protrudes into the lower chest, worsening heartburn and weakening the esophageal sphincter.

- Obesity: Excess weight puts pressure on the stomach, forcing open the esophageal sphincter and allowing stomach acids to back up.

- Overeating and eating high-fat meals puts pressure on the lower esophageal sphincter, allowing stomach acids to back up.

- Peptic ulcers can affect stomach emptying, causing a buildup of acids.

- Pregnancy: The growing belly puts pressure on the stomach; higher progesterone levels relax the muscles (esophageal sphincter), allowing stomach acids to reflux.

- Smoking increases stomach acid, weakens the esophageal sphincter, and dries up saliva, which helps dilute the stomach acid.

DOCTOR'S ORDERS

Most cases of heartburn and GERD can be treated effectively. Lifestyle and dietary modifications alone are often not enough. Over-the-counter (OTC) or prescription medications are often necessary, especially for those who have suffered for a prolonged period of time or have experienced damage to the esophagea. The most commonly used classes of drugs include the following:

- Alginic acid forms a protective seal at the top of the stomach to prevent acid reflux. It is found OTC in a product called Gaviscon.
- Antacids contain ingredients such as magnesium, aluminum, and calcium, which work quickly to neutralize stomach acids. However, they do not reduce inflammation or promote healing. Antacids are available OTC and include Tums, Rolaids, Maalox, and Mylanta.
- H2 receptor blockers reduce the production of acid and reflux. They take longer to work, but provide longer relief. Side effects include dry mouth, bowel changes, dizziness, and drowsiness. Examples include famotidine (Pepcid) and ranitidine (Zantac). They are available full strength by prescription, or in lower dosages OTC.
- Proton pump inhibitors block acid production and allow the damaged esophagus to heal. These are long-acting products and the most effective medical treatment for GERD. Examples include Losec (omeprazole), Pantoloc (pantoprazole), and Prevacid (lansoprazole). These products are well tolerated; side effects are rare and include headache and dizziness.

HOMEOPATHIC RECOMMENDATIONS

Nux vomica: This remedy relieves nausea and cramps from indigestion, especially after excessive spicy food or alcohol.

Pulsatilla: This homeopathic remedy relieves gastric discomfort such as bloating, belching, or slow digestion caused by eating too much fatty foods, cakes, or ice cream.

SHERRY'S NATURAL PRESCRIPTION

Dietary Recommendations

Foods to include:

- Aloe vera juice helps reduce acid output and is soothing to the mucous membranes. Try 1 tbsp of pure aloe vera juice two or three times daily.

- Drink caffeine-free herbal teas that contain chamomile, ginger, marshmallow, and slippery elm, herbs that are soothing and help relieve heartburn.

- Drink fluids between meals rather than with meals, which will help prevent reflux.

- Eat vegetables, non-citrus fruits, whole grains, beans, fish, and lean meat.

- Eat small, frequent meals (instead of one or two large meals), which will prevent excess production of stomach acid and is also less stressful to the esophageal sphincter. Eat slowly and chew your food thoroughly.

- Small amounts of olive and vegetable oils are fine.

- Stay upright after eating and don't eat within three hours of bedtime.

Foods to avoid:

- Alcohol, carbonated beverages, spicy foods, tomatoes, citrus fruits, spearmint, peppermint, and onions are irritating to the esophagus.

- Chocolate and coffee relax the esophageal sphincter and increase the risk of reflux.

- High-fat foods worsen symptoms because they stay in the stomach longer and increase the time the esophagus is exposed to stomach acids. Avoid or minimize cream, butter, ice cream, gravy, oils, fried foods, sausage, and processed fatty meats and cream soups.

Lifestyle Suggestions

- Lose excess weight by eating healthy and exercising regularly.

- Do not bend over, lie down, or exercise right after eating. Wait two hours after eating to exercise and three hours after eating before lying down.

- Do not wear tight belts or pants that are tight at the waist.

- Don't smoke.

- Raise the head of your bed—use pillows or a block under the head of your bed. Keeping your head higher than your stomach will help prevent acids from refluxing.

- Chewing gum after a large meal stimulates the flow of saliva, which is alkaline. This helps neutralize acid in the esophagus and prevent GERD symptoms. Avoid mint flavour.

- Lozenges containing slippery elm and marshmallow can help coat the esophagus and reduce irritation.

. . . .

BMI AND GERD

Several studies have shown a link between elevated body mass index (a scale used to determine overweight and obesity) and symptoms of GERD. The risk of GERD symptoms, such as heartburn and acid reflux, rises with BMI. Studies have also shown that losing excess weight can reduce symptoms.

. . . .

Top Recommended Supplements

Calcium carbonate: This is the main ingredient in many OTC heartburn products and is also available as a supplement. Calcium helps neutralize stomach acid and provides short-term relief. Dosage: 500 mg three times daily with meals and before bedtime.

Deglycyrrhizinated licorice (DGL): This herb soothes and coats the mucous membranes of the stomach. It helps restore the mucous lining that protects the stomach from hydrochloric acid (stomach acid). Dosage: Two to four tablets before each meal and at bedtime.

Complementary Supplements

Digestive enzymes: Improve digestion by breaking food down into smaller components. Choose a broad spectrum enzyme containing protease, lipase, and amylase to aid digestion of protein, fats, and carbohydrates, respectively. Dosage: One capsule with each meal.

Fenugreek: Contains galactomannan fibre. When consumed with a glass of water prior to food intake, the fibre binds to stomach contents forming a barrier and preventing reflux into the esophagus. It also protects the stomach. Dosage: 2–4 g daily.

Probiotics: Contain friendly bacteria, which improve digestion and gut health. Preliminary research on an infant probiotic (BioGaia) found it improved gut function and motility and reduced reflux episodes. Dosage: Varies by formulation.

FINAL THOUGHTS

To prevent or relieve the symptoms of acid reflux, consider the following:

- Work on losing excess body weight.
- Don't smoke.
- Raise the head of your bed.
- Avoid high-fat and spicy foods, alcohol, and other triggers, and don't overeat.
- Consider supplements of calcium and DGL.

ACNE

Acne is a chronic disorder of the skin's sebaceous glands (oil glands), leading to the development of comedones, also known as pimples or more commonly "zits." There are many myths surrounding acne. Acne is not caused by eating chocolate—unless you are allergic. Almost every teenager will have an occasional acne outbreak, and approximately 40 percent of teens have severe cystic acne. Even those 30 and older are affected.

During puberty hormones called androgens trigger the sebaceous glands to grow and produce more sebum (oil). Irregular shedding of skin cells lining the hair follicle can lead to clumping and cause the pores to clog. A type of bacteria called *Propionibacterium acnes,* which normally lives in the skin, invades the clogged pore and begins to grow, creating inflammation and irritation. The result is a plugged, inflamed follicle that develops into a pimple.

SIGNS & SYMPTOMS

- Cystic acne is marked by clusters of deep, painful, fluid-filled cysts; areas of the skin appear red or purple and are inflamed.

- Pitting, pockmarks, and scarring can occur with severe forms of acne, or if the lesions are picked or squeezed and become infected.

- Whiteheads, blackheads, red spots, and white, pus-filled pimples appear primarily on the face, but also on the shoulders, neck, back, chest, and buttocks.

RISK FACTORS

- Allergies: Reactions to foods, medications, or environmental chemicals
- Cosmetics or exposure to airborne grease
- Exposure to extreme temperatures
- Family history: Having a parent with acne
- Friction and sweating caused by wearing headbands, helmets, or tight collars
- Hormonal changes in teenagers, premenstrual women, and during pregnancy
- Medications: Use of hormones such as testosterone or cortisone
- Race: Caucasians are more affected than African Americans or Asians
- Stress

DOCTOR'S ORDERS

Since acne can cause scarring, those with severe cases, where there are multiple lesions or cysts, should consult a dermatologist.

Drugs used for acne work by inhibiting sebum and keratin production, reducing bacterial growth, or encouraging shedding of skin cells to unclog the pores. Most over-the-counter products contain salicylic acid, benzoyl peroxide, or sulphur. Benzoyl peroxide is the most effective. All of these products may cause redness, burning, stinging, and scaling of the skin.

Creams and gels containing tretinoin (a vitamin A derivative) or tazarotene (synthetic vitamin A) are used to slough off dead skin, clear pores, and dry acne. Accutane is an oral medication derived from vitamin A; it reduces sebum production and swelling, and minimizes acne-causing bacteria. It is effective, but must be taken for several months and may cause dry mucous membranes, muscle aches, and liver problems. It must be avoided by women who are pregnant or trying to conceive as it can cause severe birth defects.

Antibiotics (tetracycline, erythromycin, or minocycline) are sometimes prescribed for mild to moderate acne. They work for some people, but their use is limited by side effects such as upset stomach, diarrhea, sun sensitivity, and yeast infections.

Birth control pills are prescribed for women with menstrual-related acne. They reduce androgen levels and sebum production. Side effects include blood clots, bloating, cramps, spotting, liver and gallbladder disease, and increased risk of breast cancer.

HOMEOPATHIC RECOMMENDATIONS

Silicea: Silicea is for deep-seated acne that's accompanied with a general low immune resistance and swollen lymph nodes. Infected spots are slow to come to a head, and also slow to resolve, so may result in scarring. A person who needs this remedy is generally very chilly, but inclined to sweat at night.

Sulphur: Sulphur is for itchy, sore, inflamed eruptions with reddish or dirty-looking skin. Itching may be worse from scratching, and worse from any form of heat, especially bathing or washing.

Combination recommendation: Acne Formula R53 by Reckeweg

SHERRY'S NATURAL PRESCRIPTION

Dietary Recommendations

Foods to include:

• Fibre supports detoxification and elimination; flaxseed is particularly helpful as it is high in both fibre and essential fatty acids.

• Yogurt contains beneficial bacteria, which is especially important for those who have taken antibiotics.

Foods to avoid:

• Food allergies can trigger acne breakouts. Refer to Appendix D for more information.

• Sugar reduces immune function and may increase bacterial growth. Research also suggests that eating highly processed breads and cereals, which break down quickly into sugar in the body, increases the release of insulin and insulin-like growth factor, leading to excessive production of male hormones and promoting acne.

Lifestyle Suggestions

• Drink eight to ten glasses of water daily.

• Wash your face morning and evening with warm water and a gentle cleanser.

• Do not scrub hard or use abrasive cleaners as this can irritate acne.

• Go for regular facials as aestheticians can cleanse, exfoliate, and extract pores.

• Sauna or steam helps to clear pores and aids in detoxification.

• Don't pick or squeeze; this can cause tissue damage, infection, and scars.

• Minimize cosmetics use. Use only water-based and hypoallergenic skin care products. Products containing lavender, chamomile, and tea tree are beneficial.

Top Recommended Supplements

Tea tree oil: A natural antibiotic and antiseptic; try a lotion or cream with 5 to 15 percent tea tree oil. Studies have found it just as effective as benzoyl peroxide, but it is better tolerated.

Vitamin A: Essential for skin health; regulates sebum and keratin production. Dosage: 5,000–10,000 IU daily. Higher doses should be taken only under medical supervision. Women who are pregnant or trying to conceive should not exceed 5,000 IU daily.

Zinc: Promotes tissue healing, balances hormones, and reduces inflammation. Dosage: 25–50 mg daily. Choose a supplement that also contains copper (3–5 mg) because chronic use of zinc can reduce copper absorption.

Complementary Supplements

B-vitamins: Deficiencies of some B-vitamins, such as B2 and B6, are associated with acne. In general, B-vitamins are important for healthy skin. Supplementing may reduce breakouts. Try a B-complex that provides 50–100 mg of the B-vitamins.

Chasteberry (Vitex): May help premenstrual acne in women. There is limited research, but this herb is well known to help balance hormones. Try 160 mg or 40 drops of tincture daily.

Omega-3 fatty acids: Reduce inflammation and repair damaged skin cells. Try 1–3 g daily.

Vitamin C: Aids skin repair and improves collagen production. Take 500–2,000 mg daily.

Vitamin E: Essential for skin health, and may help prevent scarring. Dosage: 400 IU daily.

Note: For acne related to polycystic ovarian syndrome, please refer to that particular section of this book.

FINAL THOUGHTS

To improve acne and overall skin health, consider the following:

• Nourish your body and skin with a healthy diet, including lots of fibre, good fats, and water.
• Keep your skin clean and avoid picking blemishes.
• Skin products containing tea tree can improve acne.
• Supplements of vitamin A and zinc are helpful.
• Those with severe acne should consult a dermatologist.

ALLERGIC RHINITIS

Approximately 20 percent of Canadians—about 7 million adults and children—suffer from seasonal allergies, also known as hay fever. These allergies occur when the immune system overreacts upon exposure to allergens, substances such as trees, grass, or flower pollen. Some people have persistent, year-long allergies that are triggered by environmental factors such as house dust, mould, animal dander, dust mites, and air pollution.

The immune system responds to these otherwise harmless substances as invaders, similar to how it would react to viruses or bacteria. It produces an antibody against the allergen called immunoglobulin E (IgE), which triggers the release of inflammatory chemicals—histamine, leukotrienes, and prostaglandins. Histamine is responsible for the notorious allergy symptoms of itchy, runny eyes and nose, and sneezing; leukotrienes cause excess mucus production; and prostaglandins trigger inflammation.

Researchers do not completely understand why some people get allergies while others don't, but there are a few theories. One is the overuse of antibiotics, which causes destruction of the normal flora (bacteria) in the gut. Another is the ultra-hygienic society that we live in. With little exposure to dirt and bacteria, our immune system is primed to respond when faced with a foreign invader.

THE ORIGIN OF "HAY FEVER"

Despite the common name of "hay fever," allergies are rarely triggered by hay. The name originated in the 1800s when British doctors found that people living in rural areas experienced sneezing and itching with exposure to cut hay or grass. This reaction caused nervousness, which was referred to as "fever," hence the name "hay fever."

SIGNS & SYMPTOMS

- Cough

- Fatigue

- Headache

- Irritability

- Itchy eyes, nose, roof of mouth, or throat

- Sinus pressure and pain

- Sneezing

- Runny nose and congestion

- Watery eyes

Having allergies increases your risk of developing other inflammatory diseases such as asthma and eczema. Prolonged sinus congestion can increase the risk of sinusitis (infection or inflammation of the sinuses).

RISK FACTORS

- Exposure to cigarette smoke during first years of life
- Exposure to indoor allergens (dust or pet dander) or environmental pollution (smoke)
- Family history of allergies
- Firstborn child
- Gender (men are at greater risk)

DOCTOR'S ORDERS

There are several different types of medications that are used to manage allergy symptoms. Antihistamines block histamine release and improve symptoms of itching, runny nose, and sneezing. Benadryl (diphenhydramine) and Chlor-Tripolon (chlorpheniramine) are older antihistamines, which cause substantial drowsiness and are taken every six hours. Newer products cause less drowsiness and are taken once daily. Examples include Claritin, Aerius, Allegra, and Reactine. Side effects include dry eyes, mouth, and nose.

Decongestants relieve sinus congestion (feeling of fullness and pressure). Examples include Sudafed (pseudoephedrine) and phenylephrine. Side effects include insomnia, racing heart, increased blood pressure, and irritability. Avoid use with medications for high blood pressure, glaucoma, or prostate enlargement. Note: Decongestant nasal sprays can cause rebound congestion if used longer than three days.

Cromolyn is a drug that prevents the release of histamine. It is most effective as a preventative (before symptoms start) and is available in eyedrops and nasal spray. Singulair is a prescription drug that blocks the action of leukotrienes. It is taken once daily and may cause headaches.

Allergy shots are helpful for some people. These injections contain purified allergen extracts, which desensitize a person to allergies. They are given yearly, prior to the allergy season.

HOMEOPATHIC RECOMMENDATIONS

Allium cepa: Indications for this remedy include watery eyes and a clear nasal discharge that irritates the upper lip, along with sneezing and a tickling cough. The person usually is thirsty, feels worse indoors and in warm rooms, and is much better in fresh air.

Sabadilla: Frequent and persistent spasms of sneezing, itching in the nose with irritating runny discharge, a feeling of a lump in the throat, and watery eyes will all suggest a need for this remedy. The person may feel nervous during allergy attacks, and trying to concentrate can bring on drowsiness or a headache.

Combination recommendation: Euphorbium Compositum (nasal spray) by Heel

SHERRY'S NATURAL PRESCRIPTION

Dietary Recommendations

Foods to include:

- Fruits and vegetables provide antioxidants that support healthy immune function. Apples, red onions, red grapes, tomatoes, raspberries, and cranberries contain quercetin, a natural antihistamine.

- Green tea also contains quercetin along with flavonoids that help reduce inflammation.

- Fish and seeds (flaxseed and chia seed) provide omega-3 fatty acids that help reduce inflammation.

- Peppers, onions, and garlic help thin and reduce mucus.

- Yogurt and kefir contain probiotics that help support immune function and may help reduce allergic reaction symptoms.

- Horseradish, in particular wasabi (Japanese horseradish), and cayenne peppers act like natural decongestants and help clear the sinuses.

- Foods fortified with Wellmune (a type of beta-glucan) can support immune function, and preliminary research shows benefits for reducing allergies. This natural ingredient is added to commercial brands of juice, bars, cookies, and soups.

Foods to avoid:

- Those who are sensitive to cow's milk may find that it aggravates symptoms.

- Foods that contain artificial dyes and preservatives should be avoided.

- Foods that promote inflammation, such as refined flours, and saturated and hydrogenated fats should be avoided.

- Those with ragweed allergies may find that banana, chamomile tea, and sunflower seeds worsen symptoms.

- Those with tree pollen allergies may react to cherries, apples, carrots, and almonds.

Note: People who have seasonal allergies often have food allergies as well. Refer to Appendix D for information on how to do an elimination diet.

Lifestyle Suggestions

- Know your triggers and try to avoid them—pollen production is highest between 5 a.m. and 10 a.m., so avoid the outdoors during this time.

- Heavy rain reduces pollen in the air, making post-shower outings safer.

- Wear a mask when cutting the grass or gardening.

- Don't dry your clothes outside, as they can collect pollen.

- Use an air purifier to remove allergens from your home.

- Keep your windows closed to prevent pollen from blowing into your home.

- Use a high-efficiency particulate air (HEPA) filter on your air conditioner and furnace and change it monthly.

- Use a vacuum with a double bag and a HEPA filter.

- Don't keep cut flowers in the house, and minimize indoor plants. Wet dirt allows mould to grow.

- Nasal irrigation, such as using a Neti pot or nasal wash, can help clear pollen and mucus from your nasal passages, relieve congestion and dryness, and improve breathing. Make a salt-water solution by mixing 1 tsp of salt with 500 mL (16 ounces) purified lukewarm water. Lean forward over a sink and slowly pour the solution into one nostril and let it run out the other nostril. This can be repeated a few times daily. You can also purchase nasal wash solutions with essential oils added such as menthol, eucalyptol, thymol, camphor, and wintergreen, which help relieve congestion.

Top Recommended Supplements

Aller-7: A combination of seven plant extracts that reduces allergy symptoms when taken regularly. Dosage: 660 mg twice daily for six to twelve weeks, then 330 mg twice daily thereafter.

Butterbur: An herb that reduces inflammation and has antihistamine effects. Dosage: 50 mg twice daily. Studies used a standardized extract providing 8 mg of petasine (an active chemical) three times daily.

Probiotics: Help support healthy gastrointestinal flora, which is important for immune function. Some research shows benefits for reducing allergies, although it may take several months to notice benefits. Dosage: One to three capsules daily.

Complementary Supplements

Moducare: A mixture of plant sterols and sterolins (plant fats) that helps balance the immune system. One clinical trial found it reduced allergy symptoms. Dosage: One capsule three times daily.

Quercetin: A flavonoid with antihistamine properties. Dosage: 500 mg three times daily.

Vitamin C: Helps reduce histamine production and works well with quercetin. Dosage: 1,000 mg three times daily.

Vitamin E: Has antioxidant effects and has been shown to reduce allergic response and nasal symptoms (sneezing, itching, stuffiness, and runny nose). Dosage: 400 IU daily.

FINAL THOUGHTS

To keep allergies at bay, consider the following:

- Eat plenty of antioxidant-rich fruits and vegetables, especially garlic, onions, peppers, nuts, and seeds.
- Minimize being outdoors in the early morning and use an air purifier in your home.
- Try nasal irrigation to clear your sinuses.
- For prevention, try Aller-7 and probiotics.
- To reduce symptoms once they appear, try butterbur.

ALZHEIMER'S DISEASE

Alzheimer's disease is a chronic, degenerative disease of the brain that impairs thinking, memory, and cognitive function. It is the most common form of dementia. It is estimated that over 450,000 Canadians are affected by Alzheimer's disease. These numbers are expected to rise substantially over the next few decades due to our aging population.

Alzheimer's is not a normal part of aging, but it is more common in people as they age. The prevalence doubles every five years beyond age 65. The actual cause is not known, but its effect on brain tissue is clear: The disease causes damage and death to brain cells.

Alzheimer's was first identified by Dr. Alois Alzheimer in 1906. He described the two hallmark features of the disease—plaques (tiny dense deposits scattered throughout the brain) and tangles (structures of the brain that are twisted)—which interfere with normal brain processes and cause death of brain cells.

In a healthy brain, there are billions of neurons (nerve cells) that generate electrical and chemical signals, which help us think, remember, and feel. In those with Alzheimer's the neurons begin to die, affecting the normal signalling in the brain. A key feature of this disease is the development of plaques and tangles in the brain. The plaques consist of normally harmless proteins called beta-amyloid. It is thought that a genetic defect in these proteins may be involved in the development of the disease. Tangles refer to a twisting of internal support structures of the brain, which causes damage and death of the neurons.

Research has shown that Alzheimer's disease involves oxidative and inflammatory processes, although it is not known whether these processes are a cause or an effect of the disease or both. The ultimate result, however, is disruption of neuronal cell functioning and signalling, leading to neuronal cell death, which impairs memory and other mental abilities. There also are lower levels of some neurotransmitters, chemicals in the brain that carry messages back and forth between nerve cells. This also results in impaired thinking and memory.

Although there's no cure for Alzheimer's disease, a number of medical advances in recent years and the use of natural supplements along with dietary and lifestyle interventions can delay the progression of the disease and improve symptoms and quality of life.

SIGNS & SYMPTOMS

- Confusion and disorientation
- Depression
- Difficulty performing familiar tasks (cooking, tying your shoes)
- Difficulty with abstract thinking (e.g., dealing with numbers)
- Gradual memory loss

- Increasing forgetfulness

- Loss of judgment (difficulty solving everyday problems)

- Paranoia

- Personality changes (mood swings)

Symptoms and the progression of the disease vary among individuals. As the disease progresses, there is a decline in language skills and the ability to perform tasks. The average length of time from diagnosis of Alzheimer's to death is about eight years, but some people live beyond ten years.

RISK FACTORS

- Age: It is most common in those over the age of 65 and rarely affects those younger than age 40.

- Environmental toxicity: Pollution and smoking generate excess free radicals. Some research has connected aluminum and mercury exposure to the disease, but this has not been proven and most experts today do not believe that these metals contribute to Alzheimer's disease.

- Family history: Having a parent or sibling with the disease increases your risk as there are genetic mutations that may be inherited.

- Gender: Women are at greater risk. Twice as many women as men have Alzheimer's.

- Head injury: Some studies show that trauma to the head increases risk of Alzheimer's.

- Heart and blood vessel disease: Growing evidence suggests that those with high blood pressure, heart disease, stroke, diabetes, and high cholesterol are at increased risk.

Other factors that may increase risk include inactivity, obesity, poor diet, drug abuse, heavy and chronic alcohol use, smoking, inflammatory conditions (reflecting a possible immune system malfunction), use of hormone replacement therapy, a history of clinical depression, stress, and inadequate exercising of the brain.

DOCTOR'S ORDERS

There are no drugs that can reverse the disease, but there are a few that can help improve cognitive function and slow the cognitive decline associated with Alzheimer's, such as Aricept, Reminyl, and Exelon. These drugs improve the levels of neurotransmitters (chemical messengers such as serotonin and acetylcholine) in the brain and can delay the onset of Alzheimer's in those with mild cognitive impairment. Not everyone responds positively to these drugs; some people have to stop because of side effects such as nausea, vomiting, and diarrhea. There are also a variety of drugs that can help reduce symptoms of insomnia, anxiety, and agitation.

SHERRY'S NATURAL PRESCRIPTION

Dietary Recommendations

Foods to include:

• Malaysian palm fruit oil provides the richest source of tocotrienols (a potent form of vitamin E), which emerging evidence suggests is protective to the brain and cognitive function. Coconut oil also provides some tocotrienols. Both palm fruit oil and coconut oil are heat stable, so ideally suited for cooking. These healthy fats are also incorporated into a variety of grocery store products like peanut butter, margarine spreads, and even cookies.

• Curcumin (turmeric) has antioxidant and anti-inflammatory properties and some evidence suggests it has protective effects. This is a common ingredient in curry and can be added to stir-fry dishes and soups.

• Brightly coloured fruits and vegetables are rich in antioxidants that can neutralize free radicals. Eat more blueberries, blackberries, grapes, spinach, and broccoli.

• Eat more foods rich in vitamins B6 and B12. B6 is present in bananas, beans, and chicken breasts, and B12 is found in shellfish, salmon, trout, liver, and lean beef.

• Fish (wild, organic salmon, halibut, sole, and cod) also provide good sources of omega-3 fatty acids, a polyunsaturated fat that has been found to reduce Alzheimer's risk by reducing inflammation and protecting the nerve cell membranes.

• Olive oil is a monounsaturated fat that is also helpful.

• Vegetables that are rich in antioxidants, such as leafy greens and cruciferous vegetables, have been found to have protective benefits in a few very large clinical trials; those who ate the most vegetables had the most benefits.

• Vitamin E–rich foods such as whole grains, vegetable oils, nuts, seeds, and egg yolks are helpful. Two studies have found a lower risk of Alzheimer's disease with a higher food intake of vitamin E.

• Zinc may be deficient in those with Alzheimer's. Boost your intake by eating pumpkin seeds, black-eyed peas, wheat germ, tofu, and seafood.

Foods to avoid:

• Saturated and trans fats raise blood cholesterol levels and are associated with an increased risk of Alzheimer's. Avoid fast foods, deep-fried foods, baked goods, and margarine containing hydrogenated oils; minimize saturated fat (red meat and high-fat dairy).

Lifestyle Suggestions

• Maintain a healthy body weight. Being obese and its consequences of high blood pressure, high cholesterol, and obesity are risk factors for Alzheimer's.

• Exercising regularly helps with weight management and also increases blood flow to the brain. According to one study, regular exercise (walking 15 minutes three times per week) reduced the risk of Alzheimer's and dementia by 40 percent in individuals over age 65.

- Mental exercises: Some studies have shown that keeping your brain active, especially in later years, reduces the risk of Alzheimer's. The theory is the more you use your brain, the more synapses you create, which provide a greater reserve as you age. Read, do crossword puzzles, and play memory games.

- Eliminate risky situations at home that may cause injury or falls, such as clutter and floor mats. Grip rails in the bathroom can be helpful.

- Interact with others as much as possible to enhance communication and get necessary assistance from support groups and health care aides.

Top Recommended Supplements

Acetyl-L-carnitine: An amino acid derivative that crosses into the brain and increases the levels of acetylcholine, a brain neurotransmitter that is depleted in those with Alzheimer's. It also protects the neurons against beta amyloid. Several studies have shown that it can delay the progression of the disease. Dosage: 1 g three times daily.

Fish oils: Reduce inflammation and support and protect the nerve cell membranes. Regular consumption of fish reduces Alzheimer's risk and is important for brain function. Those who do not eat fish should consider supplements. The omega-3 DHA is particularly important for brain health. Dosage: 1–3 g daily.

Phosphatidylserine: A nutrient that is related to lecithin, which is naturally occurring in the brain. It helps support the structure and health of cell membranes. Several studies involving more than 1,000 people suggest that phosphatidylserine is an effective treatment for Alzheimer's disease and other forms of dementia. It improves both behaviour and mental function and reduces symptoms of depression. This supplement may work best when taken with DHA from fish oil. Dosage: 300 mg daily.

Vinpocetine: A compound derived from periwinkle plants. It has been widely researched for Alzheimer's disease, with most studies showing significant benefits. Dosage: 10 mg three times daily.

Complementary Supplements

Antioxidants: Oxidative stress is a factor in the development of Alzheimer's disease, and various antioxidant supplements may play a role in protecting the brain from damage caused by oxidative stress and inflammation, reducing plaque formation and slowing cognitive decline. Among those antioxidants showing preliminary but promising benefits are grape seed extract, vitamin E, coenzyme Q10, alpha lipoic acid, and glutathione.

Bacopa monnieri: An herb that has been shown to enhance several aspects of mental function. It increases availability of acetylcholine in the brain, which improves memory and cognition. Antioxidant properties help protect brain cells. Dosage: 200–450 mg daily, standardized to contain bacosides.

B-vitamins: Support neurotransmitter function. Vitamin B1 is involved in nerve transmission and may be deficient in those with Alzheimer's. Two small studies found benefits in mental function with B1 supplements. Dosage: Take 40–100 mg as part of a B-complex as they work together.

Curcumin: Shows promise for treating and preventing Alzheimer's disease. Research suggests it can target various aspects of Alzheimer's, such as lowering oxidative damage and inflammation, reducing cognitive defects, and reducing damage to neural synapses and the deposition of amyloid plaques. Dosage: 2–8 g per day.

Ginkgo biloba: Improves memory and cognitive function and may slow the progression of Alzheimer's. Some research has found it helpful in those with early stages of the disease. Dosage: 120–240 mg daily, standardized to 6 percent terpene lactones and 24 percent flavone glycosides. It may take six weeks to notice benefit.

Glycerophosphorylcholine (GPC): A key structural component of brain cell membranes that helps improve acetylcholine levels in the brain. Emerging research suggests that taking alpha-GPC significantly improves thinking skills in Alzheimer's patients after three to six months of treatment. GPC is not widely available, so check with a health care practitioner. Dosage: 1,200 mg daily.

FINAL THOUGHTS

To improve cognitive function and delay the progression of Alzheimer's, consider the following:

- Eat more fish, whole grains, vegetables, nuts, seeds, and olive oil.
- Avoid saturated fats, trans fats, and high alcohol intake.
- Get regular exercise like walking, and maintain a healthy body weight.
- Keep your brain active with games, puzzles, and exercises.
- Consider supplements of acetyl-L-carnitine, phosphatidylserine, fish oils, and vinpocetine.

ANEMIA

Derived from the Greek word meaning "without blood," anemia is a deficiency of red blood cells or hemoglobin. Every cell in our body requires oxygen to function normally. Anemia impairs the ability of blood to transfer oxygen to the tissues throughout the body. Either the body produces too few healthy red blood cells, loses too many, or destroys them faster than they can be replaced. This makes one feel very tired, both mentally and physically.

There are various forms of anemia. The most common form is iron-deficiency anemia. This affects about one in five women, most often during pregnancy. The body needs iron to produce hemoglobin, the oxygen-carrying component of red blood cells. Without adequate iron, hemoglobin levels are low.

In addition to iron, the body needs folate and vitamin B12 to produce healthy red blood cells. B12-deficiency anemia is called pernicious anemia. It is more common among the elderly and those with intestinal disorders, which impair B12 absorption.

Aplastic anemia is a rare, life-threatening disease caused by a decrease in the bone marrow's ability to produce blood cells. This may result from chemotherapy, radiation, exposure to environmental toxins, pregnancy, and lupus.

Hemolytic anemia is a condition in which the red blood cells are destroyed faster than they can be produced in the bone marrow. This may result from autoimmune disease and use of certain medications, such as antibiotics.

Sickle cell anemia is an inherited form of anemia caused by a defective form of hemoglobin that causes the red blood cells to become an abnormal (sickle) shape. These cells die prematurely, resulting in a deficiency. This form of anemia is most common among Blacks and Arabs. Thalassemia is another form of anemia caused by defective hemoglobin.

SIGNS & SYMPTOMS

- Difficulty in thinking

- Fatigue and weakness

- Frequent infections

- Headaches and dizziness

- Menstrual irregularity

- Numbness in extremities

- Pale skin and lips

- Shortness of breath

If left unchecked, anemia can lead to a rapid or irregular heartbeat (arrhythmia) because the heart works harder to compensate for the lack of oxygen in the blood. This can even lead to congestive heart failure. Untreated pernicious anemia can lead to nerve damage and decreased mental function, as vitamin B12 is important not only for healthy red blood cells but also for optimal nerve and brain function.

Some inherited anemias, such as sickle cell anemia, can be serious and lead to life-threatening complications. Losing a lot of blood quickly results in acute, severe anemia and can be fatal.

RISK FACTORS

- Alcoholism: Alcohol interferes with the absorption of folic acid

- Anorexia or bulimia

- Blood loss: Surgery, heavy menstrual periods, ulcers, and hemorrhoids

- Family history: Sickle cell anemia and thalassemia

- Medical conditions: Kidney or liver disease, cancer, autoimmune disease, malabsorption disorders such as Crohn's or celiac disease, and bariatric surgery

- Medications: Non-steroidal anti-inflammatory drugs such as aspirin and ibuprofen can cause stomach bleeding

- Poor diet: Inadequate intake of iron, folate, and vitamin B12

- Pregnancy: Iron stores are depleted by the growing baby

DOCTOR'S ORDERS

The treatment of anemia depends on the underlying cause. Iron-deficiency anemia is treated with supplemental iron. It may take several months to build back iron stores. Pernicious anemia is treated with injections of vitamin B12, and folate deficiency is treated with folate supplements. Aplastic anemia is very serious and may require blood transfusion or bone marrow transplant. Hemolytic anemia is managed with medications that suppress the immune system so that it stops attacking the red blood cells. Sickle cell anemia is treated with oxygen, intravenous fluids, and sometimes blood transfusions.

SHERRY'S NATURAL PRESCRIPTION

Anemia can be a serious condition and requires medical attention. Do not self-diagnose or begin taking iron supplements unless advised by your doctor.

The recommendations for anemia vary depending on the underlying cause. The following information is provided for anemia due to iron, folate, or vitamin B12 deficiency.

Dietary Recommendations

Foods to include:

- Iron-rich foods such as organic beef (calf liver), oysters, beans, lentils, fortified cereals, figs, egg yolks, blackstrap molasses, brewer's yeast, fortified grains, raisins, prune juice, nuts, and seeds

- Folate-rich foods such as citrus, legumes, and fortified cereals

- Dark green leafy vegetables (except spinach) are good sources of both iron and folate

- Vitamin B12 is found in meat and dairy products, fish, and eggs

- Foods rich in vitamin C, such as citrus, peppers, and berries, improve iron absorption

Foods to avoid:

- Star fruit, rhubarb, spinach, chard, beets, chives, parsley, and chocolate are high in oxalic acid, which inhibits iron absorption.

- Coffee and tea contain polyphenols, which can significantly reduce iron absorption (limit consumption to no more than three cups per day).

- Soy protein (tofu) can inhibit iron absorption.

Lifestyle Suggestions

- Have regular medical checkups and report any changes to your doctor.

- If you have iron-deficiency anemia, cook your food in cast-iron pots and pans as the food will absorb some of the iron from the cookware.

Top Recommended Supplements

Folate: Supplements are required by those deficient and women trying to get pregnant. Dosage: 800–1,200 mcg daily.

Iron supplements: Should be taken only if you have iron-deficiency anemia, as excess iron can be dangerous. Usual dosage: 50–100 mg two to three times daily on empty stomach or with a small, low-fibre snack. Iron is available in various forms, including sulphate, succinate, gluconate, and fumarate, and each varies in their proportion of elemental iron. Some forms of iron may offer greater absorption and bioavailability with less stomach irritation, including ferric pyrophosphate (SunActive Fe), iron chelates, and iron-rich mineral water (SpaTone).

Liver extracts: Made from beef, they provide a rich natural source of iron, vitamin B12, folate, and other nutrients. Dosage varies.

Multivitamin and mineral complex: Highly recommended because there are many nutrients required for healthy blood cells. Aside from iron, vitamin B12, and folate, a deficiency of vitamins A, C, E, B2, B6, or copper can lead to anemia.

Vitamin B12: Supplements are required by those who are deficient or at risk of deficiency such as the elderly, vegetarians, and those with malabsorption conditions (celiac and Crohn's). Look for a B-complex supplement that provides 1,000–2,000 mcg daily. Those with malabsorption may benefit from sublingual B12 (a small tablet placed under the tongue), which is more readily absorbed. Individuals with pernicious anemia may require B12 injections from their doctor.

Complementary Supplements

Vitamin C: Increases the absorption of iron from food. It also supports absorption of other nutrients. Dosage: 100–500 mg. Take with your iron supplement for best results.

FINAL THOUGHTS

Inherited forms of anemia can't be prevented, but they can be managed with medical treatments. Iron- and vitamin-deficiency anemia can be managed well with the following:

- Eat more leafy green vegetables, nuts, seeds, whole grains, beans, and legumes.
- Consider beef and calf liver if you are deficient in iron.
- Reduce coffee and tea intake.
- If deficient, supplement with iron, vitamin B12, and folate, along with a complete multivitamin and mineral complex.
- See your doctor and have your blood checked regularly.

ANXIETY

Everyone experiences occasional feelings of anxiety, for example, when starting a new job or speaking in front of a crowd. The excitement brought on by these situations is normal and can actually help improve performance. However, feeling anxious for no reason, or having excessive worry, fear, or dread that affects your quality of life, could signify generalized anxiety disorder (GAD). This condition is among the most common psychiatric ailments, affecting 12 percent of Canadians.

Anxiety can lead to physical, emotional, cognitive, and behavioural effects. Feelings of anxiety can cause a person to freeze with fear, which is typically followed by an urge to flee or fight, known as the fight-or-flight response (despite the fact that the response to flee occurs before the fight response). This response triggers the body to release stress hormones that prepare you to react to a perceived threat or stressful situation. The heart pumps stronger, breathing is increased, blood is shunted to the extremities to increase strength in the arms and legs, and digestion slows down so the body can reserve resources. Hundreds of years ago, this response was experienced occasionally and was vital to our survival. Today, however, stress and anxiety can be persistent and debilitating with far-reaching consequences on health, leading to high blood pressure and cholesterol, insomnia, mood swings, depression, and other health problems.

Some people experience extreme states of anxiety and worry, called panic attacks, which cause heart pounding, shortness of breath, chest pain, sweating, dizziness, and weakness. This can be scary, as the symptoms mimic the early signs of a heart attack.

There are various lifestyle strategies and supplements that can be helpful in reducing anxiety and improving emotional well-being.

TYPES OF ANXIETY

Generalized anxiety disorder is one type of anxiety disorder. Others include

Obsessive-compulsive disorder: Obsessions are persistent thoughts, ideas, impulses, or images that are intrusive and inappropriate and cause anxiety or distress. Compulsions are repetitive behaviours (such as hand washing or checking things) or mental acts (such as counting or repeating words) that occur in response to an obsession or in a ritualistic way.

Phobias: A phobia is a significant and persistent fear of objects or situations, such as flying.

Post-traumatic stress disorder: Symptoms of post-traumatic stress disorder include flashbacks, persistent frightening thoughts and memories, and anger or irritability in response to a terrifying experience in which physical harm occurred or was threatened (such as rape, child abuse, or war).

SIGNS & SYMPTOMS

Signs and symptoms vary among individuals and in severity, and may include

- Diarrhea
- Difficulty concentrating
- Edginess
- Excessive worry
- Fatigue
- Headache
- Irritability
- Muscle tension
- Racing heart, palpitations
- Restlessness
- Shortness of breath
- Sleep disturbance

Generalized anxiety disorder is diagnosed when there is excessive anxiety and worry about a number of events or activities over a period of at least six months.

RISK FACTORS

- Alcohol or drug abuse
- Chronic illness (diabetes, low blood sugar, depression, thyroid disorder)
- Diet (excessive sugar and caffeine)
- Family history of anxiety disorder
- Food allergies
- Personality disorders
- Smoking
- Stress (family, work, financial problems)
- Trauma

DOCTOR'S ORDERS

Doctors typically prescribe medications and/or psychotherapy to treat anxiety disorder. Benzodiazepines are the main class of anti-anxiety drugs and include alprazolam (Xanax), clonazepam (Rivotril), diazepam (Valium), and lorazepam (Ativan). These drugs work quickly (30 to 60 minutes) to ease anxiety and promote relaxation. However, they are addictive and have numerous side effects, including drowsiness, loss of coordination, dizziness, and impaired memory. Buspirone (Buspar) is a different type of anti-anxiety drug that is less addictive, but it still has side effects, including headache, nervousness, and insomnia.

Antidepressants may be used for anxiety that is associated with depression. They work by altering the activity of neurotransmitters (chemical messengers) in the brain. Examples include citalopram (Celexa), fluoxetine (Prozac), paroxetine (Paxil), and venlafaxine (Effexor). These drugs may take four to six weeks to work and are not effective for everyone (some experience worsened anxiety). Other side effects include nervousness, headache, nausea, sexual dysfunction, sleep disturbance, and changes in appetite and weight.

Professional counselling can help a person develop tools and coping skills to deal with stress and anxiety. One form of therapy that is highly effective for anxiety disorder is cognitive behaviour therapy. A therapist works with you to identify distorted thoughts and beliefs that trigger anxiety, and you learn to replace negative thoughts and reactions with more positive ones, so that you view and cope with life's events differently.

HOMEOPATHIC RECOMMENDATIONS

Aconitum napellus: This remedy helps when a panic attack comes on suddenly with very strong fears (even fear of death).

Argentum nitricum: This remedy may relieve apprehension or stage fright accompanied by agitation and a feeling of being chronically rushed.

Arsenicum album: This remedy is indicated for those who are deeply anxious about their health and extremely concerned with order and security. It may also help those who are restless or fidgety, or who anxiously pace around. These people may also have digestive problems or asthma attacks accompanied by anxiety.

Calcarea carbonica: This remedy may be indicated for those who become overwhelmed from too much work and start to fear a breakdown.

SHERRY'S NATURAL PRESCRIPTION

Dietary Recommendations

Eating small, frequent meals will help promote good blood sugar balance. Drink lots of water and decaffeinated beverages such as herbal teas (lemon balm, passion flower, and chamomile are known for their calming properties) or vegetable juices. Green tea is also helpful, as it contains L-theanine, an amino acid that has a calming effect.

Foods to include:

• Low-glycemic carbohydrates (high-fibre, slow-release carbohydrates, like whole grains such as brown rice, wheat bran, and oats) help to keep blood sugar balanced and prevent the lows that can contribute to anxiety. These foods also provide serotonin, a brain chemical that induces a calm feeling.

- Whole grains and leafy green vegetables contain B-vitamins, which are essential to the nervous system and help the body with stress.

- Foods rich in magnesium (brewer's yeast, broccoli, sea vegetables, nuts, salmon, and molasses) promote calming and muscle relaxation.

Foods to avoid:

- Caffeine and alcohol can trigger and worsen anxiety. Go off caffeine slowly to avoid withdrawal symptoms, which can worsen anxiety.

- Sugary foods cause fluctuations in blood sugar, which may cause mood swings and worsen symptoms of anxiety. Avoid refined carbohydrates (white bread, baked goods), candy, condiments (ketchup, salad dressings, and peanut butter), and snack foods.

Note: Food allergies can trigger symptoms of anxiety disorder. An elimination diet can help identify food allergies. Refer to Appendix D.

Lifestyle Suggestions

- Don't dwell on the past and things you can't change. Learn to let things go.

- Look for the positive in a situation rather than focusing on the negative.

- Practise positive affirmations, messages that make you feel empowered and good about yourself. Say them to yourself and post them on your fridge or mirror as a reminder.

- When feeling anxious, calm yourself by going for a walk; closing your eyes and taking slow, deep breaths; meditating; or having a bath with mineral salts.

- Get adequate rest, which is crucial for the nervous system.

- Spend time with family and friends who are supportive. Talk about your fears and problems, as sharing your feelings can be relieving.

- Get regular exercise. Walking, cycling, yoga, tai chi, and Pilates are great ways to reduce stress and anxiety.

- Acupuncture helps promote calming and relaxation.

- Try biofeedback. There are specific programs and techniques that can help reduce stress and anxiety, such as the Institute of HeartMath (www.heartmath.org).

HOW TO REDUCE ANXIETY

Controlled breathing techniques can help ease anxiety and panic attacks. When feeling anxious, go to a quiet place where you can sit down and close your eyes. Take a slow, deep breath and hold it for four seconds, then exhale slowly for four seconds. Repeat this several times until you feel calmer and more relaxed.

Top Recommended Supplements

B-vitamins: Essential for nervous system function; a deficiency can cause depression and anxiety. Look for a product that provides 50–100 mg of the B-vitamins. Some studies have found benefits with higher doses of a vitamin B3 derivative (niacinamide).

Fish oil: Important for brain and nervous system health. Recent research shows benefits for reducing inflammatory compounds associated with depression and anxiety. Dosage: 1–3 g daily. Choose a product with a 7:1 ratio of EPA:DHA.

Magnesium: Promotes calming and relaxation; levels may be depleted in those with stress and anxiety. Dosage: 200 mg three times daily. It may cause loose stools, so combine with calcium. A 2:1 calcium to magnesium ratio is recommended to offset that effect.

L-theanine: An amino acid naturally present in small amounts in green tea. A patented and clinically studied supplement form of L-theanine called Suntheanine has been shown to reduce stress, promote calming and relaxation, and improve sleep quality without causing drowsiness, memory loss, or addiction. Dosage: 50–200 mg daily.

Complementary Supplements

Passion flower: An herb that promotes relaxation; studies support benefits for reducing anxiety and nervousness. Dosage: 4–8 mg of dried herb daily or 5–10 mL of tincture three to four times daily.

Relora: A combination of magnolia and phellodendron that reduces stress without causing drowsiness. It is non-addictive. Dosage: 250 mg three times daily.

Valerian: An herb with relaxing and calming properties. It causes drowsiness, so it can be helpful for those with insomnia due to anxiety. Dosage: 300–500 mg of an extract an hour before bed.

FINAL THOUGHTS

To help deal with anxiety, keep the following in mind:

- Adopt a positive attitude and practise positive affirmations.
- Eat a healthy diet with whole grains, vegetables, and magnesium-rich foods.
- Get adequate rest and exercise regularly to reduce stress and anxiety and improve mood.
- Take a supplement with B-vitamins, magnesium, and fish oil regularly.
- To reduce anxiety and stress try a supplement that contains Suntheanine.

ARTHRITIS (RHEUMATOID)

"Arthritis" is a term used to describe conditions that cause joint inflammation. There are over 100 forms of arthritis. Rheumatoid arthritis (RA) is the second most common form of arthritis and affects about 300,000 Canadians, or one in 100.

RA is an autoimmune disease. The immune system produces antibodies that attack healthy joints, causing inflammation in the lining of the joints and pain. Chronic, uncontrolled inflammation leads to damage and destruction of the cartilage and joint tissues (bones, tendons, and ligaments) and the formation of scar tissue. Those with severe RA often suffer with deformity, reduced joint mobility, and pain that limits normal daily activities.

There are several lifestyle modifications and supplements that can help ease the pain and inflammation of RA and improve quality of life.

SIGNS & SYMPTOMS

The symptoms of RA vary from person to person, but typically affect the fingers, wrists, knees, ankles, and toes. It may start gradually or as a sudden, severe attack causing

- Flu-like symptoms (fatigue, weakness, and loss of appetite)
- Joint pain, stiffness, and warmth
- Swollen, red joints

Some people have continuous symptoms and others go through periods of remission followed by flare-ups. Severe cases of RA can cause red skin lumps (rheumatoid nodules) on the elbows, ears, nose, knees, toes, or scalp and deformity of the joints.

RISK FACTORS

- Age: It can strike at any age; however, most people develop RA between ages 25 and 50.
- Gender: Women are three times more likely than men to develop RA.
- Family history: This may increase risk, but is not absolute; some people with a family history never get the disease, and others with no history will get it.
- Smoking cigarettes over a long period of time can cause RA.
- Environment: Infection (bacterial or viral), stress, food allergies, or toxin exposure may trigger the onset in those who are susceptible.

DOCTOR'S ORDERS

Non-steroidal anti-inflammatory drugs (NSAIDs), such as ibuprofen, naproxen, and indomethacin, are commonly prescribed to reduce pain and inflammation, yet they should be used cautiously because they can cause many serious and life-threatening side effects including kidney and liver damage, stomach ulcers, and bleeding. One class of these drugs (COX-2 inhibitors) has been linked to an increased risk of heart attacks. Ironically, long-term use of these drugs can worsen joint health by accelerating the breakdown of cartilage. Use the lowest possible dose for short-term relief. Contact your doctor if you have stomach pain, cramping, or dark stools as these are signs of stomach bleeding.

Corticosteroids like prednisone are used to reduce pain and inflammation, but are not recommended for long-term use as they can cause bruising, thinning of bones, cataracts, weight gain, a round face, and diabetes.

Disease modifiers such as methotrexate, Plaquenil, and Imuran are taken to halt inflammation, slow the progression of RA, and control the immune system response. These drugs can cause serious side effects, such as nutrient deficiencies, blood disorders, and increased risk of infection.

Surgery to remove inflamed tissue and replace joints may be done for severe cases.

CAUTION: NSAIDs can cause serious and life-threatening side effects such as stomach ulcers and bleeding, increased gut permeability, water retention, and kidney damage. One class of these drugs (COX-2 inhibitors) has been linked to an increased risk of heart attacks. Use the lowest possible dose for short-term relief. Contact your doctor if you have stomach pain or cramping or dark stools as these are signs of stomach bleeding.

HOMEOPATHIC RECOMMENDATIONS

Bryonia: This remedy can be helpful for stiffness and inflammation with tearing or throbbing pain, made worse by even the smallest motion. The condition may have developed gradually, and is worse in cold, dry weather. Discomfort is aggravated by being touched or bumped, or from any movement. Pressure brings relief because it stabilizes the area. Typically, the person wants to stay completely still and not be interfered with.

Rhus toxicodendron: Rheumatoid arthritis, with pain and stiffness that is worse in the morning and worse on first motion, but better from continued movement, is the indication for Rhus tox. Hot baths or showers and warm applications improve the stiffness and relieve the pain. The condition is worse in cold, wet weather. The person may feel extremely restless, is unable to find a comfortable position, and needs to move constantly.

Combination recommendation: Zeel by Heel

SHERRY'S NATURAL PRESCRIPTION

Dietary Recommendations

An elimination diet as outlined in Appendix D can help identify food allergies that could be triggering inflammation.

Foods to include:

• Cold-water fish, olive oil, chia seed, flaxseed, and hemp, which are rich in essential fatty acids, can help reduce inflammation.

- Asparagus, cabbage, garlic, and onions contain sulphur, which is beneficial for the joints.

- Pineapple contains the enzyme bromelain, which can help reduce inflammation.

- Pomegranate contains antioxidants (polyphenols) with anti-inflammatory effects. Preliminary research suggests benefits for reducing RA symptoms, including inflammation.

- Ginger contains compounds that help reduce inflammation. Add fresh ginger root to soups, stews, and stir-fries.

- Several studies have found that the antioxidants in green tea (catechins) can reduce chronic joint inflammation and slow cartilage breakdown.

There is some evidence that a vegan (eliminating all animal products) diet can help reduce inflammation and improve symptoms of RA.

Foods to avoid:

- Nightshade vegetables (potatoes, tomatoes, peppers, eggplant) contain a substance called solanine, which can trigger pain and inflammation; preliminary studies have found benefits in avoiding these foods.

- Processed, fast, and deep-fried foods contain trans fatty acids, which trigger inflammation.

- Red meat, milk, cheese, and deep-fried foods contain saturated fats, which trigger inflammation.

- Sugar and refined carbohydrates, which are high on the glycemic index, may worsen symptoms.

- Alcohol and caffeine may worsen symptoms.

Lifestyle Suggestions

- Acupuncture may help reduce pain and stress and improve quality of life.

- Physical therapy, such as ultrasound and laser therapy, is beneficial for pain and inflammation.

- Light activities that are not stressful on the joints, such as swimming, cycling, and stretching (yoga), help to improve joint mobility and overall health.

- Hot paraffin baths, therapeutic mud treatments, baths with Epsom/mineral salts, and sauna can reduce pain and inflammation.

- Apply hot or cold packs/compresses to the affected joints. Both are helpful.

- Light massage with botanical oils (camphor, eucalyptus, pine needle, or rosemary) can help reduce pain and promote relaxation.

- Assistive devices, such as canes, walkers, and joint supports, offer support and reduce joint strain.

Top Recommended Supplements

Curcumin: A spice from the turmeric plant, curcumin is an antioxidant and has been shown in studies to have anti-inflammatory effects comparable to cortisone and to help reduce pain. It also helps protect cartilage against destruction and promote cartilage regeneration. Dosage: 300–400 mg three times daily.

Fish oil: Contains beneficial omega-3 fatty acids (EPA and DHA), which have been shown in studies to reduce the pain and inflammation associated with arthritis. These "good" fats work in part by boosting levels of prostaglandins, which are hormone-like substances that have anti-inflammatory activity. Dosage: The typical dosage is 3–9 g of EPA and DHA daily, although higher amounts have been used in some studies. Look for a product that provides at least 400 mg EPA and 200 mg DHA per capsule.

GLA: An omega-6 fatty acid found in black currants, borage, and primrose oil. Several small studies have found that it can reduce RA symptoms such as tender joints and swelling. Dosage: 1400 mg daily.

Complementary Supplements

Boswellia: A tree resin used in traditional Ayurvedic/Indian medicine; several studies show that it reduces pain and inflammation, similar to NSAIDS, but does not cause stomach irritation. Dosage: 400–800 mg three times daily.

Capsaicin: A hot pepper extract that reduces pain, capsaicin is available in creams; look for a product with 0.025–0.075 percent capsaicin (Zostrix or Menthacin); wash hands after application to avoid getting the product in the eyes.

Celadrin: A patented blend of fatty acids, Celadrin reduces inflammation and pain, lubricates joints, and promotes healing. Celadrin is available in capsules or as a cream. Dosage: 1,500 mg daily; apply the cream twice daily.

Vitamin D: Levels of vitamin D are often deficient in those with RA (as well as those with other autoimmune diseases). Mounting research suggests benefits in supplementing, especially among those who have low levels. Dosage range: 1,000–10,000 IU.

FINAL THOUGHTS

RA is a chronic condition with many underlying factors. The key is to control inflammation and pain, which will help to prevent joint damage and loss of mobility. The main points to keep in mind are as follows:

- Eat more fish, chia, olive oil, and pineapple and drink green tea.
- Minimize red meat, dairy, sugar, and refined/processed foods.
- Do light exercises and stretching daily.
- Reduce stress and pain with acupuncture, mineral baths, paraffin treatments, and massage.
- Consider curcumin, fish oils, or GLA for a first-line natural approach for RA.

ASTHMA

Asthma is a chronic inflammatory disease of the bronchial tubes (airways) of the lungs. Exposure to an asthmatic trigger initiates the release of inflammatory compounds that cause the lining of the airways to become inflamed and irritated, and the cells in the lungs to produce extra mucus, narrowing the airways. The muscles that surround the bronchial walls start to twitch and tighten, further narrowing the airways and causing difficulty breathing. In some cases, breathing may be so laboured that an asthma attack becomes life-threatening. Asthma affects about 3 million Canadians and it is estimated that six out of ten people with asthma do not have good control over their disease. Every year about 500 people die from asthma.

Researchers believe that asthma results from a combination of environmental and genetic factors. You are more likely to develop asthma if you have a parent with the disease and if you're sensitive to environmental allergens. Common allergens include pollen, animal dander, dust mites, smoke, and chemicals, such as dyes, perfumes, and preservatives in food like sulphites. Being exposed to an allergen may cause irritation and swelling in various areas of the body, such as the nose, eyes, skin, and lungs. Allergens can make asthma symptoms worse by increasing inflammation in the airways and making them more sensitive.

There are a number of factors that can trigger an asthma attack in those with the disease, such as having a respiratory infection, gastroesophageal reflux disease (GERD), exercise, stress, and exposure to cold air.

Asthma is a chronic but manageable condition. While medication may be necessary, there are also lifestyle approaches and nutritional supplements that can help control the inflammation and reduce the severity and frequency of attacks.

SIGNS & SYMPTOMS

- Disturbed sleep

- Shortness of breath and difficulty breathing

- Tightness in the chest

- Wheezing and coughing

The signs and symptoms can range from mild to severe. Some people have only occasional asthma attacks that are mild and short-lived, while others experience chronic coughing and wheezing and severe attacks.

RISK FACTORS

- Exposure to occupational triggers, such as chemicals used in farming, hairdressing, and in paint, steel, plastics, and electronics manufacturing

- Exposure to second-hand smoke

- Family history

- Having multiple respiratory infections as a child
- Having a mother who smoked while pregnant
- Living in a large urban area (exposure to environmental pollutants)
- Low birth weight
- Obesity

ASTHMA AND ANTIBIOTICS

According to recent research, taking antibiotics before one year of age can increase the likelihood of developing asthma later in life by as much as 50 percent. This risk appears to be highest for infants who receive multiple courses of broad spectrum antibiotics. Researchers speculate that because these antibiotics kill a wide range of bacteria (good and bad), they disrupt the natural microflora in the gut, resulting in impaired immune function. (*Pediatrics,* 2011, 127(6): 1125–1138)

DOCTOR'S ORDERS

The medical treatment of asthma often involves use of bronchodilators, which relax the bronchial muscles and open up the airways, and anti-inflammatory drugs to reduce swelling in the airways.

Quick-acting bronchodilators, also called "rescue" medications, include salbutamol (Ventolin) and ipratropium (Atrovent). These drugs can stop an asthma attack and relieve symptoms of coughing, wheezing, chest tightness, and shortness of breath. These medications should be carried with you at all times so that you have them handy when you feel an attack coming on. There are also long-acting bronchodilators, such as salmeterol (Serevent Diskus), which are used to control moderate and severe asthma and to prevent nighttime symptoms.

Anti-inflammatory medications (steroids), which help relieve the swelling of tissue, are used for those with moderate to severe asthma. They are available in tablets (prednisone) and inhalers such as fluticasone (Flovent), budesonide (Pulmicort), and beclomethasone (Beclovent). They may take a few hours or even days to work, so they are not to be used as rescue medications. Long-term use of these drugs can cause serious side effects, including cataracts, osteoporosis, muscle weakness, decreased resistance to infection, and thinning of the skin. The inhalers are safer than oral steroids, but they may still increase risk of osteoporosis when taken over the long term and can cause thrush and coughing. Using a spacer device (AeroChamber) will help improve delivery of the medication to your lungs and can reduce the risk of thrush and mouth irritation. Another drug used to reduce inflammation is montelukast (Singulair). Those with exercise-induced asthma may need only a bronchodilator when exercising. For asthma triggered by allergies, injections to desensitize you to the allergen can be given.

HOMEOPATHIC RECOMMENDATIONS

Arsenicum album: This remedy is usually indicated for those whose asthma tends to be aggravated while lying down but is less active when the sufferer sits up.

Pulsatilla: This remedy may help asthmatic individuals who wheeze when they get too warm (especially in a stuffy room), after eating rich foods like cheese or ice cream, or when emotional turmoil brings on difficult breathing.

Spongia tosta: This remedy is recommended for those with laboured breathing that produces a sawing-like sound with a concomitant cough that is often barking.

SHERRY'S NATURAL PRESCRIPTION

Dietary Recommendations

Foods to include:

• Dark green, yellow, and orange vegetables and fruits contain antioxidants (carotenoids) that help reduce inflammation and allergies. Citrus fruits and berries contain vitamin C, which also reduces inflammation and has antioxidant properties.

• Eat small, frequent meals to keep pressure off your diaphragm.

• Fish, chia seed, and flaxseed contain fatty acids that reduce inflammation.

• Garlic and onions have anti-inflammatory properties.

• Green tea contains antioxidants that reduce inflammation.

• Research suggests that the Mediterranean diet, which includes more monounsaturated fats than saturated fats; lots of fish, vegetables, fruit, nuts, and grains; and minimal dairy, is associated with a lower incidence of asthma and less asthma symptoms in those with the disease.

Foods to avoid:

• Sensitivity to dairy products derived from cow's milk is common in those affected and can worsen asthma symptoms, causing wheezing, coughing, chest tightness, and excessive mucus production.

• Food additives, dyes, and preservatives can trigger asthma attacks in certain people.

• Frozen drinks and extremely cold foods can cause the muscles in your airways to tighten.

• Salt has been shown to worsen asthma.

• Try an elimination diet (Appendix D) to determine if you have any food sensitivities that could be triggering your asthma.

Lifestyle Suggestions

• Identify and avoid indoor and outdoor allergens and irritants. Keep your house clean and as dust-free as possible. Control pet dander by having your pets groomed regularly and vacuuming your carpets and furniture.

• Avoid second-hand smoke.

- Manage your stress, because stress can trigger an attack. Try yoga, tai chi, stretching, or breathing exercises.

- Acupuncture may help to reduce asthma symptoms in some people.

- Monitor your breathing using a peak flow meter and treat an attack as soon as possible to prevent it from becoming severe.

- Maintain a healthy body weight as being obese can impair lung function.

- Regular exercise can strengthen your lungs so that they don't have to work so hard. Aim for at least 30 minutes of moderate intensity activity each day. Gradually build up your intensity level. During cold months, exercise indoors or wear a face mask to warm the air you breathe. Be aware that if your asthma is not under control, exercise can trigger an attack.

- Use an air purifier with a HEPA filter to clean the air you breathe and remove allergens. Change the filters in your furnace and air conditioner regularly.

- Keep the humidity in your home and office low as high humidity can increase the growth of moulds.

Top Recommended Supplements

The supplements listed here can be helpful for managing mild to moderate cases of asthma. However, you should never stop taking your asthma medications unless advised to do so by your doctor.

Boswellia: An herb that reduces inflammation. Some research has shown that it can reduce the frequency of asthma attacks and improve lung function and breathing. Dosage: 300 mg three times daily.

Pycnogenol: An extract from pine bark that has potent antioxidant and anti-inflammatory properties. Some research has shown that it can significantly improve lung function and asthma symptoms. One of these studies involved children and found that it reduced the need for rescue medication. Dosage: Adults should take 100 mg daily; children should take 1 mg per pound of body weight per day.

Vitamin C: Reduces bronchial inflammation, spasms, and the response to allergies. Several studies have shown benefits for reducing the severity and frequency of asthma attacks. Dosage: 1,000 mg daily. To avoid upset stomach, choose a buffered vitamin C such as calcium ascorbate.

Complementary Supplements

Butterbur: An herb that contains compounds (petasins) that inhibit inflammatory chemicals responsible for symptom aggravation in asthmatics. Some research suggests it can also reduce the frequency and severity of attacks. Dosage: 50–75 mg twice daily.

Fish oil: May help reduce the inflammation that triggers and worsens asthma. There is also evidence that it can reduce exercise-induced asthma. Dosage: 1–3 g daily of EPA and DHA.

Magnesium: Helps relax the bronchial tubes and improve lung function. Studies have found that asthmatics have low levels of this mineral. Supplements may help to prevent asthma attacks by reducing bronchial spasms and relaxing bronchial muscles. Dosage: 300–400 mg daily with meals.

FINAL THOUGHTS

To improve the management of asthma, consider the following:

- Eat more fruits, vegetables, garlic, onions, and fish, and drink plenty of water.
- Get regular exercise and manage your stress.
- Monitor your breathing with a peak flow meter and see your doctor regularly.
- Use an air purifier and keep your home as clean as possible. Avoid second-hand smoke and other known irritants.
- Consider supplements of boswellia, pycnogenol, and vitamin C.

ATHLETE'S FOOT

Athlete's foot (*Tinea pedis*) is a common fungal infection that affects 20 percent of the population at any given time. These fungi, called dermatophytes, infect the skin of the foot, which may result in an intensely itchy, red, scaly rash on the soles of the feet and between the toes. The fungi that cause athlete's foot are highly contagious and grow in warm, moist environments, so it may be picked up easily by walking barefoot in public areas such as bathrooms, swimming pools, saunas, showers, and locker rooms. Athlete's foot is difficult to get rid of because in socks and shoes, feet provide the ideal environment for the fungi to thrive. If you are exposed to the fungi that cause athlete's foot, you may be contagious, even if you don't develop athlete's foot. Once you have had athlete's foot, you are more susceptible to re-infection. Thus, it is important to have a holistic strategy for prevention and to eradicate infections.

SIGNS & SYMPTOMS

- Discomfort that can range from mild to severe
- Heels that crack, scale, or peel
- Infected toenails that may thicken, become yellow/brown, flake, or crumble
- Intense itching, inflammation, or stinging on the soles of the feet or between the toes (usually the third, fourth, and fifth toes)
- Painful sensations when rubbed or scratched
- Sores or blisters
- Thick, dry skin on the feet

RISK FACTORS

- Affects adults and children, and men more often than women
- Direct contact with fungi in public areas (shower floors, wet towels)
- Person-to-person contact with someone with infected skin
- Warm, moist environments such as wet socks, tight shoes, and sweaty feet will encourage growth
- Weakened immunity such as diabetes or HIV/AIDS

RINGWORM AND JOCK ITCH

Ringworm and jock itch are caused by the same type of fungus that causes athlete's foot. This fungus can grow anywhere on the skin but most commonly occurs in moist areas such as the feet, groin and underarm. A fungal infection that causes a circular patch of red skin is known as ringworm. Fungal infections can spread when people touch or scratch the infected area and then touch another part of their body without washing their hands. Be sure to wash your hands regularly while treating an athlete's foot infection. Also, after a bath or shower, use a different towel to dry an infected area than for the remainder of your body. Wash towels in hot water and dry them immediately after each use.

DOCTOR'S ORDERS

Although athlete's foot has obvious signs and symptoms, consult with your doctor for a proper diagnosis because symptoms could be masking a more serious condition.

Most cases of athlete's foot may be treated with a prescription or over-the-counter antifungal medication in the form of an ointment, lotion, powder, or spray. For mild conditions, a cream such as terbinafine (Lamisil), clotrimazole (Lotrimin), or miconazole (Micatin) may be used. Even in mild cases, athlete's foot can be difficult to kill. Most antifungal medicines only limit the growth of the fungal infection, which then allows the fungus to gradually die out as the body sheds infected skin. Follow the medication's instructions precisely for optimum effect.

Avoid using anti-itch creams, such as hydrocortisone. Although these products may relieve the itching, they can worsen the infection.

A solution of 1 percent potassium permanganate dissolved in hot water is a good alternative to antifungal drugs. This can be purchased at a pharmacy.

For severe cases, such as when the fungal infection spreads to the nails, a doctor may prescribe an oral medication such as itraconazole (Sporanox), fluconazole (Diflucan), or terbinafine (Lamisil). These drugs can have serious side effects, especially on the liver, and should be used only under close doctor supervision.

SHERRY'S NATURAL PRESCRIPTION

Some people seem to be naturally resistant to athlete's foot while others find it to be a persistent problem. A diet that promotes immune system health and proper hygiene will go a long way toward prevention.

Dietary Recommendations

The body's ability to ward off infections depends on the health of the immune system. While there are no foods that directly treat athlete's foot, eating a healthy diet that supports the immune system and detoxification is crucial to prevention and effective treatment.

Foods to include:
- Fibre-rich foods such as whole grains, chia seed, and ground flaxseed support detoxification.
- Filtered water, green tea, and green drinks support detoxification.
- Garlic helps fight fungal infections.
- Yogurt with active cultures provides beneficial bacteria that help prevent overgrowth of fungus.

Foods to avoid:

• Alcohol weakens the immune system.

• Sugar hampers immune function, so limit candy, sweets, soft drinks, and refined starches.

Lifestyle Recommendations

• Wear waterproof shoes or sandals in all public places such as swimming pools and showers.

• Dry your feet and toes thoroughly.

• Wear cotton socks and change socks frequently. Sprinkle baby powder or cornstarch between toes to prevent moisture.

• Wear comfortable, well-ventilated shoes or sandals.

• Avoid socks and shoes made of synthetic materials, which promote sweaty feet.

• Don't wear someone else's shoes.

• Wash all clothes, towels, and bed linens that come in contact with infected skin in hot, soapy water separate from other items.

• For sweaty feet, soak daily for 30 minutes in a footbath with baking soda or salt.

Top Recommended Supplements

Tea tree oil: Has a long history of use for treating skin infections. It contains compounds that have disinfectant, antibacterial, and antifungal properties. It is used topically as a solution or in a cream. Three studies have shown that it is effective for treating athlete's foot. Dosage: Apply a topical solution that contains 25–50 percent tea tree standardized to contain 10 percent cineole and at least 30 percent terpinen-4-ol. Use twice daily for four weeks. Creams containing tea tree can also be used at a 10–50 percent concentration. Do not take tea tree orally. Discontinue use if skin becomes irritated.

Complementary Supplements

Garlic: Has antifungal properties. Dosage: 600 mg of aged garlic extract daily.

Vitamin C: Supports proper immune function. Dosage: 500 mg twice daily.

FINAL THOUGHTS

To prevent and manage athlete's foot, consider the following:

• Eat a healthy diet including whole grains, yogurt, and garlic.
• Wear waterproof shoes in public areas and don't share shoes or socks.
• After bathing, dry your feet thoroughly and apply powder.
• Wear cotton socks and properly fitted shoes that don't promote sweaty feet.
• Consider tea tree oil solution for the treatment of athlete's foot.

ATTENTION-DEFICIT/HYPERACTIVITY DISORDER (ADHD)

Attention-deficit/hyperactivity disorder (ADHD) is a chronic neurobehavioural disorder that arises in childhood and may continue into the teen years and adulthood. Children and adults with ADHD may appear inattentive or distracted, hyperactive, and/or impulsive (act without thinking). These symptoms affect the way they interact with the world, negatively impacting their ability to function, concentrate, and excel in school or at work, and affect their efforts to form strong personal relationships. Because the symptoms of ADHD are disruptive and difficult to deal with for other people, children and adults with ADHD are often unfairly judged and suffer from low self-esteem as a result. Children with ADHD are more likely to have a learning disorder and develop a behavioural disorder. Teens and adults with ADHD are at greater risk for self-destructive behaviours.

ADHD is the most commonly diagnosed mental health problem among children. A recent national study reported that up to 23 percent of Canadian children show symptoms of ADHD, including hyperactivity, impulsivity, and inattentiveness, more commonly among boys (boys tend to be more hyperactive while girls tend to be more inattentive). Children with ADHD begin to show signs of their condition before the age of four, but it is often not diagnosed until the school years when their inability to conform to school expectations and achieve academic standards becomes apparent.

There has been a great deal of research on ADHD, but the actual cause is not known. There are many misconceptions about the disorder. It does not result from poor parenting skills or low income status. It is thought that ADHD may result from structural changes in the brain such as alterations in neurotransmitter levels. Environmental and dietary factors may also be involved.

Brain scans of some people with ADHD have shown smaller basal ganglia and reduced frontal lobe activity. Basal ganglia, or nerve clusters, are involved in routine behaviours, and the frontal lobes are involved in planning and organizing, attention, impulse control, and inhibition of responses to sensory stimulation.

It is thought that those with ADHD may have low levels of neurotransmitters (chemical messengers) such as dopamine and norepinephrine. Dopamine is involved in controlling emotions and reactions, concentrating, reasoning, and coordinating movement. An abnormally low level of dopamine can cause the three primary symptoms of ADHD: inattention, impulsiveness, and hyperactivity.

ADHD IN THE CLASSROOM

"Learning disabilities are the only major disability area where the existence of the condition is treated with skepticism and where the person who has the condition is blamed for his or her situation."

—ADHD Foundation of Canada website

SIGNS & SYMPTOMS

The hallmark symptoms of ADHD, whether in children or adults, are hyperactivity, impulsiveness, and inattention. Children may be diagnosed with ADHD if they exhibit significant and disabling symptoms at home and at school for at least six months. Not all children with ADHD are hyperactive or impulsive but may have disabling inattentiveness or easy distractibility. Girls are more likely to suffer from the primarily inattentive form of the disorder (often referred to as ADD) and are often never diagnosed. Many adults with ADHD were never properly diagnosed as children and they often suffer serious problems in their life if they don't obtain proper treatment.

Signs of hyperactivity:

• Cannot play independently or quietly

• Cannot sit still or fidgets when sitting

• Restless, jittery, and always moving

• Talks excessively in a loud voice

Signs of impulsiveness:

• Frequently interrupts and blurts out responses

• Impatient, cannot tolerate waiting or line-ups, becomes agitated

• Unable to control impulses, and acts before thinking (such as crossing the street without looking, making rude comments, or exhibiting dangerous or inappropriate behaviour)

• May not be able to control frustration and anger

Signs of inattentiveness:

• Cannot focus or concentrate; easily distracted

• Does not pay attention to what he or she has been told

• Has a hard time finishing large or involved tasks without frequent reminders to stay on task

• Is not well organized; may appear forgetful or careless

• May appear to daydream and not listen

The above symptoms mean a child with ADHD may have difficulty developing healthy social skills and friendships. Other symptoms may include mild to severe sleeping and eating problems.

ADHD IN ADULTS

The symptoms of hyperactivity, impulsiveness, and inattentiveness are present in adults, but may be more difficult to identify. Here are some of the criteria that doctors use when diagnosing ADHD in adults:

• A childhood history of ADHD

• Anger and stress management issues

- Difficulty having strong personal relationships, or frequently has negative interactions with people and co-workers

- Difficulty in controlling impulsive behaviour (reckless driving, drug and alcohol abuse, other addictions, frequent job changes, financial problems)

- Difficulty in relaxing; restlessness

- Inability to focus on tasks and cannot make deadlines or complete assigned work

- Forgetful about daily activities (failure to make appointments and commitments)

RISK FACTORS

- Heredity: There are known genes associated with ADHD; having a parent with ADHD triples your risk of developing the disorder; identical twins are both likely to be affected.

- Low birth weight

- Childhood illness or infection may increase risk (strep, ear infections, meningitis, encephalitis)

- Infant or childhood exposure to environmental toxins: preservatives, food additives, heavy metals (lead and mercury)

- Infants who experience brain trauma during pregnancy or delivery, or after birth

- Maternal smoking, drug or alcohol use, or exposure to toxins (lead)

- Poor nutrition of child or mother during pregnancy

ENVIRONMENTAL TOXINS AND ADHD

Preschool children exposed to certain environmental toxins, particularly lead and PCBs, are at increased risk of developmental and behavioural problems, many of which are similar to those found in children diagnosed with ADHD. Exposure to lead, which is found mainly in paint and pipes in older buildings, has been linked to disruptive and even violent behaviour and to a short attention span. Exposure to PCBs in infancy may also increase a child's risk of developing ADHD.

DOCTOR'S ORDERS

There is no definitive way to diagnose ADHD. If a child exhibits symptoms of ADHD, the parents, caregivers, and teachers involved with the child will be asked to fill out a variety of questionnaires regarding the child's behaviour. A complete physical examination is also done to rule out other conditions. In some cases, a psychological assessment is done.

The typical medical approach to the management of ADHD is the use of psycho-stimulant drugs, which boost levels of neurotransmitters (dopamine) in the brain. Although these drugs help relieve symptoms in some children, they don't cure ADHD and they can cause troubling side effects, such as difficulty falling or staying asleep, loss of appetite and weight, and upset stomach. Some children develop jerky muscle movements, such as grimaces or twitches (tics). These drugs may also cause reduced growth rate in children and may negatively impact brain development.

The most commonly prescribed medications for treating ADHD include the following:

- Dextroamphetamine/amphetamine (Adderall)
- Dextroamphetamine (Dexedrine)
- Methylphenidate (Ritalin or Concerta)

Atomoxetine (Strattera) is a non-stimulant medication for ADHD that is believed to provide the brain with a steady supply of norepinephrine.

Sometimes children with ADHD are prescribed antidepressants if they do not respond to stimulants. These drugs also cause a variety of unpleasant side effects such as sleeping problems, dry mouth, irregular heartbeat, and changes in appetite. The younger the child, the more susceptible he or she is to the side effects.

Counselling and family and school support are other key parts of treatment. It can be demanding and frustrating for parents dealing with a child with ADHD and equally difficult for the child. A holistic strategy that incorporates counselling along with nutritional and lifestyle strategies, patience, and perseverance are essential. Drug therapy should be considered only as a last resort.

SHERRY'S NATURAL PRESCRIPTION

Dietary Recommendations

A nutritious, whole foods diet is essential for the management of ADHD. Some individuals with ADHD have food allergies or sensitivities that can cause inflammation in the gut and worsening of ADHD symptoms. The most common allergens are wheat, yeast, dairy, corn, soy, and food additives (preservatives, dyes, and chemicals). To determine potential food allergies, consider an elimination diet as outlined in Appendix D.

Foods to include:

- Cultured dairy, such as yogurt and kefir, contains beneficial bacteria that support intestinal health and immune function, and aids in the elimination of toxins.

- Eat fresh organic fruits and vegetables as tolerated, and whole grains (brown rice, whole oats, millet, amaranth, and quinoa).

- Ensure adequate protein intake. Choose free-range poultry, wild fish, beans, and legumes.

- Include healthy fats such as extra-virgin olive oil, hemp oil, or flaxseed oil. Palm and coconut oil are suitable for cooking. Use ghee (clarified butter) instead of regular butter or margarine.

- Medicinal food blends, such as Learning Factors (by Natural Factors), contain a blend of essential nutrients and protein to help support proper brain function and overall health.

Foods to avoid:

- Avoid fast foods, processed foods, and junk foods, such as hot dogs, burgers, french fries, snack cakes, cookies, and sugary breakfast cereals, which are high in sugar, refined starch, saturated and trans fats, and preservatives and are also low in nutritional value.

- Read labels and avoid foods that contain ingredients such as additives, flavour enhancers (MSG), artificial sweeteners (aspartame, saccharin), colourings, dyes, and preservatives such as nitrates, sodium benzoate, sulphites, BHA, and BHT. If you have trouble reading or pronouncing an ingredient, chances are you should avoid that food.

Lifestyle Suggestions

Here are some suggestions for helping children with ADHD both at home and at school.

At home:

- Provide support, patience, and love. Children with ADHD exhibit behaviour that can be trying. Despite this, they need as much positive feedback as possible as they work toward correcting these problems.

- Provide structure and realistic expectations. Children with ADHD need to know what's expected of them and they need these expectations to be enforced. Be consistent.

- As your child develops better coping mechanisms and social skills, he or she will be better able to cope with demanding situations. Until then, avoid triggers for bad behaviour such as line-ups, restaurants, and so on.

- Avoid overstimulation or keep stimulating activities to under two hours.

- Facilitate the organization of personal belongings. Keep bins that are clearly labelled and a white board with the weekly agenda in plain sight.

- Make physical activity a priority and limit their TV, video game, and computer time to less than two hours per day.

- Keep any discussions clear and brief.

At school:

- Discuss your child's ADHD with school administration and all teachers or aides who interact with your child. If the school or teacher is unresponsive, do not give up.

- Be assertive. You are your child's best advocate. Don't be shy to ask the school for what your child needs such as reading or writing aids or occupational therapy.

- Create a personal learning program suited to your child. School boards call these programs by different names, but they describe what accommodations your child warrants in the classroom and also typically enable the school to apply for financial support for resources and teaching aids.

- Have your child sit close to the front of the class or teacher's desk, beside model students and away from distractions.

- Have the teacher give your child responsibilities in the classroom that allow him or her to move around with purpose.

- Break large tasks down into manageable assignments. Have a daily agenda and create clear expectations and consequences for classroom behaviour.

Top Recommended Supplements

There are many supplements that can provide nutritional support to children with ADHD. These supplements may be taken in conjunction with prescription medications, but always discuss any supplements with your doctor or pharmacist before giving them to a child on medication.

Essential fatty acids: Essential for proper development and function of the brain, eyes, and nerves; deficiency is common in children with ADHD. The omega-3 fatty acids EPA and DHA (from fish oil) are particularly important for brain function and the proper release of neurotransmitters, such as dopamine. The omega-6 fatty acid GLA also provides benefits by reducing inflammation in brain cells. A recent review of 10 clinical studies found that those who took omega-3 fatty acids experienced modest improvements in certain symptoms like inattentiveness and hyperactivity. Research done on a specific blend of fatty acids called Equazen eye q (which provides a 9:3:1 ratio of EPA:DHA:GLA) has shown that it can improve concentration levels in children and adolescents with ADHD. Typical dosage: 558 mg EPA, 174 mg DHA and 60 mg GLA.

Multivitamin and mineral formula: Children with ADHD may be deficient in certain nutrients, which can hamper proper brain function and affect behaviour. The B-vitamins, vitamin C, magnesium, selenium, iron, and zinc are necessary for the brain and nervous system and for the production of neurotransmitters, and there is evidence that these nutrients may be deficient in those with ADHD. In particular, some research has found benefits with zinc, magnesium, and vitamin B6 supplements for improving ADHD symptoms. Choose a product that is free of chemical additives and dyes.

Probiotics: Beneficial bacteria that support intestinal health, aid digestion of nutrients and elimination of toxins, and support immune function. Children with ADHD may be depleted in beneficial bacteria and have overgrowth of the fungus *Candida albicans,* which can affect behaviour and cognitive function. Dosage: For children over the age of four, give a product that provides at least 10–20 billion live cells daily. Use half that amount for those under age four. Probiotic supplements are available in capsules, chewable tablets, and powders. Some require refrigeration.

L-theanine: An amino acid that helps reduce anxiety, stabilize mood, and improve behaviour, concentration, and sleep quality. The clinically studied supplement form is called Suntheanine. Typical dosage: 200 mg two to three times daily for children eight years or older, and half this dosage for children as young as four years.

Complementary Supplements

American ginseng: Has antioxidant properties, supports immune function, improves resistance to stress, and supports cognitive function (learning, attention, and memory). One small study of a combination of American ginseng and ginkgo biloba (AD-FX) found benefits for improving behavior. Dosage (AD-FX): For adults and children seven years and older, one to two capsules twice daily for two months, then one capsule twice daily thereafter.

Melatonin: Some research has found melatonin supplements helpful in improving sleep in children with ADHD who are taking stimulant drugs. Dosage: 1–5 mg at bedtime.

RESEARCH HIGHLIGHT

A recently published study examined the impact of L-theanine (Suntheanine) in 98 boys ages 8 to 12 with ADHD. The objective of this study was to measure the potential benefits of L-theanine on sleep quality. This study found that 200 mg of L-theanine chewable tablets twice daily was safe and effective in improving sleep quality in boys with ADHD. (*Alternative Medicine Review,* 2011, 16(4): 348–354)

FINAL THOUGHTS

To improve the management of ADHD, consider the following:

- Encourage a healthy diet of organic vegetables and whole grains, free-range poultry, wild fish, beans, healthy oils, and cultured dairy.
- Avoid or minimize fast foods, processed foods, junk foods, preservatives, and other chemicals.
- Counselling and school support can help both the family and child.
- Consider supplements of essential fatty acids, multivitamin/minerals, L-theanine and probiotics.
- Give a child with ADHD patience, support, and love.

AUTISM (AUTISM SPECTRUM DISORDERS)

Autism is a neurodevelopmental disorder marked by mild to severe delays in communication and social skills and repetitive behaviours. There is a broad range of symptoms and degree of severity with autism, hence the medical name autism spectrum disorders (ASDs). One milder form of the disorder is known as Asperger syndrome. Other developmental disorders that fall under the ASD umbrella are Rett syndrome, PDD-NOS (pervasive developmental disorder not otherwise specified), and childhood disintegrative disorder. Signs and symptoms usually appear before age three and continue throughout life. Some children learn to cope with their unique needs while others need a lifetime of support.

In addition to problems with communication and general social interactions, children with autism are often disengaged from the world around them and may develop unusually focused interests. Intelligence also varies greatly with children with autism, from below average to genius.

Autism is the most common neurological disorder affecting children and one of the most common developmental disabilities affecting Canadians. Autism strikes one in every 110 Canadian children and occurs three to four times more often in boys than in girls. The incidence of autism has been rising by 10 to 17 percent annually.

The actual cause of autism is not known, but genetics appear to play a role; up to 20 sets of genes have been identified. There also appears to be abnormalities in several regions of the brain that affect behaviour and communication. This may result from a combination of genetics and environmental factors, such as toxins and heavy metals, which cause inflammation and oxidative stress in the brain.

Researchers are also looking into the gut–brain link. Many children with autism have digestive problems (diarrhea and constipation) and there are reports showing that symptoms of autism are worsened by certain dietary factors, particularly milk or wheat products. It is thought that food sensitivities may cause alterations in the normal gut flora (bacteria), which impair the absorption of essential nutrients, thus affecting normal development.

Another factor that has been implicated in causing ASD is the use of vaccines, particularly those containing thimerosal, a preservative that contains mercury. This preservative was widely used in vaccines prior to the mid-1990s; however, since numerous safety concerns were raised manufacturers have removed it from single-dose vaccines. There are still a few multi-dose vaccines that contain small amounts of thimerosal, including some types of the influenza vaccine and the hepatitis B vaccine. Overall, the issue of vaccination has been a subject of great debate, yet researchers have not found a definitive link.

There is no cure for autism, but early diagnosis and treatment can help improve quality of life for children with an ASD.

SIGNS & SYMPTOMS

The signs and symptoms of autism vary widely and are grouped into three different areas: behaviour, language, and social skills.

Behaviour

• Inability to cope with changes in routines or unexpected situations

• May fidget or exhibit repetitive movements, such as head banging or rocking

• May become inconsolable or explosive

• May develop strict patterns of behaviour and become upset if they can't be followed precisely

• May develop narrow interests that exclude them from others

• May be unusually fixated on or highly sensitive to noise, light, movement, sound, touch, and textures

• May use toys, books, and games in unusual ways

• May have picky eating habits

• May suffer from digestive problems such as upset stomach and diarrhea

Language

• Abnormal tone or rhythm (may speak in a robotic way)

• Cannot participate in conversations; most expression is one-way

• Delayed or non-existent use of language

• Inappropriate language and expressions; makes odd noises

• Loss of previously acquired words

• Unusual speech patterns, repeated words or phrases

Social Skills

• Cannot maintain eye contact

• Difficulty making and keeping friends

• May be inattentive or appear to not be listening

• May prefer to be alone, engaged in solo play longer than is age appropriate

• May react negatively to being in large group settings, or being touched or bumped

• May not understand or be able to correctly interpret non-verbal communications such as facial expressions

• May blurt out inappropriate comments; appears thoughtless, insensitive

• Rigid; may have strict rules of conduct and react negatively when parents, siblings, or others "break the rules"

SIGNS OF AUTISM IN INFANTS AND TODDLERS

If your infant or toddler does the following, see your doctor:

- Does not make eye contact or interact as expected with parents, family, pets, or surroundings

- Does not make baby noises by the first year

- Does not make hand gestures, point, or wave by the first year

- Does not say single words by 16 months

- Does not make two-word phrases by two years of age

- Experiences loss of language or social skills at any time

- Reacts in an unusual way or negatively to touch, sounds, movement, or light

RISK FACTORS

- Difficulty or trauma during pregnancy or childbirth (breech position); premature birth

- Digestive system problems

- Environmental exposure: Heavy metals such as lead and other toxins

- Heredity: Those who have a child with ASD have a 1 in 20 chance of having a second child with the disorder

- Low Apgar score after birth (a test done right after birth that measures a baby's heart rate, breathing, activity and muscle tone, grimace response, and appearance)

- Parental history of schizophrenia, depression, or bipolar disorder

DOCTOR'S ORDERS

Currently, there is no definitive way to diagnose autism. If signs and symptoms exist, a doctor will do a complete examination and medical history of the child and family. If no other condition is found, the child is usually sent to a developmental specialist or team of specialists that includes doctors, psychologists, physiotherapists, speech and language therapists, and occupational therapists. Usually the child is screened over the series of appointments, and parents, caregivers, and teachers are asked to fill out a variety of questionnaires regarding language and social interactions.

Treatments for autism may include special schools or programs tailored for children with autism; behavioural therapy and social skills training; speech, occupational, and physical therapy; and prescription medications that address symptoms such as anxiety, anger management, and repetitive movements.

SHERRY'S NATURAL PRESCRIPTION

Dietary Recommendations

Children with autism vary so greatly that broad dietary recommendations are not possible. However, it is critical to try to get these children to eat a healthy diet with as much nutrition and variety as possible. This is easier said than done because they can be highly sensitive to taste and texture and eat only a handful of foods. Be patient and prepared for a lot of experimenting. Exposing children to different foods and encouraging trying new foods is an important social skill for them to learn.

Foods to include:

- Cultured dairy, such as yogurt and kefir, contains beneficial bacteria that support intestinal health and immune function, and aid in the elimination of toxins.

- Ensure adequate protein intake (free-range poultry, wild fish, beans, and legumes)

- Include fresh organic fruits and vegetables as tolerated, and whole grains (brown rice, whole oats, millet, amaranth, and quinoa).

- Include healthy fats such as extra-virgin olive oil, hemp oil, or flaxseed oil. Coconut oil is suitable for cooking. Use ghee (clarified butter) instead of regular butter or margarine.

- Medicinal food blends, such as Learning Factors (by Natural Factors), provide essential nutrients, protein, and nutraceuticals to support proper brain function.

Foods to avoid:

- Processed, refined, and fast foods contain lots of sugar, starch, and saturated and trans fats, and are low in nutritional value.

- Read labels and avoid foods that contain ingredients such as additives, flavour enhancers (MSG), artificial sweeteners (aspartame, saccharin), colourings, dyes, and preservatives such as nitrates, sodium benzoate, sulphites, BHA, and BHT. These chemicals can be a problem for those with autism. If you have trouble reading or pronouncing an ingredient, chances are you should avoid that food.

- Food allergies may contribute to symptoms of autism. Common allergens include gluten (a protein found in wheat, rye, and barley) and casein (found in dairy). Many children with autism improve significantly on a strict gluten- and casein-free diet. While scientific studies are lacking, many families report that children have improved behaviour and overall health following this approach. To rule out potential sensitivities, try an elimination diet as outlined in Appendix D.

Lifestyle Suggestions

- Social skills training is imperative; visit your local learning disability association for guidance.

- Increase social skills opportunities; find daycares, schools, camps, and clubs for children with autism spectrum disorders.

- Massage therapy may be helpful. In a review of four randomized, controlled trials, researchers found that massage therapy may help improve symptoms, such as language and social abilities.

- Regular exercise is important to developing gross and fine motor skills (though autistic children may not cope well on a typical sports team, so look for individual sports such as martial arts and swimming).

- Water therapy, music, art, and the use of animals, may be helpful.
- Expose your child to new activities in safe settings (always prepare your child for a new activity and advise the teacher or coach of your child's needs).
- The importance of family support cannot be overemphasized; families of children with autism need a huge amount of emotional support.
- Seek out as many government support programs as your province has available.

Top Recommended Supplements

Essential fatty acids: Essential for proper development and function of the brain, eyes, and nerves; deficiency is common in children with autism spectrum disorders. The omega-3 fatty acids EPA and DHA (from fish oil) are particularly important for brain development and function. Research suggests that supplements that provide EPA, DHA, and GLA can help improve symptoms of ASD. Typical dosages: 558 mg EPA, 174 mg DHA, and 60 mg GLA.

Multivitamin and mineral formula: Children with autism may be deficient in certain nutrients, which can hamper proper brain and nervous system function. In particular, the B-vitamins (especially B6), vitamin C, magnesium, selenium, and zinc are necessary for the brain and nervous system and production of neurotransmitters. Choose a product that is free of chemical additives and dyes.

Probiotics: Beneficial bacteria that support intestinal health, aid digestion of nutrients and elimination of toxins, and support immune function. Children with autism may be depleted in beneficial bacteria and have overgrowth of the fungus *Candida albicans,* which can affect behaviour and cognitive function. Dosage: For children over the age of four, give a product that provides at least 1 billion live cells daily. Use half that amount for those under age four. Probiotic supplements are available in capsules, chewable tablets, and powders.

Complementary Supplements

Carnosine: A substance manufactured in the human body, it is composed of the amino acids alanine and histidine. Carnosine is highly concentrated in the brain, nervous system, eyes, and muscle tissue. One preliminary study found that supplements of 400 mg twice daily significantly improved symptoms of ASD.

Phosphatidylserine: An essential component of all cell membranes that is highly concentrated in the brain and supports proper function of the brain and nervous system. Dosage: 300–500 mg daily.

FINAL THOUGHTS

To improve the management of ASD, consider the following:

- Encourage a healthy diet of organic vegetables and whole grains, free-range poultry, wild fish, beans, healthy oils, and cultured dairy.
- Avoid or minimize fast foods, processed foods, junk foods, preservatives, and other chemicals.
- Encourage regular exercise and try massage and acupuncture.
- Counselling, social skills programs, and school support can be very helpful.
- Consider supplements of essential fatty acids, multivitamin/minerals, and probiotics.

BACK PAIN

Back pain is one of the leading reasons for doctors' visits and missed workdays. Over 80 percent of adults experience low back pain sometime during their life, and it can range from mildly uncomfortable to completely debilitating.

We rely on our back for almost every move we make. It takes a great deal of stress and is particularly vulnerable to injury. The area most at risk of injury is the lower back, or lumbar region, because it has the greatest curve and supports most of the body's weight. Because the back is a complex network of bones, joints, muscles, ligaments, discs, and nerves, inflammation or injury to any of these parts can cause acute or chronic pain. The most common cause of back pain is improper or heavy lifting or a sudden awkward movement.

Often back pain will resolve within a few weeks, with or without medical attention. There are numerous drugs that are used to reduce pain and inflammation, but they can cause a range of unpleasant side effects. There are also many natural treatments, including supplements, acupuncture, and chiropractic, that can offer significant benefits for reducing pain and improving healing.

SIGNS & SYMPTOMS

- Pain, aching in the lower or middle back
- Radiating pain to the hips or neck

RISK FACTORS

- Arthritis: Spondylosis is a type of arthritis affecting the spine as a result of the degenerative changes in the spine that often come with aging
- Constipation
- Heavy or improper lifting
- Herniated disc occurs when a disc in the spinal column bulges out and presses on a nerve; if the disc impinges the sciatic nerve, the condition is called sciatica, which causes sharp, shooting pain through the buttocks and back of the leg
- Inactivity (poor muscle strength and flexibility)
- Injury (car accident or a fall)
- Obesity and pregnancy
- Osteoporosis
- Tumour or infection of the spine

DOCTOR'S ORDERS

The treatment of back pain depends on the underlying cause. If it is acute pain due to strain or lifting, a short period of rest may help. However, being inactive for longer than that can do more harm than good. Light activity, such as walking and stretching, can actually speed healing and recovery.

Depending on the cause and severity of your pain, your doctor may recommend physiotherapy. Physiotherapists offer a range of treatments, such as heat, ice, ultrasound, electrical stimulation, and muscle-release techniques, to reduce pain. They also advise on specific exercises to increase your flexibility, strengthen your back and abdominal muscles, and improve your posture. Exercise can help pain from recurring.

Medications, such as pain relievers, anti-inflammatories, and muscle relaxants, may be recommended. Some of these medications, such as the opiates (codeine, morphine, and derivatives) are highly addictive and can cause serious side effects. Always use the lowest possible dose to minimize side effects and don't rely on medications over the long term unless you have a chronic problem and are under close medical supervision.

Surgery is always considered a last resort for dealing with severe back pain caused by a herniated disc.

HOMEOPATHIC RECOMMENDATIONS

Aesculus: Helpful for pain in the very low back that feels worse when getting up from a sitting position and worse when getting up from stooping. It is especially indicated for people with low back pain who also have a tendency toward venous congestion (such as congested return blood flow, varicose veins, and hemorrhoids).

Arnica montana: This remedy relieves uncomplicated lower back aches and stiffness from overexertion or minor trauma. It works best in topical gel or cream form.

Bryonia: This remedy is helpful for back pain after injury and back aches during illness. It is especially indicated when back pain is worse from even the slightest motion. If changing position, coughing, turning, or walking brings on a sharp, excruciating pain, this remedy is the one to try.

Rhus toxicodendron: This remedy is recommended when the pain is worse on initial movement and improves with continued motion. The type of aching and stiffness that this remedy alleviates is further aggravated in cold damp weather but relieved by warm applications, baths or showers, and massage. Also recommended for neck and shoulder pain.

SHERRY'S NATURAL PRESCRIPTION

Dietary Recommendations

Foods to include:

• Eat a high-fibre diet, as constipation can worsen back pain.

• Fish and flaxseed contain essential fatty acids, which can help reduce pain and inflammation.

• Fruits and vegetables contain essential vitamins and minerals that help your body cope with stress (back pain).

• Herbal teas with ginger or green tea provide antioxidants that help reduce inflammation.

Foods to avoid:

- Fast foods and processed foods are typically high in saturated fats, sugar, and calories, which can affect your ability to manage your weight.

- While alcohol may temporarily make you feel better, it can worsen inflammation and lead to nutrient deficiencies that can negatively affect nerves, muscles, and bones.

●●●

SMOKING AND BACK PAIN

While many smokers feel that smoking lessens pain, it actually has the opposite effect. Studies have found that smoking can actually contribute to back pain and worsen the likelihood of developing a herniated disc. It is thought that smoking causes malnutrition of spinal discs, which in turn makes them more vulnerable to mechanical stress. Smokers also have diminished oxygen levels in their spinal tissues, which can hinder the healing process.

●●●

Lifestyle Suggestions

- Exercise regularly to strengthen your muscles and improve flexibility. Having strong abdominal and back muscles helps to reduce the risk of injuries, and having good flexibility in your hips and legs will take the strain off your back. Walking, swimming, Pilates, yoga, and stretching are good choices.

- Don't smoke, as this can worsen pain and prevent healing.

- Wear a back support or brace if you are doing heavy lifting.

- Maintain a healthy body weight to reduce strain on your back muscles.

- Studies have shown that acupuncture, chiropractic, osteopathic treatments, and massage are effective therapies for easing back pain.

- Apply cold and then heat to your back to soothe sore and inflamed muscles. If you have just strained your back, apply ice (wrapped in a towel) for 10 to 20 minutes several times a day. Use ice as long as spasms persist. Then you can apply heat using a heating pad or hot water bottle for 20 minutes.

- Use a topical cream that contains capsaicin (such as Zostrix HP), a hot pepper extract that reduces pain at the nerves. Four studies have found significant benefits for reducing lower back pain. Look for a product that contains 0.025 to 0.075 percent capsaicin and apply three times daily. Do not apply to broken skin. Wash your hands after applying this cream as it can cause burning.

- When standing for long periods of time, alternate placing each foot on a low footstool to take some pressure off your lower back.

- If your job involves sitting, use a chair with good lower back support and arm rests. Keep your knees and hips level and use a foot rest.

- Medium–firm mattresses are best for those with back pain. To recover from a back ache, put a pillow under your knees when lying on your back or between your knees when on your side to ease the pressure on your back.

- Use proper form when lifting.

....

PROPER LIFTING TECHNIQUE

When lifting objects, keep your back straight, bend only at the knees, and let your legs do the work. Hold the object close to your body and avoid lifting and twisting at the same time. Have a partner help you when lifting heavy objects.

....

Top Recommended Supplements

Devil's claw: Reduces inflammation and back pain, particularly due to osteoarthritis. Several studies have found benefits. Dosage: Look for a product that provides 60 mg of harpagoside (active constituent) and take twice daily. Avoid using if you have heartburn, ulcers, or gallstones.

Fish oil: Reduces pain and inflammation. Studies have found it helpful for reducing symptoms of arthritis, back pain, and neck pain. Dosage: 3–6 g daily of combined EPA and DHA.

White willow: Reduces pain and inflammation. Studies have found it effective for treating low back pain. The active component is salicin, which is similar to aspirin, only it is better tolerated. Dosage: 60–240 mg salicin daily.

Complementary Supplements

Boswellia: Reduces pain and inflammation due to arthritis. Dosage: 400–600 mg of a product that contains 40–60 percent boswellic acid three times daily.

California poppy: Preliminary research suggests it can reduce pain and improve sleep in those with both acute and chronic pain. Dosage: 2–3 g at bedtime. Look for a product standardized to 0.5 percent isoquinoline alkaloids. It can be combined with devil's claw to reduce inflammation.

Curcumin: Reduces inflammation and pain, particularly in arthritis. Dosage: 300–400 mg three times daily.

Enzymes: Bromelain, chymotrypsin, papain, and trypsin are proteolytic enzymes that have been shown in some studies to help reduce inflammation and pain caused by trauma, surgery, sports injuries, and arthritis. Follow product directions.

S-adenosylmethionine (SAMe): Reduces inflammation and pain and improves joint mobility in those with arthritis and degenerative joint disease. Some studies have even shown SAMe to be as effective as anti-inflammatory drugs. Dosage: 400–1,200 mg daily.

FINAL THOUGHTS

When dealing with back pain, remember the following:

- For acute injuries, apply cold and then heat, and do light exercises.
- To prevent injuries, exercise to increase strength and flexibility, use proper lifting techniques, and use proper form for sitting and standing.
- Acupuncture, chiropractic, and massage can help relieve back pain.
- For pain relief, use a cream containing 0.025 to 0.075 percent capsaicin and apply three times daily.
- Supplements of devil's claw, fish oils, and white willow offer benefits for reducing pain and inflammation. Boswellia, curcumin, enzymes, and SAMe may also offer benefits.

BAD BREATH (HALITOSIS)

Bad breath, known medically as halitosis, is a common condition that affects over 50 percent of the population. While it can be embarrassing and annoying, bad breath is not just a cosmetic problem—it can signify an underlying health problem.

Approximately 90 percent of cases of bad breath originate from problems in the mouth. Poor oral hygiene (not brushing or flossing regularly or properly) allows bacteria to grow and feed on food particles in the mouth. Bacteria emit sulphur gases, which not only cause bad breath but also damage the tissues in the mouth, leading to inflammation of the gums (periodontitis). If left untreated, the bacteria continue to grow and cause gum recession, tooth decay, and even worse-smelling breath. The treatment of bad breath depends on the underlying cause. In most cases, dietary, lifestyle and supplementary approaches can help the situation.

FRESH BREATH THROUGH THE AGES

The ancient Greeks chewed tree resin and the Mayans chewed chicle (sap from the sapodilla tree) to keep their breath fresh. Early American settlers made chewing gum from spruce sap and beeswax. In 1848, John B. Curtis made and sold the first commercial chewing gum, called the State of Maine Pure Spruce Gum.

SIGNS & SYMPTOMS

- Unpleasant odour in the mouth and breath
- Unpleasant taste in the mouth

RISK FACTORS

- Constipation
- Diabetes (fruity odour in breath caused by ketoacidosis)
- Diet (garlic, onions, fish)
- Dieting and fasting
- Dry mouth (due to medications, radiation therapy, sleeping with your mouth open)
- Gum disease
- Infection in the mouth, throat, sinuses, or lungs
- Kidney or liver disease
- Poor oral hygiene (food caught between teeth)
- Smoking
- Tooth decay

MORNING BREATH

We all have it, but did you know that this occurs because saliva flow is decreased when we sleep? Sleeping with your mouth open also causes dry mouth. Good saliva flow is important because the oxygen in saliva kills bacteria.

DOCTOR'S ORDERS

For bad breath caused by problems in the mouth, your dentist will advise you to improve oral hygiene: Brush at least twice daily, floss daily or use an interdental cleaner to remove food between teeth, and have regular checkups. When brushing, don't forget to brush your tongue, as it can trap large amounts of bacteria.

If the cause of bad breath is a lung, throat, or mouth infection, an antibiotic may be prescribed. If it is due to constipation or poor digestion, which can lead to the release of toxins into the breath, a laxative or fibre supplement may be recommended.

SHERRY'S NATURAL PRESCRIPTION

Dietary Recommendations

Foods to include:

- Fruits, vegetables, and whole grains are high in fibre, which aids digestive function and prevents constipation.

- Adding parsley to your foods or chewing on parsley after a meal is a natural way to deodorize your breath. Parsley contains chlorophyll, which neutralizes odour. Chlorophyll is also found in green vegetables, alfalfa, and watercress.

- Chewing on fennel seeds after a meal can aid digestion and reduce bacteria in the mouth.

- Vitamin C is important for oral health; the best food sources are citrus, peppers, berries, spinach, cabbage, kale, and broccoli.

- Cranberries and cranberry juice contain powerful antioxidants that reduce bacterial adhesion to the gums. Choose low-sugar juice.

Foods to avoid:

- Foods that move slowly through your digestive tract are more likely to cause constipation and bad breath, such as red meat, fried foods, and processed foods.

- Sulphur compounds found in meat, eggs, and dairy products interact with bacteria in your mouth, causing bad breath.

- Coffee and alcohol cause dry mouth and allow odour-causing bacteria to thrive.

- Foods high in sugar (candy, soft drinks, baked goods) promote tooth decay.

Note: Garlic, onions, and spicy food are commonly blamed for bad breath. However, food is only a temporary cause of the problem. The food we eat is digested and absorbed into the bloodstream. The pungent compounds in some foods like onions and garlic can cause odours to be transferred to the lungs and expelled by our breath. This continues until the food is eliminated.

Lifestyle Suggestions

• Brush your teeth after meals to remove food particles, especially after drinking coffee or eating sulphur-containing foods such as milk products, fish, eggs, and meat. Be sure to brush your tongue or use a tongue scraper to remove bacteria from the surface of the tongue. Change your toothbrush every three to four months.

• Antibacterial mouthwash and toothpaste can help reduce bacteria in the mouth and on the teeth. Research shows that those containing cetylpyridinium chloride and those with chlorhexidine can prevent production of odours that cause bad breath. Zinc chloride has also been found to reduce odorous sulphur compounds in the mouth, and some research has shown it can lessen halitosis. Zinc can be found in some toothpastes and mouthwashes. Other natural mouthwashes contain ingredients like tea tree or eucalyptus oil, which have antibacterial and antiseptic properties. Avoid products containing alcohol as it can dry out your mouth.

• If you wear removable dentures, take them out at night and clean them thoroughly before replacing the next morning.

• Drink lots of water to prevent dry mouth and flush food particles out of your teeth and mouth.

• Quit smoking—tobacco is a major cause of bad breath, teeth stains, and gum disease. It also negatively affects the taste of food and irritates the gums.

• Chewing gums and mints with xylitol help reduce bacteria and prevent dry mouth by stimulating saliva. Make sure there is no added sugar in the gum. Look for CulturedCare Probitoic Gum, which contains the probiotic BLIS K12 that has been shown in research to control the bacteria that causes bad breath.

• Peppermint tea, mints, and gum also help to freshen breath, stimulate flow of saliva, and reduce bacteria in the mouth after meals.

Top Recommended Supplements

Chlorophyll: A component of green plants, chlorophyll helps neutralize odour. Dosage: 1 tsp of liquid or one to two capsules after meals.

Coenzyme Q10: A deficiency of coenzyme Q10, an antioxidant that is important for gum health, has been linked to gum disease, and studies have found that supplements can help promote healing of the gums and improve oral health. Dosage: 50–200 mg daily.

Probiotics: Friendly bacteria that help to reduce the formation of bad bacteria that cause bad breath. Look for probiotic lozenges; use as directed.

Complementary Supplement

Vitamin C: Essential for healthy gums and teeth; levels may be deficient in those with gum disease and in smokers. Dosage: 250–500 mg daily.

FINAL THOUGHTS

To prevent bad breath and maintain good oral hygiene:

• Brush and floss daily and have regular dental visits.
• Use mouthwash and toothpastes containing zinc, tea tree oil, or eucalyptus.
• Drink lots of water and eat parsley and cranberry.
• Don't smoke.
• Chew gum with xylitol or peppermint and take supplements of chlorophyll, coenzyme Q10, and probiotics for gum health.

BLADDER INFECTION

Bladder infections, also known as urinary tract infections (UTIs), are a common problem, especially among women. In fact, they are the second most common infection in women and the most common complication of pregnancy. Men can get them too, although this is rare.

Normally the urine is sterile and does not contain any bacteria, viruses, or fungi. However, an infection can develop when these bugs enter the urethra (the tube that carries urine out of the body) and travel up into the bladder. This leads to inflammation of the bladder (cystitis) and unpleasant urinary symptoms. Over 90 percent of UTIs are caused by *Escherichia coli* (*E. coli*), a bacteria present in high amounts in the colon and rectal area.

If a bladder infection is not treated properly, it can spread to the kidneys and become very serious. Some people get recurrent bladder infections. This is often due to a structural abnormality in the urethra or bladder affecting the flow of urine.

SIGNS & SYMPTOMS

- Blood in the urine
- Cloudy or strong-smelling urine
- Low-grade fever
- Frequent urge to urinate
- Pain and burning upon urination
- Discomfort in the pelvic area, abdomen, or lower back
- Passing small amounts of urine

Note: Back pain, fever, chills, nausea, and vomiting are possible signs that the infection has spread to the kidneys. Seek immediate medical attention.

RISK FACTORS

UTIs are much more common in women because of the following:

- Anatomy: The female urethra is shorter and closer to the rectal area, making it easier for bacteria to enter during sex or after elimination.
- Pregnancy: The growing baby presses on the bladder, preventing it from completely emptying. When urine is left to stagnate in the bladder, the risk of developing infection increases.
- Menopause: A decline in estrogen leads to thinning of the urinary tract, making it easier for bacteria to enter.
- Other risk factors include
  - Dehydration: The urine becomes more concentrated.
  - Catheter use: Insertion and removal can allow bacteria to enter.

- Enlargement of the prostate gland in men: Puts pressure on the urethra and prevents the bladder from completely emptying.

- Weak immune system: Conditions such as diabetes, AIDS, cancer, and stress can weaken the immune system, affecting its ability to fight off infection.

DOCTOR'S ORDERS

Treatment of a bladder infection often requires antibiotics, such as Bactrim or Noroxin. Antibiotics are sometimes given preventatively to those who suffer frequent, recurrent UTIs. While often necessary, there are various drawbacks to the use of antibiotics, including side effects such as diarrhea, stomach upset, and yeast overgrowth. Overuse of antibiotics causes resistance—the bugs become stronger than the drugs, leaving people vulnerable to attack by bacteria. Antibiotic therapy can also be expensive. Therefore, these drugs should be used only when absolutely necessary. Cranberry (discussed below) has emerged as an effective preventative for those at risk of recurrent infections, without the side effects and risks associated with antibiotics.

To relieve the pain and burning, a drug called phenazopyridine (Pyridium) may be prescribed. This is given for two to three days; it contains a dye and will cause discoloration of the urine and feces.

SHERRY'S NATURAL PRESCRIPTION

For those at risk of bladder infections, or those who suffer recurrent infections, preventative measures, including lifestyle changes and supplements, can be very helpful.

Dietary Recommendations

Foods to include:

- Drink eight or more glasses of water daily to help flush bacteria out of your bladder. Eat foods high in water such as watermelon and celery.

- Cranberry juice contains antioxidants called condensed tannins or proanthocyanidins, which prevent bacteria from adhering to the bladder walls. Many studies have shown that cranberry juice prevents bladder infections. Pure cranberry juice is best, but it is quite tart. You can sweeten it with stevia, which is a natural, low-calorie, plant-based sweetener. Juice cocktails are an alternative that offer better taste and tolerability, but contain less juice and have added sugar. Drink three 8-ounce glasses daily.

- Blueberries contain the same beneficial antioxidants as cranberries and may offer bladder benefits.

- Garlic strengthens the immune system response and helps fight infection.

- Pineapple contains the enzyme bromelain, which may enhance the action of antibiotics used to fight bladder infections.

- Yogurt with active cultures promotes good immune health and may play a role in UTI prevention. It also helps restore microflora balance and reduces the risk of diarrhea, upset stomach, and yeast infections when taking antibiotics for a UTI.

Foods to avoid:

• Caffeine has diuretic properties, which promote fluid loss, making the urine more concentrated. Minimize or avoid consumption of coffee, soda pop, and caffeinated beverages.

• Alcohol is dehydrating and reduces immune function.

• Refined sugar and flour may hamper immune function.

• Spicy foods may aggravate symptoms.

Lifestyle Suggestions

• Drink at least eight glasses of water daily or more if you are exercising or spending time in the sun. Dehydration concentrates the urine and increases the risk of infection.

• Urinate regularly as you feel the need. Holding in urine concentrates bacteria.

• Ladies, after going to the bathroom, wipe from front to back to prevent bacteria around the rectum from entering the urethra. Don't use feminine deodorant sprays in the genital area.

• Cleanse your genital area before and after sex and keep the genital area dry. Wear cotton underwear, which allow the skin to breathe; change clothing promptly after swimming.

• Support immune function by exercising regularly, getting adequate sleep, and minimizing stress.

• Consider acupuncture. Some evidence suggests that acupuncture can help prevent infections in women who suffer from recurrent UTIs.

Top Recommended Supplements

Cran-Max: Studies show that it prevents bladder infections by preventing bacterial adhesion to the bladder wall. Dosage: 500 mg daily for prevention.

Complementary Supplements

Probiotics: Support immune function, help fight off infections, and are essential for those on antibiotics because they restore the friendly bacteria destroyed by antibiotics. They can be used orally or vaginally for prevention. Dosage: One to three capsules daily.

Vitamin C: Acidifies urine, making it more difficult for bacteria to grow; inhibits the growth of *E. coli*; supports the immune system. Preliminary evidence found it helpful in preventing UTI in pregnant women. Dosage: 100–500 mg daily.

FINAL THOUGHTS

A bladder infection is an uncomfortable problem that requires immediate treatment. To prevent a bladder infection:

• Drink plenty of water and void regularly.
• Eat cranberries, blueberries, and their juices.
• Keep the genital area clean and dry.
• Get regular exercise and adequate sleep.
• For prevention, consider Cran-Max, probiotics, or vitamin C.

BRONCHITIS

Bronchitis occurs when the lining of the bronchial tubes (airways that lead to the lungs) become infected and inflamed. Acute bronchitis most commonly occurs following a respiratory infection. In fact, about 95 percent of cases are caused by a viral infection, such as influenza, parainfluenza, or the common cold virus. It can also develop due to exposure to cigarette smoke or pollution, or in those who have gastroesophageal reflux disease caused by backflow of acids into the lungs. Acute bronchitis caused by a viral infection often clears up on its own in a week or two without lasting effects.

Long-term exposure to lung irritants (particularly cigarette smoke) can lead to continual inflammation and thickening of the lining of your bronchial tubes, which is called chronic bronchitis. People with chronic bronchitis have a persistent productive cough and shortness of breath. It is an ongoing, serious disease that typically worsens over time. One of the best ways to improve this condition is to quit smoking.

If you have a cold or flu and symptoms persist beyond a few weeks, consult with your doctor.

SIGNS & SYMPTOMS

Acute bronchitis:

- Chest and sinus congestion (due to respiratory tract infection)

- Cough with yellowish-grey or green phlegm

- Fatigue

- Shortness of breath

- Sore throat

Chronic bronchitis:

- Chronic shortness of breath

- Continual need to clear your throat

- Persistent coughing: You're generally considered to have chronic bronchitis if you cough most days for at least three months a year in two consecutive years.

- Wheezing

If left untreated, bronchitis can lead to pneumonia in those at risk (the elderly, smokers, and those with respiratory disease such as asthma). Those with chronic bronchitis who smoke are at increased risk of lung cancer above and beyond the normal risk that a smoker faces.

RISK FACTORS

- Compromised immune function (the elderly, infants, and young children)

- Gastroesophageal reflux disease: Stomach acids that persistently back up into your esophagus may cause a chronic cough and bronchial irritation

- Pollution and occupational exposure to chemicals that irritate the lungs, such as fumes from ammonia, strong acids, chlorine, hydrogen sulphide, sulphur dioxide, or bromine

- Smokers and those in contact with second-hand smoke

DOCTOR'S ORDERS

If you have acute bronchitis, your doctor will advise you to rest, drink fluids, and allow your body to recover. Since most cases of acute bronchitis are caused by a viral infection, antibiotics offer little benefit unless your doctor suspects a bacterial infection or you are at risk of this. Taking an antibiotic when not necessary can lead to resistance and secondary infections, such as thrush, yeast, and urinary tract infections, so it is important to ask your doctor if antibiotics are necessary if one is prescribed.

Cough suppressants are not recommended because coughing helps the lungs remove irritants. However, if your cough disrupts your sleep, then you may want to take a cough medicine at bedtime. Over-the-counter options include the cough suppressants dextromethorphan (DM) and codeine (low dose available without a prescription but kept behind the pharmacy counter), and guaifenesin (an expectorant that helps thin the mucus).

For severe cases of bronchitis, your doctor may prescribe an inhaler to reduce inflammation and help you breathe.

HOMEOPATHIC RECOMMENDATIONS

Causticum: A deep, hard, racking cough and a feeling of chest congestion can indicate a need for this remedy.

Pulsatilla: If you are experiencing a sensation as if a weight is on your chest, you may respond to this remedy. Other symptoms include a cough that tends to be dry and tight at night but loose in the morning, bringing up thick yellow mucus.

SHERRY'S NATURAL PRESCRIPTION

Dietary Recommendations

Foods to include:

- Drink lots of fluids (water, juice, and tea). Herbal teas, such as Throat Coat, which contains marshmallow and licorice, can help relieve sore throat. There is some evidence that chicken soup can help reduce symptoms of congestion and sore throat and speed healing.

- Essential fatty acids—which are found in fish, flaxseed, and olive oil—may help reduce inflammation.

- Fruits and vegetables are rich in antioxidants and nutrients that can help support immune function and reduce free radical damage. Studies have shown that increasing fruit and vegetable consumption may reduce the risk of developing bronchitis.

- Honey can help soothe a sore throat and ease cough. Buckwheat honey (dark amber colour) has been studied and found to be comparable to DM cough syrup.

- If you take antibiotics, increase your consumption of yogurt and cultured dairy products (kefir), which contain beneficial probiotics (friendly bacteria).

- Onions, garlic, and ginger have anti-inflammatory properties and immune benefits.

••

RESEARCH HIGHLIGHT

Eat your fruit and fish. Researchers at Harvard did a study of 2,112 teenagers and found an association between good lung function and levels of dietary intake of fruit and fish rich in omega-3 fatty acids. Teens who ate less of these foods (two servings of fruit per week and less than 22 mg of omega-3 fatty acids per day) had higher rates of asthma, wheezing, and symptoms of chronic bronchitis such as cough and phlegm. (*Chest,* 2007, 132: 238–245)

••

Foods to avoid:
- Cow's milk allergy has been linked to bronchitis in children. Dairy products may increase mucus formation in those with a sensitivity.

- Sugar can hamper immune function. Avoid adding sugar to foods and minimize high-sugar foods (candy, soft drinks, and sweets).

Lifestyle Suggestions
- To prevent contracting or spreading a virus, avoid rubbing your eyes, nose, or mouth and wash your hands frequently.

- Get plenty of rest to allow your body to recover from the infection.

- Avoid smoking and exposure to second-hand smoke. Tobacco is damaging to the lungs and increases your risk of chronic bronchitis and emphysema.

- For a sore throat, gargle with warm salt water and try lozenges that contain one or more of the following ingredients: slippery elm, marshmallow, vitamin C, zinc, eucalyptus, or menthol.

- For dry nose, try a nasal lubricant, such as Secaris, or a saline nasal spray.

- Use an air purifier and humidifier (vaporizer) in your room. Air purifiers remove bacteria, viruses, and dust from the air, cleaning the air you breathe. A humidifier adds moisture to the air, and warm, moist air helps relieve coughs and loosens mucus in your airways. But be sure to clean the humidifier according to the manufacturer's recommendations to avoid the growth of bacteria and fungi in the water container. Research shows that adding a mixture of essential oils of cineole from eucalyptus, d-limonene from citrus fruit, and alpha-pinene pine to your vaporizer can help to clear congestion and improve breathing.

- Massage therapy to the back and chest can help break up phlegm.

Top Recommended Supplements
Echinacea: Helps support immune function, and studies show that it can reduce the severity and duration of cold symptoms. It may also help prevent a cold from developing

into bronchitis. Look for echinacea purpurea. Dosage: 300–600 mg capsules twice daily or 2–4 mL tincture four to six times daily at the first sign of a cold for seven to ten days. Some products combine echinacea with astragalus, which also has antiviral and antibacterial properties.

N-acetylcysteine (NAC): An amino acid derivative with antioxidant properties that helps break up mucus and reduce cough. Numerous clinical trials have found it beneficial for reducing symptoms in both acute and chronic bronchitis. Dosage: 300–600 mg once or twice daily.

North American ginseng: Helps to prevent colds and flu and lessen symptoms, so it may help reduce these respiratory infections from leading to bronchitis. Look for COLD-FX, a patented extract of polysaccharides derived from North American ginseng that has been clinically studied. Dosage: 200–300 mg twice daily.

Complementary Supplements

Aged garlic extract: Contains antioxidant compounds that help support immune function. When taken regularly, it may help prevent colds and flu that lead to bronchial infections. Dosage: 600 mg daily.

Fish oils: Contain essential fatty acids that help reduce inflammation. One study in children found that daily fish oil supplements reduced the risk of recurrent respiratory tract infections. Dosage: Children should take 15 mg EPA plus DHA per pound of body weight per day; adults should take 1–3 g EPA plus DHA daily.

Vitamin C: Supports immune function, helps prevent oxidative damage to the lungs, and may help speed recovery. Studies have shown that it can reduce the severity and duration of the common cold, which may reduce the likelihood of complications like bronchitis. Dosage: 200–1,000 mg daily.

Vitamin E: An antioxidant that helps prevent oxidative damage to the lungs caused by environmental pollution and cigarette smoke exposure. Dosage: 400 IU daily.

FINAL THOUGHTS

To improve healing of bronchitis and prevent it from occurring, consider the following:

- Eat more fruits, vegetables, fish, onions, garlic, and ginger.
- Drink lots of fluids, especially water and herbal teas.
- Avoid smoking and being around smoke and other irritants.
- Use an air purifier and humidifier in your home.
- Consider supplements of echinacea, NAC, and North American ginseng (COLD-FX).

BURNS

Whether they are the result of sunburn or a scalding pan, skin burns can be frightening and painful. They also may lead to serious complications, so proper treatment is critical.

Your skin is made up of three layers—the epidermis (outer layer of the skin), the dermis (under the epidermis, containing blood vessels, hair follicles, and connective tissue), and the subcutis (the final layer of skin containing adipose tissue and storage of nutrients). The skin provides a first line of defence against all forms of external toxins and bacteria, but this protective barrier may be burned at temperatures higher than 120°F (49°C). Skin burns occur from exposure to extreme heat such as the sun, fire, boiling water, hot beverages, cooking heat, steam, and hot objects such as an iron. Other causes of burns include chemicals, electricity, lightning, or radioactive material.

Depending on the cause and length of exposure, burns can range from mild to severe and can potentially be fatal. Burns are classified according to their degree of severity and the amount of skin affected:

- **First-degree burns** damage the epidermis. These burns may be painful, but can usually be self-treated. They heal quickly and rarely cause scars.
- **Second-degree burns** damage the epidermis and dermis, and can cause acute pain, blisters, and scarring. Depending on the extent of the burn and subsequent tissue damage, second-degree burns may be self-treated, but must be diligently watched and treated to avoid infection.
- **Third-degree burns** severely damage the epidermis, dermis, and subcutis. They may affect muscles, bones, nerves, and blood vessels, requiring extensive treatment, skin grafts, and therapy. Because of the risk of shock and infection, third-degree burns are always considered a life-threatening medical emergency.

There are a variety of lifestyle recommendations and also natural products that can help relieve the pain and promote skin healing for first-degree and minor second-degree burns. Third-degree burns need to be managed by your doctor to reduce the risk of infection and serious complications.

SIGNS & SYMPTOMS

- First-degree burns: Mild pain where contact occurred for 24 to 48 hours, inflammation, redness, soreness
- Second-degree burns: Lingering pain, inflammation, redness, and blistering
- Third-degree burns: Skin may become white, brown, red, or black and quite swollen; unlike first- or second-degree burns, damage to the subcutis may mean there is no immediate pain; other symptoms include shock, dizziness, nausea, vomiting, fever, cold, and stiffness.
- Some burns may not leave visibly physical symptoms: Exposure to smoke may burn the lungs; electrical burns may cause more internal than external damage. These are also considered medical emergencies because the extent of the damage is unseen by the naked eye and must be assessed.

- Age: Children and the elderly have thinner skin, putting them at higher risk of burns.
- Chemicals, electrical wiring, lightning
- Lifestyle: Certain high-risk jobs or habits (such as drug or alcohol consumption)
- Most burns are caused by accidents in the home: boiling water, hot objects, hot oil
- Sun exposure or tanning beds

DOCTOR'S ORDERS

You should call a doctor if your burn is larger than the size of your palm or if it is painful; if your burn is on your face, hands, or genitals; if you have symptoms of infection, including fever, vomiting, chills, swelling, and stiffness; or if your burn is not healing. Third-degree burns always demand immediate medical attention.

The goals of burn treatment are to speed wound healing, prevent infection and scars, relieve pain, and restore the patient to normal health. As such, doctors may employ a variety of antimicrobial and antibiotic agents, as well as pain relievers and dressings to achieve these goals. For extensive burns, extensive treatment is needed, which may include lengthy hospital stays to ensure that infection does not occur, and outpatient appointments for therapy.

HOMEOPATHIC RECOMMENDATIONS

Apis mellifica: This remedy relieves minor burns that present superficially and is indicated for pink, swollen skin with itching, burning pain.

Cantharis: This remedy effectively relieves more moderate injury such as blisters from burns or friction.

Urtica urens: When a burn is mild and the primary symptoms are redness and stinging pain, this remedy often brings relief. It can be useful for sunburn when the pain is still prickly and stinging.

SHERRY'S NATURAL PRESCRIPTION

For minor burns, there are natural ways to promote and support wound healing.

Dietary Recommendations

A healthy diet is critical for effective burn treatment to replace vital nutrients, promote wound healing, and reduce the risk of infection and scars.

Foods to include:

- Drink plenty of water and electrolyte drinks to replace lost fluids. Caffeine-free herbal teas are also fine.

- Eat brightly coloured fruits and vegetables for vitamins A, C, and E and other bioflavonoids, which promote skin healing and reduce inflammation.

- Ensure adequate protein intake to aid in skin repair. Eat lean poultry, fish, beans, nuts, and seeds.

- Essential fatty acids, which are found in fish, chia seed, and flaxseed, help reduce inflammation.

Note: Those with severe burns need to increase total caloric intake because as the body tries to repair itself, it burns calories at a faster rate.

Foods to avoid:

- Salty foods promote dehydration. Minimize eating chips, snack foods, deli meats, and other high-salt foods.

- Saturated fat can worsen inflammation and depress the body's immune system, delaying recovery.

- Sugar impairs immune function and slows skin and tissue regeneration. Minimize sweets, soft drinks, candy, and other high-sugar foods.

Lifestyle Suggestions

To prevent the risk of burns:

- Wear sunscreen every day with a minimum of SPF 15; wear wide-brimmed hats to shield your face.

- Be mindful at all times about burn hazards in the home and your environment.

- Reduce the hot-water tank temperature to 120°F (49°C).

- Turn the handles of cooking pots and pans inward to avoid bumping.

- Get an automatic shut-off iron; unplug curling irons when not in use.

- Teach your children burn safety and first-aid treatment.

- Keep a first-aid and burn kit in your home that contains fresh gauze and antibacterial agents.

- Follow all precautions for electrical equipment.

To manage a minor burn:

- Gently cool and clean the area with cold water or cold wet compresses for at least 15 minutes. Do not apply ice because this can further damage the skin.

- Cool compresses soaked in chamomile tea can help promote healing.

- Apply a topical anaesthetic cream, such as Polysporin Burn Cream or Calendula. Honey can also promote healing and reduce infection. Do not cover with butter or any type of petroleum-based cream because they retain heat, slow healing, and increase risk of infection.

- Cover with a dry, sterile dressing. Do not wrap tightly.

- Do not break blisters or pick skin. Blisters keep infections out of the wound.

- Cleanse the wound daily with antiseptic solution or gauze soaked in green tea and change the dressing.

- Avoid exposing the burned area to the sun or hot water until it has healed.

Top Recommended Treatments

Antioxidants: Studies have shown that oral supplements of vitamins A, C, E, zinc, and selenium can help protect the skin from sunburn due to free radical–producing ultraviolet rays. These vitamins also help promote skin healing after a burn. Topical vitamin C and E, when used along with sunscreen, has also been shown to reduce sunburn. Preliminary research on a patented tomato lycopene complex called Lyc-O-Mato has shown it can reduce the risk of UV damage when skin is exposed to sun.

Honey: Honey is hygroscopic (attracts and absorbs moisture), which has proven helpful in the treatment of wounds and first-degree burns because it retains the plasma released by a wound allowing for reabsorption. Studies show that raw honey and gauze applied to a burn can speed healing and reduce risk of infection. Consult with your health care provider prior to use.

Complementary Treatments

Aloe vera gel: Cooling, helps relieve pain and inflammation, and also has anti-inflammatory properties. It is commonly used to manage burns and has a long history of use to promote wound healing, although the scientific research is lacking. Use aloe vera from a plant (split open a leaf) or get pure aloe gel at a health food store or pharmacy. Dosage: Apply two or three times daily.

Calendula cream: Soothing, has anti-inflammatory properties, and may help promote tissue repair. Dosage: Apply three times per day.

Ornithine alpha-ketoglutarate (OKG): Manufactured from two amino acids, ornithine and glutamine, it is used to stimulate the body to build muscle and tissue. Studies have shown that it can speed recovery. It is not widely available, so check specialty health food stores or practitioner offices. Dosage: 5–25 g (as a powder) daily as directed.

FINAL THOUGHTS

Here are some important points to keep in mind for treatment of minor burns:

- For minor (first-degree and small second-degree) burns, cool skin in cold water then seek medical attention.
- Raw honey can speed healing of minor burns and reduce the risk of infection.
- Antioxidants can help protect against sunburn and help promote wound healing after a burn.
- Eat a healthy diet with lots of fresh fruits and vegetables, whole grains, and fish. Increase calorie intake during the healing process and drink lots of liquids.
- Consider OKG supplements to speed healing.

CANCER

Cancer is one of the most feared diseases, and rightfully so—it is the leading cause of death worldwide. In Canada, about 24 percent of women and 29 percent of men will die from cancer. Cancer has become an age-related phenomenon: 42 percent of new cancer cases and 59 percent of cancer deaths will occur among those who are at least 70 years old. However, aging does not cause cancer. Rather, in many cases it is generally thought that our lifetime exposure to factors that increase our risk, such as smoking or eating a poor diet, leads to the development of cancer. And as we age our cellular repair mechanisms tend to be less effective.

Cancer is the uncontrolled growth of abnormal cells in our body. Our bodies are made up of millions of cells grouped together to form tissues such as muscles, skin, bones, and organs. Cancer occurs when there is an abnormal growth of cells, which can form lumps or tumours or can spread through the bloodstream and lymphatic system to other parts of the body. Tumours can be either benign (non-cancerous) or malignant (cancerous). Benign tumour cells stay in one place in the body and are not usually life-threatening.

Malignant tumour cells are able to spread to nearby tissues and invade other parts of the body, which is a process called metastasis. When a malignant tumour spreads, it often causes swelling of nearby lymph nodes. Finding cancer early and getting treatment before it spreads can greatly help improve your chances of survival.

While we think of cancer as one disease, it is actually a group of more than 100 different diseases. It can involve any tissue of the body and have many different forms in each body area. Most cancers are named for the type of cell or organ in which they start. For example, if it starts in the liver it is called liver cancer. The four most common types of cancer in Canada are breast, prostate, lung, and colon.

A great deal of research has focused on the underlying causes of abnormal cell growth. We do know that certain factors, such as free radical damage, genetics, diet, and lifestyle, are involved. While many of us may blame our family history, only about 5 to 10 percent of cancers are attributed to faulty genes. Having a family history may increase your risk of certain cancers, but researchers feel that whether or not those genes are "switched on" may depend largely on lifestyle and environment. These critical yet often overlooked factors play a role not only in prevention but also in the treatment and recovery from cancer.

STARTLING CANCER STATISTICS

According to the Canadian Cancer Society, an estimated 177,800 new cases of cancer and 75,000 cancer deaths occurred in Canada in 2011. Based on current incidence rates, 40 percent of Canadian women and 45 percent of Canadian men will develop cancer during their lifetimes.

Cancer is a very broad subject and it is beyond the scope of this chapter to discuss each type and make individualized recommendations. The goal here is to provide you with information on known risk factors for the most common forms of cancer, how to reduce your risk of getting cancer, and how to improve your chances of survival if you have cancer. If you have been diagnosed with cancer, it is critical that you consult with your health care provider to create an individualized program. In many cases, dietary and lifestyle strategies and supplements can be taken along with your other treatments. Certain supplements, however, could interact with chemotherapy or other medical treatments, so it is important to work with your health care provider.

SIGNS & SYMPTOMS

Cancer does not happen overnight. It may take months or years before there are any signs or symptoms, and these symptoms can vary greatly depending on the location of the cancer. Here are some key things to look for:

- A lump or area of swelling under the skin, or bloating in the pelvic area

- A mole that is asymmetrical, has an irregular border, is dark in colour, or grows in size or thickness

- Change in bowel or bladder habits

- Difficulty swallowing, upset stomach, nausea, or vomiting

- Persistent cough, hoarseness, or a cough that brings up blood

- Persistent low-grade fever

- Rectal bleeding or blood in the urine or stool

- Recurrent infections or wounds that do not heal

- Unexplained pain, especially in the bones, breasts, or pelvic area

- Unexplained vaginal discharge or bleeding

- Unexplained weight loss and loss of appetite

- Unusual fatigue, headaches

RISK FACTORS

- According to the World Health Organization, about 30 percent of cancer deaths are due to five leading behavioural and dietary risks: high body mass index, low fruit and vegetable intake, lack of physical activity, tobacco use, and alcohol use.

- Becoming sexually active at a young age or having multiple partners increases the risk of cervical cancer.

- Exposure to environmental toxins such as tobacco, pollution, dioxins, asbestos, heavy metals (arsenic, lead, nickel), and radiation (X-rays), and handling of petroleum products. Smoking is responsible for 22 percent of all cancer deaths. Chlorinated drinking water increases the risk of bladder cancer. Some substances used in pesticides are classified as known, probable, or possible carcinogens.

- Excessive sun exposure or sunburn during childhood increases the risk of skin cancer.

- Genetics: Family history of cancer increases risk.

- Heavy alcohol consumption increases risk.

- High insulin levels (hyperinsulinemia) and insulin resistance increase risk.

- High intake of saturated fat, trans fats, and high-glycemic foods (refined starches and sugar); low intake of fibre; consumption of pesticides or food additives; and nutritional deficiencies (lack of antioxidants) increase risk.

- Lack of exercise increases your risk of several types of cancer.

- Obesity increases risk of breast, endometrial, cervical, ovarian, and gallbladder cancer for women and colon and prostate cancer for men.

- Poor liver function can increase risk. The liver plays a key role in removing toxins.

- Stress hampers immune function and may increase the risk of cancer (particularly breast cancer). Stress may also worsen recovery in those with cancer.

- Use of the hormones estrogen and progestin (HRT) increase the risk of breast cancer; risk is greatest with higher dosages for long periods of time (longer than five years).

- Weakened immune function, exposure to viruses (hepatitis, HPV), and fungal infections increase risk.

Exposure to many different risk factors may increase a person's risk more than the risk associated with each individual toxin or chemical alone, so it is important to avoid as many known risk factors as possible. As you see from this list, many of the known risk factors are within our control.

DOCTOR'S ORDERS

The treatment of cancer depends on the location, stage of cancer, your existing health status, and many other factors. Today there are numerous options for medical treatment including chemotherapy, radiation, surgery, and hormone therapy.

There are a variety of important screening tests that can help in the early detection of cancer:

- Breast self-exams, mammograms, and thermography scans
- Digital rectal exams
- Pap test (for cervical cancer) and pelvic exam
- Prostate exam and prostate specific antigen (PSA) test
- Skin exam
- Testicular exams

See your doctor yearly for a thorough health examination and blood work, and discuss any changes in your health or unexplained new symptoms.

SHERRY'S NATURAL PRESCRIPTION

Numerous studies have shown that good nutrition and various lifestyle measures can significantly reduce the risk of cancer. For those who have cancer, a good nutritional program can help prevent weight loss, aid digestion, support immune function, boost energy levels, and aid recovery. Supplements can also play an important supportive role.

Dietary Recommendations

Foods to include:

- Boost your fibre intake. Aim for 25–38 g daily of soluble and insoluble fibre. Eat 2 tbsp of chia or milled flaxseed every day to aid detoxification and elimination. Flaxseed contains lignans (plant-based compounds) that may slow the growth of prostate cancer.

- Choose free-range poultry and wild (not farmed) fish, beans, and legumes.

- Choose healthy fats such as olive oil and flaxseed oil.

- Drink green tea, which is a potent antioxidant. Studies have linked drinking green tea to a lower risk of several cancers. Green tea has also been shown to improve survival in those with cancer.

- Drink lots of purified water.

- Eat cancer-fighting foods such as broccoli, cabbage, cauliflower, Brussels sprouts, kale, tomatoes, onions, and carrots. These foods contain various compounds that have anti-cancer properties.

- Eat cancer-fighting herbs and spices like ginger, garlic, cayenne, rosemary, oregano, and curcumin.

- Eat lots of vegetables and fruit (7 to 10 servings daily). Those highest in antioxidants include berries, grapes, plums, peppers, kale, spinach, and beets. Choose organic produce as much as possible to avoid ingestion of pesticides. Foods that contain the highest amounts of pesticide residue include peaches, strawberries, apples, spinach, nectarines, celery, pears, cherries, potatoes, peppers, and raspberries. If organics are not available or are cost prohibitive, wash your produce with lots of water and scrub the skins. This will also help eliminate harmful bacteria.

- Eat small, frequent meals, which are easier on digestion and also help improve blood sugar control.

- Fermented soy products (tofu, tempeh, and miso) appear to have cancer-fighting properties. Studies have found associations between higher soy consumption and lower incidence of hormone-related cancers such as prostate, breast, and uterine cancer.

- Ginger tea may be helpful for managing nausea caused by chemotherapy.

- Yogurt and fermented dairy can aid digestion and intestinal function.

Consider doing a detoxification program, such as a juice cleanse. See Appendix C for more information.

Foods to avoid:

- Reduce intake of saturated fat to less than 10 percent of total calories by limiting red meat and choosing low-fat dairy products. Avoid trans fats (found in many processed/snack foods and fried foods) completely. Read labels carefully.

- Avoid preservatives (nitrates and sulphites) and chemical food additives.

- Deli meats (bologna, salami) and hot dogs are full of nitrates and other chemicals that are associated with cancer and poor health.

- Eating charred meat (BBQ) and well-done meat has been associated with increased risk of breast cancer because of the creation of carcinogenic compounds. Marinating meat helps prevent the formation of these carcinogens. Marinades that contain olive oil, vinegar, garlic, mustard, lemon juice, rosemary, oregano, and curcumin are ideal. Meat should be marinated for at least two hours.

- Minimize alcohol, as it is hard on liver and immune function. Heavy drinking increases the risk of cancers of the mouth, esophagus, breast, colorectal, and stomach. If you drink, limit yourself to one or two drinks daily and choose red wine as it contains antioxidants that may offer cancer-protecting properties.

- Minimize eating sugar and refined starches, which quickly raise blood sugar and insulin levels, increasing the risk of insulin resistance, which is associated with increased risk of certain cancers.

Lifestyle Suggestions

- According to the Canadian Cancer Society, 35 percent of all cancers can be prevented by being active, eating well, and maintaining a healthy body weight.

- Get regular exercise. Regular exercise is known to reduce the risk of several types of cancer and it can also improve energy and well-being in those undergoing cancer treatment. Aim for one hour of moderate-intensity activity each day, such as walking, cycling, or swimming.

- Don't smoke, and avoid second-hand smoke and highly polluted areas.

- Manage your stress. Try yoga, meditation, or breathing techniques.

- Drink purified water. Several long-term studies have found that drinking chlorinated tap water increases the risk of cancer, particularly bladder cancer.

- Do not microwave food in plastic containers; use glass or ceramic. Only store food in plastic containers designed for that purpose and cool food prior to storing in plastic containers.

- Minimize exposure to dangerous phthalates (see next page). Ask manufacturers about non-vinyl flooring alternatives, and consider other types of materials such as natural flooring and fabric shower curtains.

- Use stainless steel cookware. All non-stick cookware is made up of a chemical called PTFE (polytetrafluoroethylene). When heated to high temperatures (greater than 572°F/300°C), they can create fumes that contain a suspected cancer-causing chemical, tetrafluoroethylene-TFE.

- Don't spray pesticides on your lawn—look into natural methods of weed control. Don't let your children or pets on lawns that have recently been sprayed with pesticides as they can inhale the fumes and absorb the chemicals through their skin. Signs are posted when lawns are sprayed.

- Massage and acupuncture may be helpful for reducing pain, anxiety, stress, and nausea associated with chemotherapy.

- Find humour in life. Laughing can help promote relaxation, improve coping, and reduce anxiety. Laughter also has a beneficial effect on the immune system and can improve your pain threshold.

- Have a positive outlook. This can help reduce fear and anxiety, and there is evidence that positive thoughts, affirmations, and beliefs can make a difference in treatment outcomes.

PHTHALATES: CANCER-CAUSING PLASTICS

Phthalates (pronounced THA-lates) are a group of chemicals often called "plasticizers," which are used in a variety of products, including polyvinyl chloride (PVC) products. Phthalates are added to PVC products to make them soft and flexible. Phthalates are associated with a number of health problems, including liver abnormalities, cancer, and fertility problems. There are many different types of phthalates. The most widely used is DEHP, which is found mostly in PVC plastics (vinyl flooring and medical plastics such as IV bags and tubes). DINP is another phthalate, which is also used in PVC plastics, including children's toys. Canadian guidelines suggest that DEHP and DINP shouldn't be used in items that are likely to be placed in children's mouths, but manufacturers aren't legally bound by these guidelines. Many suppliers of baby bottles use phthalate-free substances such as polypropylene (recycling code 5), but be sure to check with the manufacturer or use glass bottles. For nipples and pacifiers, choose those made of silicone or latex. In cosmetics, such as nail polish and perfume, DBP, DEP, and DMP are the phthalates most often used. Health Canada has set new regulations that will limit the amount of phthalates in consumer products.

Top Recommended Supplements

It is critical that you consult with a qualified natural health care practitioner for advice on supplements for cancer. There aren't any known cancer cures, but certain supplements can help improve energy and well-being, support immune function, and support the body during chemotherapy and radiation. There are also supplements that may help in the prevention and the treatment of cancer. Some of the supplements that have been researched and are generally considered safe are noted here, but this is by no means a complete list. Your health care provider will be in the best position to advise you on which supplements can benefit your particular situation.

Coriolus versicolor: A type of mushroom extract used in traditional Chinese medicine that has been shown in many studies to support immune function and enhance the effectiveness of various forms of standard cancer therapy. The two main active components are polysaccharide-K (PSK) and polysaccharopeptide (PSP), which are thought to work by stimulating the body's own cancer-fighting cells. This product may also be helpful in cancer prevention. Dosage: The typical dosage for use as an adjunct to standard cancer treatment is 2–6 g daily.

Ginseng: Both American and Korean ginseng may offer benefits for reducing fatigue, nausea, and vomiting, and improving well-being in those undergoing cancer treatment. American ginseng has been shown to reduce fatigue in those with breast, lung, colon, and other forms of cancer. It may also increase the effectiveness of treatment for breast cancer. Panax ginseng has been shown to improve energy and well-being in those with cancer. Regular use of Korean ginseng was found to lower overall cancer risk. Dosage: Varies depending on product used; follow label instructions or the advice of your health care provider.

Indole-3 carbinol: An antioxidant naturally present in cruciferous vegetables. There is some evidence that it can fight hormonally related cancers such as breast and cervical cancer in several ways: converting cancer-promoting estrogen to a safer form, blocking the effects of estrogen on cells, directly killing or inhibiting cancer cells, and reducing free radicals, which promote cancer by damaging DNA. Dosage: 300–600 mg daily.

IP6 (inositol hexaphosphate): A supplement derived from rice bran. Animal research and preliminary human studies have shown that it has significant anticancer effects. It can help in the prevention of cancer and has growth-regulating effects on various cells and tissues, including those of the colon, breast, and prostate. It may also help reduce the side effects of chemotherapy. Dosage: 4–8 g daily. Look for Inocell, a clinically studied brand of IP6.

Multivitamin/mineral complex: Ensures that your body gets essential nutrients to support immune function and overall health. Certain nutrients have cancer-protecting properties and may play a role in prevention, including calcium, folic acid, selenium, lycopene, and vitamins A, C, D, E, and K. Look for a product that provides a full range of nutrients and is free of dyes and artificial chemicals. Consider extra antioxidants, as it is difficult to obtain therapeutic dosages from a multivitamin. Antioxidant nutrients and herbs may offer benefits for those undergoing chemotherapy and radiation by improving response to the therapy and reducing its toxic effects They also play a role in cancer prevention and in inhibiting angiogenesis (tumour growth/spread). Examples include grape seed extract, quercetin, milk thistle, green tea, and ginkgo biloba. It is important to consult with your health care provider for proper dosage and guidelines.

Vitamin D: A number of studies have found a correlation between vitamin D levels and cancer. In particular, low levels have been associated with an increased risk of developing breast, colon, and prostate cancer. The amount in most multivitamins may be inadequate; most health authorities recommend adults take at least 1,000 IU daily.

Complementary Supplements

Aged garlic extract: Offers cancer-protecting and therapeutic benefits: supports immune function and detoxification and has antioxidant, anti-inflammatory, and anti-cancer properties. Dosage: 600 mg twice daily. Much higher amounts have been used in some studies.

Curcumin: Has preventive and therapeutic anticancer properties. There is also some evidence that it may stop the growth of certain cancers (breast, prostate, and colon). Dosage: As advised by a health care provider.

Fish oils: Reduce inflammation and help to reverse the weight loss associated with poor appetite. Dosage: 1–3 g daily.

Green drinks: Contain barley and wheat grass, chlorella, spirulina, and other plants that support detoxification and overall health. Follow label directions.

Melatonin: Helps improve immune function and sleep in those with cancer. There is also some evidence that it can reduce growth of cancer cells. Dosage: 3–10 mg at bedtime.

Probiotics: Replenish friendly bacteria that are depleted by treatment with chemotherapy and antibiotics. Probiotics aid digestion, support immune function and detoxification, and assist in nutrient absorption. They may also help to minimize diarrhea and upset stomach caused by chemotherapy and radiation. Dosage: 1 billion live cells twice daily.

FINAL THOUGHTS

To improve the management of cancer, consider the following:

- Eat lots of vegetables (broccoli, cabbage, tomatoes, garlic, and onions), whole grains, milled flaxseed, and yogurt. Choose free-range poultry and wild fish. Drink green tea.
- Reduce saturated fat, sugar, and alcohol. Avoid trans fats and chemical food additives.
- Get regular exercise, reduce stress, and don't smoke.
- Avoid exposure to pesticides, phthalates, and other carcinogens.
- Take a multivitamin/mineral complex and consult with your health care provider for advice on which supplements may help your individual situation.

CANKER SORES

Canker sores, known medically as aphthous ulcers, are small ulcers or lesions that develop inside the mouth, typically inside the cheeks or at the base of the gums. Canker sores are not contagious and they are not transmitted by a virus (like cold sores). Several factors contribute to the development of canker sores including mouth injuries (such as biting the inside of your cheek or wearing braces), food sensitivities, consumption of spicy or acidic foods, deficiencies of certain nutrients, infection with *Helicobacter pylori*, hormonal changes, alterations in oral bacteria, inflammatory and autoimmune diseases, and stress.

Canker sores are painful but they typically go away on their own in a week or two. Check with your doctor or dentist if you have unusually large or painful canker sores or canker sores that don't seem to heal.

SIGNS & SYMPTOMS

Canker sores appear as small round sores inside the mouth with a white or yellow centre and a red border. They are painful and there may be a tingling or burning sensation before the sore appears. More severe canker sores can be large and deep and associated with significant swelling in the tissue around the sore.

RISK FACTORS

Anyone can develop canker sores, especially when there is mouth trauma. Here are some of the other known risk factors:

• Gender: Canker sores are more common in women.

• Family history: About one-third of people with recurrent canker sores have a family history. It is thought that this association may be due to genetics or to inherited allergies, lifestyle habits, and shared environmental factors.

• Medical conditions such as celiac disease, inflammatory bowel disease, Behcet's disease (an inflammatory condition), and immune system diseases including HIV/AIDS.

• Nutrient deficiencies: People low in vitamins B1, B2, and B6, folic acid, iron, and zinc.

DOCTOR'S ORDERS

Small and minor canker sores often go away within a week or so and don't require medical treatment. Over-the-counter products that contain an anaesthetic (benzocaine) can help relieve discomfort. Examples of these products include Anbesol and Orajel.

If the sores are larger or painful or you have multiple sores, your doctor may prescribe a steroid oral gel (Kenalog or Orabase) or anti-inflammatories such as ibuprofen (Advil or Motrin) to reduce pain and inflammation. The drug cimetidine, which is typically used for stomach ulcers, may also help speed healing of canker sores.

HOMEOPATHIC RECOMMENDATIONS

Arsenicum album: Indicated when symptoms include burning, painful mouth sores, in particular when they occur following episodes of anxiety leading to fatigue.

Borax: Indicated for canker sores that occur inside the cheeks and present like small blotches of white plaque. Especially suitable for young children.

Mercurius solubilis: If you experience a bad, bitter taste in the mouth along with canker sores, this remedy may help.

Nux vomica: If canker sores break out after you overindulge in sweets, strong spicy foods, stimulants, or alcoholic beverages, then nux vomica (also known as Colubrina) is the indicated remedy. These sores are often small, and you may also present with a thick coat on your tongue.

SHERRY'S NATURAL PRESCRIPTION

There are a number of dietary, lifestyle, and supplemental approaches to managing and preventing canker sores.

Dietary Recommendations

Foods to include:

• Eat lots of fruits, vegetables, and whole grains to help prevent nutritional deficiencies.

• Garlic and onions may be particularly helpful for supporting immune system health and reducing inflammation.

• Yogurt contains beneficial bacteria that support immune health and may also help speed healing of canker sores.

Foods to avoid:

• Acidic foods such as citrus, pineapple, tomato products, soft drinks, and spicy foods can cause further irritation and pain.

• Abrasive foods such as chips, pretzels, and anything with sharp, rough edges can irritate the sores.

• Chocolate, nuts, tea, and coffee are common triggers. To determine if food allergies or intolerances are contributing to your canker sores, refer to Appendix D.

Lifestyle Suggestions

• Suck on ice to help numb the pain and reduce inflammation.

• Brush your teeth gently and use a toothpaste that reduces nerve sensitivity, such as Sensodyne.

• Rinse your mouth with warm salt water after eating.

• Make a paste with baking soda and a little bit of water and apply to the sore between meals.

• Try CulturedCare Probiotic Gum to restore beneficial bacteria in the mouth.

To prevent canker sores:

- Be gentle when brushing and flossing. Use a soft bristle brush and don't scrub hard.

- Avoid toothpastes and mouth rinses that contain sodium lauryl sulphate because this chemical can trigger canker sores.

- Don't talk while you are eating; this can increase the risk of biting the inside of your cheek.

- If you wear braces, use dental wax to put over the braces to cover the sharp edges.

- Reduce stress. Try relaxation techniques such as deep breathing, visualization, or meditation to promote calming.

Top Recommended Supplements

Aloe vera: Contains compounds (polysaccharides) that help promote skin healing by anti-inflammatory, antimicrobial, and immune-stimulating actions. There is some evidence that aloe vera gel applied directly to a canker sore can speed healing. Dosage: Apply four times daily.

Licorice: Has soothing and wound-healing properties. A mixture of powdered deglycyrrhizinated licorice (DGL) mixed with warm water has been found to shorten healing time. DGL is a type of licorice that has the glycyrrhizic acid, which is the part of the plant that can cause elevated blood pressure, removed. Dosage: Mix 200 mg powdered DGL with 200 mL warm water. Swish for two minutes and then spit out. The same benefits may also be found using chewable DGL tablets.

Multivitamin/mineral complex: A deficiency of vitamins B1, B2, and B6, folic acid, zinc, and iron have been associated with recurrent canker sores. A multivitamin/mineral complex can prevent deficiencies and ensure adequate intake. Dosage: Take daily; choose a product based on your age, gender, and health needs.

Complementary Supplements

Myrrh: The resin (oil) from this plant has a long history of use for wound healing. It has anti-inflammatory and anaesthetic properties, so it helps reduce swelling and provide relief from pain. Mix five drops of myrrh oil with 60 mL (2 ounces) warm water and swish in mouth for one to two minutes twice daily.

Probiotics: May help in the prevention of canker sores by supporting immune system health and improving levels of beneficial bacteria in mouth. Some benefits have been found with topical and oral probiotic supplements of *Lactobacillus acidophilus*. Choose a product with at least 1.5 billion active cultures and take daily.

FINAL THOUGHTS

To speed healing of canker sores, consider the following:

- Avoid acidic, spicy, and abrasive foods.
- Eat more vegetables, non-acidic fruits, and yogurt.
- Use ice to reduce pain and inflammation and try a paste of baking soda and water between meals.
- Take a daily multivitamin/mineral complex to prevent nutritional deficiencies.
- Try aloe vera gel or DGL topically to speed healing.

CARPAL TUNNEL SYNDROME

Carpal tunnel syndrome (CTS) is a condition marked by pain, inflammation, and numbness in a small opening in the wrist that protects the main nerve (the median nerve) and tendons that run from your forearm to your hand. This nerve is sensitive to pressure. Repetitive wrist movements that cause inflammation or anything that narrows the space of the carpal tunnel and puts pressure on the nerve can lead to CTS. This condition is becoming increasingly common because of the types of jobs that people do today, particularly computer work, which leads to strain and pressure on the wrist. Bone spurs and arthritis can also cause swelling of the carpal tunnel and narrowing of this space, which place pressure on the nerve.

SIGNS & SYMPTOMS

The symptoms of CTS often start gradually and worsen over time, causing

- Aching and pain in the wrist that may extend up your arm and into your palm or fingers
- Numbness and tingling in your fingers or hand, which may be temporarily relieved by shaking your hand
- Weakness in your hands

RISK FACTORS

- Rheumatoid arthritis or other inflammatory conditions that exert pressure on the median nerve
- Diabetes or other chronic conditions (alcoholism) that increase the risk of nerve damage
- Fluid retention, which is common in pregnancy, obesity, and kidney disease, may increase the pressure within the carpal tunnel, stressing the median nerve
- Gender: Women are three times more likely to develop CTS because the carpal tunnel is smaller in women
- Genetics (being born with a narrow carpal tunnel)
- Injury: Stress or force placed on the wrist area; bone spurs; wrist fracture or dislocation can reduce the size of the carpal tunnel leading to excess pressure on the nerve
- Pregnancy or hormonal changes that cause fluid retention
- Repetitive use (working on computers, machinery, an assembly line, or with power tools), particularly when done for an extended period without rest
- Smokers often have worse symptoms and slower recovery

DOCTOR'S ORDERS

Depending on the severity of the condition, there are a variety of options your doctor may recommend, such as wearing a wrist splint to provide support to the area and protect against further damage and injury. Non-steroidal anti-inflammatory drugs, like ibuprofen, may be prescribed to reduce pain and inflammation. However, these drugs can cause a range of serious side effects and are not safe for long-term use. Stronger drugs called corticosteroids may be injected into the area to reduce inflammation. Neither of these drug classes promote healing, nor are they beneficial unless CTS is caused by underlying inflammation. For more severe forms of CTS, surgery may be done to cut the ligaments pressing on the nerve. This usually results in significant improvement, but there may still be some residual numbness, pain, stiffness, or weakness.

SHERRY'S NATURAL PRESCRIPTION

Dietary Recommendations

Foods to include:

- Beans, brewer's yeast, bananas, egg yolks, walnuts, and whole grains (wheat germ) contain vitamin B6, which is important for nerve function.

- Fish contains omega-3 fatty acids, which have anti-inflammatory properties. Fish also provides some vitamin B6. Vegetarian sources of omega-3s include chia seed and flaxseed.

- Vegetables and fruits contain vital antioxidants and nutrients that can help reduce inflammation and speed healing.

Foods to avoid:

- Minimize salt (processed foods and your salt shaker) as it can cause fluid retention, which can worsen CTS.

- Saturated fat can impair circulation.

Lifestyle Suggestions

- Give your hands and wrists a break. When working on your computer or doing repetitive movements, take a break every 20 minutes and do some gentle stretches. Alternate tasks to reduce the amount of repetitive movements and try to modify your activities as much as possible.

- Wear a wrist splint for support, especially when lifting or doing repetitive movements.

- Use proper form. For example, your keyboard should be at elbow height or slightly lower. Incorrect posture can cause strain on the neck and shoulders, which can worsen CTS. An occupational therapist can help by assessing your needs and making recommendations.

- Avoid using force with your hands. When working on a cash register or computer, hit the keys softly. Use a wide pen with a soft grip so that you don't have to squeeze the pen tightly.

- Warm paraffin wax treatments and hydrotherapy can help ease the symptoms.

- Massage, chiropractic, acupuncture, laser, and physiotherapy are very beneficial.

- Yoga and stretching can help improve posture and strength and promote relaxation.

- Don't smoke—it reduces blood flow to the median nerve.

Top Recommended Supplements

Fish oil: Contains omega-3 fatty acids that have anti-inflammatory and antioxidant properties which may help reduce symptoms of CTS. Dosage: 1–3 g daily.

Vitamin B6: There is some evidence that vitamin B6 can reduce the pain and symptoms of CTS. It may be particularly helpful in those with a B6 deficiency. Dosage: 100 mg two to three times daily. B6 is usually safe up to 500 mg daily; higher dosages can damage sensory nerves and cause numbness in the hands and feet.

Complementary Supplements

Arnica: An herb that reduces pain and inflammation. One study found it particularly helpful in relieving pain after surgery. It is available in homeopathic tablets and as topical creams and ointments.

Calcium and magnesium: These are important minerals for nerve and muscle function. Dosages: 500 mg calcium and 250 mg magnesium two to three times daily.

Curcumin: An herb with anti-inflammatory properties. Dosage: 300 mg three times daily.

Serrapeptase: A proteolytic enzyme that helps reduce inflammation and shows promise for treating CTS. Follow label instructions.

FINAL THOUGHTS

To prevent CTS or reduce the symptoms if you already have it, consider the following:

- If you work on a computer or do repetitive wrist and arm movements, use proper form, take frequent breaks, wear a support, and avoid strong force.
- Eat more beans, whole grains, fish, and chia seed.
- Consider fish oil and vitamin B6 supplements as a first line of defence.
- Use topical products with arnica to reduce pain and inflammation.
- Acupuncture, massage, and chiropractic are helpful.

CATARACTS

Cataracts are cloudy spots that develop on the normally clear lens of the eye. Initially they might not be noticeable; however, as they progress, cataracts cause gradual clouding and loss of vision.

Cataracts are the leading cause of blindness in North America. They are most common among older adults. In fact, over 2.5 million Canadians have cataracts and about half of Canadians over the age of 65 have visual impairment due to cataracts. This can affect normal daily activities, making it difficult to read, drive a car, and walk safely.

In most people cataracts occur because of age-related changes in the lens. The lens is composed mainly of protein fibres and water. With age, the lens undergoes changes; it becomes thicker, less flexible, and less transparent. The protein fibres break down and begin to clump together, creating cloudy spots on the lens, which become progressively worse. Cataracts tend to develop slowly in both eyes at the same time unless they are caused by an injury that affects only one eye. Cataracts that become completely white, known as overripe (hypermature) cataracts, can cause inflammation, pain, and headache.

Cataracts are not considered a "normal" part of aging, yet they do primarily affect older adults, likely due to lifetime exposure to free radicals from smoking, chemicals, UV light, and other factors that damage the lens.

There are other potential causes of cataracts. Infants may be born with cataracts if their mother contracted German measles (rubella) during pregnancy. They can also develop secondary to diabetes, injury, heavy metal poisoning, use of certain medications, and other factors as listed below.

Most cataracts develop slowly and, for the majority of people, it is possible to delay and even prevent cataracts with lifestyle modifications and supplements. However, once a cataract has developed, it cannot be reversed; at this point surgery is the only option to restore vision.

SIGNS & SYMPTOMS

- Cloudy, blurred vision; double vision
- Fading or yellowing of colours
- Halos around lights
- Poor night vision
- Sensitivity to light and glare

RISK FACTORS

- Advanced age
- Diabetes, high blood pressure, and obesity
- Exposure to radiation
- Family history

- Heavy metal poisoning

- Injury, trauma, or surgery to the eye

- Poor diet (a deficiency of antioxidants such as vitamins C and E, beta carotene, and selenium)

- Smoking

- Excessive alcohol intake

- Use of corticosteroids (cortisone, prednisone)

- UV light exposure

DOCTOR'S ORDERS

Once a cataract is fully developed, the only way to remove it is through surgery. An ophthalmologist replaces the clouded lens with a clear lens implant. In some cases the cataract is removed and vision is corrected with glasses or contact lenses rather than with an implant.

SHERRY'S NATURAL PRESCRIPTION

Dietary Recommendations

Foods to include:

- Several studies have found that diets high in vitamins C and E and carotenoids can help prevent cataract development by reducing free radical damage. Foods particularly high in vitamin C include berries (acai, blueberry, and cranberry), cherries, tomatoes, peppers, carrots, grapes, mangos, and citrus fruits. Kale, collard greens, spinach, and broccoli are great sources of the carotenoids lutein and zeaxanthin, which lower the risk of cataracts and macular degeneration. Foods rich in vitamin E include wheat germ, nuts, and leafy green vegetables.

- Fish provide omega-3 fatty acids, which have antioxidant properties and reduce inflammation. Some research has found that consuming fish three times a week has a protective effect.

Foods to avoid:

- Fast food and processed foods contain hydrogenated (trans fats) and saturated fats, which generate free radicals.

- Limit alcohol consumption, as it impairs the liver's ability to detoxify harmful chemicals from the diet and environment.

Lifestyle Suggestions

- Get regular eye exams at least every other year. While this won't prevent cataracts, early detection gives you a chance to take steps to slow or prevent their development.

- Don't smoke. Smoking is a known risk factor because it generates damaging free radicals. Avoid smoky environments and people who smoke, as second-hand exposure can be just as damaging.

- Wear proper-fitting sunglasses with UV protection and wide-brimmed hats to shield your eyes from the sun's damaging rays. Sunglasses should be worn year-round when driving or outdoors, as the sun's UV light can still be damaging even during colder months.

- Improve the lighting in your home and use a magnifying glass for reading.

- Maintain a healthy body weight. Obesity is associated with increased risk of cataracts.

Top Recommended Supplements

Supplements cannot improve cataracts once you have them, but they may play a role in prevention.

Carotenoids: Beta carotene and lutein are important antioxidants in the eye; numerous studies have shown that they protect against cataracts by shielding the eye against light damage. Supplements may be particularly beneficial for smokers. Dosages: 25,000 IU of beta carotene; 6 mg of lutein.

Vitamin C: A major antioxidant in the lens; essential for healthy vision and to protect the eye against free radicals. Levels in the eye decrease with age. Some research has shown that supplements of vitamin C may lower the risk of cataracts. Dosage: 500–1,000 mg daily.

Vitamin E: Activates glutathione, which is an important antioxidant in the eye. Low blood levels of vitamin E have been linked to increased risk of cataracts and some research suggests protective benefits with supplements. Dosage: 400 IU daily.

Complementary Supplements

B-complex: Vitamins B2 and B3 protect glutathione in the eye, and some evidence shows protective benefits with supplements. Dosage: 50–100 mg of a B-vitamin complex.

Bilberry: Rich in antioxidant flavonoids, which are protective to the lens. Dosage: 240–480 mg daily.

FINAL THOUGHTS

To delay the onset of cataracts and preserve your vision, consider the following:

- Get regular eye exams.
- Boost antioxidant and carotenoid intake by eating lots of berries, carrots, peppers, kale, collard greens, spinach, and broccoli, and eat more fish.
- Wear sunglasses with UV protection and wide-brimmed hats when outdoors or driving.
- Don't smoke, and avoid exposure to second-hand smoke.
- Consider supplements of vitamins C and E and carotenoids.

CELIAC DISEASE (GLUTEN INTOLERANCE)

Celiac disease is a digestive disorder caused by an abnormal immune reaction to the consumption of gluten, a protein found primarily in wheat, barley, rye, and triticale. Celiac disease is much more common than once thought—it is estimated to affect one in 100 to 133 Canadians. However, only about 3 percent of these individuals have been diagnosed.

When a person with celiac disease eats gluten-containing food, the immune system reacts by producing antibodies, which attack the villi in the small intestine, reducing their ability to absorb nutrients. Over time, the reduced absorption of nutrients leads to malnutrition and vitamin, mineral, and essential fatty acid deficiencies. This can damage the health of every organ and body system and increase the risk of many diseases, such as osteoporosis and depression.

The cause of celiac is not known; however, three factors are typically present in those who develop the disease: genetic predisposition, a diet containing gluten, and a triggering event. Possible triggers include introduction of grains into a baby's diet, puberty, pregnancy, menopause, stress, viral or bacterial infection, and trauma (accident, surgery).

There is no cure for celiac disease, but the condition can be managed by following a gluten-free diet for life. Supplements can play an important role in restoring health.

SIGNS & SYMPTOMS

Symptoms of celiac vary greatly and may include the following:

• Abdominal cramps and bloating

• Anemia

• Chronic diarrhea or constipation

• Dental and bone disorders (osteoporosis)

• Fatigue

• Headaches (including migraines)

• Infertility

• Irritability and depression

• Joint pain

• Muscle cramps

• Skin rash or mouth sores

• Stunted growth in children

• Tingling in the legs and feet

• Weight loss

Note: Dermatitis herpetiformis is an itchy, blistering skin disease that also results from gluten intolerance. It typically affects the elbows, knees, and buttocks.

DANGERS OF CELIAC DISEASE

Individuals with undiagnosed celiac disease or those who do not adhere to a gluten-free diet are at greater risk of developing osteoporosis; cancer of the intestines, mouth, esophagus, or bowel; and neurological diseases (seizures and nerve damage).

RISK FACTORS

- Existing autoimmune disease, such as lupus erythematosus, type 1 diabetes, rheumatoid arthritis, or thyroid disease, is a risk factor.
- Family history: Having a family member with celiac increases your risk by 10 to 20 percent.
- Celiac disease is more common in Caucasians and those of European ancestry and is quite rare among those of Asian and Indian descent.

DOCTOR'S ORDERS

Your doctor will recommend a strict gluten-free diet and a consultation with a dietitian to learn what this entails. Once gluten is removed from the diet, the villi start to heal and intestinal inflammation subsides. Complete healing and regrowth of the villi may take several months in younger people and as long as two to three years in older people. For severe cases that don't respond to dietary changes, medications such as prednisone are temporarily used to suppress the immune response.

SHERRY'S NATURAL PRESCRIPTION

Dietary Recommendations

A strict gluten-free diet is crucial for those with celiac disease. Even a small amount of gluten can damage the intestine and illicit an immune reaction. Read all food labels carefully; look for products labelled gluten-free. If in doubt, contact the manufacturer. When eating out, ask to speak directly to the chef as service staff may not be familiar with gluten and the many possible hidden sources. Cross-contamination can occur if gluten-free foods are prepared in unwashed bowls previously containing gluten, or cooked in the same pots or deep-fryer.

Foods to include:
- Lean meats, fish, and poultry; fruits, vegetables, corn, potato, rice, and soy.
- Healthy fats (fish, nuts, and chia and flaxseeds) are very important to help restore essential fatty acids, which are often depleted in those with celiac disease.
- Gluten-free, fibre-rich grains such as amaranth, buckwheat, quinoa, millet, pure uncontaminated oats, rice bran, and sorghum. Flours made from these grains can be substituted in recipes.

Foods to avoid:
- Foods containing wheat, barley, rye, bulgur, kamut, spelt, and triticale, such as breads, pasta, cereals, baked goods, crackers, and pies.

- Watch for hidden sources of gluten—prepared and processed foods, such as sauces, dressings, marinades, and coating agents.

- Watch for food that is cooked or fried in the same oil as gluten-containing items.

- Most beers and some wine coolers contain barley malt.

Note: Dairy should be limited initially as damage to the intestines reduces the ability to digest lactose (dairy sugar). After the intestines have healed, dairy consumption can resume.

OATS AND GLUTEN

The safety of oats in those with celiac is controversial. Several small studies investigated this matter. These studies used pure oats, free of gluten contamination, and the amount per day was limited. The Canadian Celiac Association has stated that consumption of pure, uncontaminated oats is safe in the amount of 50–70 g per day (1/2–3/4 cup of dry rolled oats) by adults and 20–25 g per day (1/4 cup of dry rolled oats) by children with celiac disease.

Note: Some individuals may not tolerate even pure oats, in which case they should be completely avoided.

Lifestyle Suggestions

- To promote healing and support immune function, it is important to get adequate rest, reduce stress, and strictly adhere to the gluten-free diet.

- Be aware that gluten can be present in supplements, drugs, and even toothpaste.

Top Recommended Supplements

Digestive enzymes: May be depleted in those with celiac; they aid proper digestion of food and are particularly important in newly diagnosed individuals. Once the intestines have healed, enzymes may not be necessary. Look for a broad spectrum product containing lipase, amylase, and protease along with DPP IV, an enzyme that has been shown to aid in the breakdown of gluten. Enzymes are not to replace a gluten-free diet but rather to aid digestion, and in the case of DPP IV to mitigate the effects of hidden gluten in the diet. Take as directed before meals.

Essential fatty acids: Highly recommended to correct deficiencies, reduce inflammation, and promote healing of intestinal cells. Look for a product that provides both omega-3 (fish) and GLA, an omega-6 (borage, primrose) fatty acid. Dosage: 1–3 g daily.

Multivitamin and mineral complex: This is absolutely essential to correct deficiencies and promote healing. The most common deficiencies include calcium, magnesium, iron, zinc, vitamins D and K, and folic acid. Even those who are stable, on a gluten-free diet, and in remission may still have nutrient deficiencies and would benefit from a supplement. Those with severe malnutrition and deficiencies may require higher than typical amounts. Consult with a health care provider for recommendations.

Complementary Supplements

Fibre: Often deficient in a gluten-free diet because of the elimination of many grains, so supplements can help improve bowel function and prevent constipation. Look for a product that contains a combination of gluten-free soluble and insoluble fibres.

Glutamine: An amino acid that supports the immune system and gastrointestinal health and may help repair damage to intestinal lining. Dosage: 3–30 g daily as advised by your health care practitioner.

Green food supplement: Provides vitamins, minerals, and fibre; improves energy and recovery. Ensure that the product is gluten-free.

Probiotics: Support intestinal health, restore normal flora, and improve bowel function. Look for a product that is non-dairy and stable at room temperature, and provides at least 1 billion live cells. Take one to three capsules daily.

FINAL THOUGHTS

To improve health and reduce complications from celiac disease, consider the following:

- Adhere to a strict gluten-free diet.
- Eat a healthy diet, including fruits, vegetables, lean protein, healthy fats, and gluten-free grains.
- To promote healing, get adequate rest and reduce stress.
- Take a quality multivitamin/mineral complex, essential fatty acids supplements, and enzymes.
- Consider fibre, probiotics, glutamine, and green food supplements to complement your diet.

Celiac Disease (Gluten Intolerance)

CERVICAL DYSPLASIA

Cervical dysplasia is a condition in which cells on the surface of the cervix become pre-cancerous or cancerous. There are various grades of cervical dysplasia, which are classified based on the degree and extent of the abnormal cell growth. Low-grade cervical dysplasia progresses very slowly and typically resolves on its own. High-grade cervical dysplasia tends to progress quickly and usually leads to cervical cancer.

The primary cause of cervical dysplasia is infection with human papillomavirus (HPV). HPV is the most prevalent sexually transmitted infection, with an estimated 79 percent infection rate over a lifetime. Although HPV is responsible for most cases, the majority of women that develop HPV infection will not develop cervical dysplasia or cancer. Factors that may contribute to the progression from cervical dysplasia to cancer include smoking, long-term use of birth control pills, and nutritional deficiencies. Risk factors are discussed below.

It is estimated that up to 50 percent of severe cases of cervical dysplasia progress to cancer within 10 years. In Canada in 2011, it was estimated that 1,300 new cases of cervical cancer and 350 deaths occurred. This is unfortunate because cervical cancer is largely preventable. With early identification, treatment, and consistent follow-up, nearly all cases of cervical dysplasia can be cured and cervical cancer can be prevented. Most cervical cancer deaths occur in women who have not had a Pap smear.

SIGNS & SYMPTOMS

There are usually no symptoms of cervical dysplasia and it is detected only during a Pap smear. In some cases woman may notice the following:

- Abnormal bleeding

- Genital warts (only 1 percent of women with HPV have visible genital warts)

- Low back pain

- Spotting after intercourse

- Vaginal discharge

Note: These symptoms are not unique to cervical dysplasia and may indicate a more serious condition such as cervical cancer.

RISK FACTORS

- Being born to a mother who took diethylstilbestrol (DES) to become pregnant or to sustain pregnancy

- Genital warts

- Having a sexual partner whose former partner had cervical cancer

- History of a sexually transmitted disease (such as herpes)

- Human papillomavirus (HPV) infection
- Long-term use (five years or more) of birth control pills, which contain estrogen
- Multiple sexual partners
- Nutritional deficiencies in folate, vitamin A, beta carotene, selenium, vitamin E, and vitamin C
- Sexual activity at a young age (less than 18 years)
- Giving birth before age 16
- Smoking
- Suppressed immune function (HIV, organ transplant, or use of chemotherapeutic medications)

DOCTOR'S ORDERS

Regular Pap tests are essential to detect changes in cervical cells and prevent cervical cancer. Every woman should have an annual Pap test beginning at age 18 and continuing on past menopause. Many women stop having this done later in life, which is dangerous since the highest incidence of cervical cancer is among those over age 65.

A vaccine for prevention of HPV infection recently became available and is recommended for young girls prior to becoming sexually active. The vaccine targets two of the more than 15 strains of the virus that cause HPV. It is suggested that the vaccine use may reduce the risk of cervical cancer by 70 percent, but its overall efficacy and benefits have been questioned and its use has been associated with some serious side effects.

The treatment of early stage cervical dysplasia is highly successful, although the lifetime recurrence rate is 20 percent. For early stages of cervical dysplasia, doctors may simply recommend frequent monitoring, as pre-cancerous changes may disappear on their own. Treatment of more advanced stages involves surgical removal of abnormal tissue. The most commonly used procedures include laser therapy, cryo-cauterization (use of extreme cold to destroy abnormal tissue), and loop excision (using a wire loop to remove tissue).

THE PAP TEST

The Pap test, named after Dr. Georgios Papanicolaou, the inventor, screens for cervical dysplasia and cancer. Your doctor takes a small scraping of cells in the cervical area for analysis by a laboratory. All women should have this test done regularly beginning at age 18 or when you become sexually active. It takes only a few minutes, is almost painless, and could save your life.

SHERRY'S NATURAL PRESCRIPTION

As there are various lifestyle and nutritional factors implicated in cervical dysplasia, it is possible to make adjustments and improve the health of your cervical cells and reduce your risk of dysplasia and cancer. These natural therapies do not replace the need for regular medical examinations and doctor's supervision.

Dietary Recommendations

Foods to include:

- Increase intake of whole grains, fresh vegetables, and fruits. Several population-based studies have suggested that eating a diet rich in nutrients from fruits and vegetables may protect against the development of cervical cancer. These foods are high in antioxidants, which fight free radical damage. They also contain vitamin C, folate, and beta carotene, which have been found to be deficient in those who develop cervical dysplasia. Choose organic as much as possible to avoid pesticide ingestion.

- Eat liver-supporting foods such as beets, carrots, onions, garlic, leafy greens, artichokes, apples, and lemons to support detoxification.

- Broccoli, cauliflower, Brussels sprouts, cabbage, and other cruciferous vegetables contain indole-3-carbinol, which helps with detoxification and elimination of estrogen.

- Flaxseed, soy, beans, and legumes contain phytoestrogens, which may help reduce the impact of other hormones.

- Green tea contains polyphenols, which have been found to inhibit growth of cancer cells and reduce cervical dysplasia.

Foods to avoid:

- Alcohol, caffeine, refined foods, food additives, sugar, and saturated fats may affect hormone balance and impair immune function.

- Regular, non-organic meat may contain hormones and chemicals that act as estrogen-mimickers.

Lifestyle Suggestions

- Have a Pap test beginning at age 18 or when you become sexually active. A second test should be done after one year, and if normal repeated every three years thereafter until age 69. If you have an abnormal test, your doctor will advise you to have more frequent screenings.

- Minimize exposure to environmental estrogens or xenoestrogens (phthalates, parabens, and dioxins), which are present in pesticides, plastics, and certain skin care products. Read labels and check with manufacturers.

- Don't smoke, and avoid second-hand smoke.

- Sexually active women should use a barrier method, such as condoms or a diaphragm, for protection against sexually transmitted diseases.

- Get regular exercise. This is a natural way to enhance immune function and prevent disease. Try walking, cycling, or aerobics.

- Reduce stress. Try yoga, Pilates, stretching, acupuncture, or massage.

Top Recommended Supplements

Green tea: Helps prevent cancer growth. One study also found that daily supplements of green tea providing 200 mg of EGCG (the antioxidant component) significantly reduced or eliminated abnormal cells in those with cervical dysplasia. Look for a supplement providing 200 mg EGCG.

Indole-3-carbinol: A compound found naturally in cruciferous vegetables that aids in detoxification of estrogen, protects liver function, and may protect against hormonal cancers. Studies have shown that supplements can reduce the formation of carcinogenic forms of estrogen and improve lesions in those with cervical dysplasia. Dosage: 200–400 mg daily.

Complementary Supplements

Beta carotene: Some research suggests that a deficiency in beta carotene increases the risk of cervical dysplasia and cancer, and that supplements may promote a regression or decline in the signs of cervical dysplasia. Dosage: 25,000–50,000 units (15–30 mg) daily.

B-vitamins: There is evidence that women with low dietary intakes of vitamins B1, B2, B6, B12, and folic acid are at greater risk of developing cervical dysplasia, and those with higher intakes of these nutrients from food and supplements are at lower risk. These vitamins may protect against cellular changes that lead to dysplasia, but they have not been shown to reverse changes that have occurred. Look for a broad spectrum B-complex and take daily for prevention.

Calcium D-glucarate: Helps the liver detoxify and eliminate excess hormones, particularly estrogen. Not specifically studied for cervical dysplasia, but may help by reducing the harmful effects of estrogen. Dosage: 300–500 mg daily.

Vitamin C: Deficiencies have been associated with cervical dysplasia. It is not known whether supplements can reverse this condition. However, it is known that vitamin C supports immune function and is an antioxidant that protects against cellular damage. Dosage: 500 mg daily.

FINAL THOUGHTS

To improve cervical health and reduce your risk of cervical dysplasia and cancer, consider the following:

- Have a regular Pap test and discuss the results with your doctor.
- Eat organic vegetables, fruits, whole grains, legumes, and flaxseed.
- Minimize red meat, dairy, alcohol, caffeine, and refined foods.
- Avoid exposure to smoke and environmental estrogens; practise safe sex.
- Top recommended supplements are indole-3-carbinol and green tea. Also consider beta carotene, B-vitamins, calcium D-glucarate, and vitamin C.

CHRONIC FATIGUE SYNDROME

Chronic fatigue syndrome (CFS) is a condition marked by profound fatigue, weakness, and flu-like symptoms that may last from months to years. The term myalgic encephalomyelitis (ME) is often used in conjunction with CFS.

CFS has become known only in the past few decades and is a mysterious condition because there is no obvious cause, no clear tests to make a diagnosis, and few (if any) medical treatment options available. This condition has become increasingly common in Canada. It is estimated to affect over 120,000 Canadians, causing a significant impact on a person's physical and emotional well-being with annual lost productivity estimated at over $2.5 billion.

The exact cause of CFS is not known. It is now generally accepted that ME/CFS is an umbrella term for a diverse group of disorders and that one particular cause may not be found.

Some of the possible causes that have been suggested include the following:

- Chemical sensitivities or toxic exposure
- Chronic inflammation
- Chronic low blood pressure
- Hormonal imbalance—low cortisol, DHEA, or thyroid levels
- Hypoglycemia—low blood sugar
- Immune system dysfunction
- Infection with a cold, virus (Epstein-Barr virus or human herpesvirus 6), or yeast (Candida albicans)
- Iron-deficiency anemia
- Stress

While there are many mysteries surrounding CFS, there are various lifestyle approaches and nutritional supplements that can help minimize symptoms and improve quality of life in those suffering with this condition.

DIAGNOSIS FOR CFS

The Canadian consensus guidelines for ME/CFS diagnosis requires the concurrent presence for at least six months of five major criteria: disabling fatigue, post-exertional malaise or fatigue, sleep dysfunction, pain, and two or more neurological/cognitive symptoms. In addition there must be two of autonomic, neuroendocrine, and immune manifestations.

SIGNS & SYMPTOMS

Primary signs and symptoms:
- Fatigue
- Extreme exhaustion after normal exercise or exertion
- Headache of a new type, pattern, or severity

- Loss of memory or concentration
- Pain that moves from one joint to another without swelling or redness
- Painful and mildly enlarged lymph nodes in your neck or armpits
- Sleep disturbance
- Sore throat
- Unexplained muscle soreness

Other signs and symptoms:

- Abdominal pain
- Alcohol intolerance
- Bloating
- Chest pain
- Chronic cough
- Diarrhea
- Dizziness
- Dry eyes and mouth
- Earache
- Irregular heartbeat
- Jaw pain
- Morning stiffness
- Nausea
- Night sweats
- Psychological problems, such as depression, irritability, anxiety disorders, and panic attacks
- Shortness of breath
- Tingling sensations
- Weight loss

RISK FACTORS

- Age: CFS can occur at any age, but it is most common in those aged 40 to 50.
- Gender: CFS is more common among women, but sex is not a proven risk factor. It is thought that women are more likely to report the symptoms.
- Obesity
- Inactivity
- Stress

DOCTOR'S ORDERS

There is no specific drug treatment for chronic fatigue syndrome—lifestyle measures are often tried first. Medications may help certain symptoms. However, the side effects may be worse than the symptoms of the condition. These medications include anti-depressants (Paxil, Zoloft, and Wellbutrin), anti-anxiety drugs (Xanax and Ativan), anti-inflammatory drugs (Motrin), allergy drugs (antihistamines), and sleeping pills. Interestingly, while antidepressants are often given, evidence that they actually improve the core symptoms of CFS is lacking.

HOMEOPATHIC RECOMMENDATIONS

Causticum: Soreness, weakness, and stiffness in the muscles, which feel worse from being cold and overused, suggest a need for Causticum. The forearms often feel stiff, unsteady, and very weak. The muscles of the legs can feel contracted and raw. Problems tend to be worse when the weather is dry and better in rainy weather, but the person doesn't like getting wet. Warm applications often relieve discomfort.

Ranunculus: This remedy is helpful for inflammation of muscle tissue resulting in stiffness, especially when the neck and back are involved. Stabbing pains and soreness may be felt near the spine and shoulder blades, especially on the left.

Combination recommendation: Sportenine by Boiron

SHERRY'S NATURAL PRESCRIPTION

Dietary Recommendations

Foods to include:

• Fish provides omega-3 fatty acids that reduce inflammation. Vegetarian sources of omega-3s include chia seed, flaxseed, and nuts.

• Vegetables, fruits, and whole grains are rich in essential nutrients for immune function and optimal health. Choose organic produce to avoid harmful pesticides.

• Yogurt contains beneficial bacteria that support immune function and digestion.

Food to avoid:

• Processed and fast foods contain additives, preservatives, and other chemicals that may trigger allergic reactions and stress the body, worsening symptoms.

• Caffeine and alcohol can affect sleep quality and cause irritability and anxiety.

• Refined flour and sugar can affect immune function and cause blood sugar imbalances, which may worsen hypoglycemia.

Sensitivities to gluten, wheat, or dairy can worsen symptoms in some people. Consider an elimination diet (Appendix D) to determine if food sensitivities are affecting your health.

Lifestyle Suggestions

• Reduce stress—promote relaxation with meditation, yoga, stretching, or breathing exercises.

CHRONIC VENOUS INSUFFICIENCY

Chronic venous insufficiency (CVI) is a common condition of poor circulation that affects up to 40 percent of Canadians. CVI occurs when there is damage to or an absence of the one-way valves in the veins. Without functioning valves to prevent the backflow of blood, the blood pools in the veins, causing them to enlarge and the blood pressure in the veins to stay elevated.

CVI can be congenital (you are born with it) or it can result from a blood clot, which damages the vein walls and valves. It often starts with the failure of a single valve, which creates a high-pressure leak in the venous system. The vein dilates, leading to failure of other nearby valves. After a series of valves have failed, the affected veins can no longer direct blood upward toward the heart. Blood pools in the veins, causing them to enlarge. This scenario often continues as increasing numbers of valves fail under the strain and high pressure, and more and more veins become affected.

SIGNS & SYMPTOMS

The symptoms of CVI are worse during the day while you are upright and include the following:

- Burning and itching

- Enlarged veins (varicose veins)

- Heavy, aching legs

- Leg swelling

- Pain and pressure

- Restless legs

If the swelling is not controlled, inflammation occurs in the skin and tissues beneath the skin. The skin may develop reddish-brown spots called lipodermatosclerosis. Over time, the skin thickens and becomes hard, leathery, dry, and itchy. If a break in the skin occurs, a venous ulcer or chronic sore may develop.

RISK FACTORS

- Advanced age: Women over 50 and men over 70 years

- Chronic constipation: Increases venous pressure

- Gender: Women are at greater risk

- Inactivity: Long periods of standing with little movement can increase venous pressure and weaken the vein walls and valves

- Lack of activity/movement: Minimizes the pump action of the calf muscles, causing higher venous pressure

- Obesity: Carrying excess weight increases venous pressure

- Pregnancy: Due to hormonal changes and carrying extra weight
- Previous vein problems: A history of deep vein thrombosis (DVT), which damages the valves causing backflow and increased venous pressure
- Smoking: Causes damage to the valves and veins
- Having varicose veins or a family history of varicose veins

DOCTOR'S ORDERS

Medical treatment is aimed at improving blood flow and preventing pooling of blood and further damage to the valves and veins. Options include the following:

Ablation/sclerotherapy/laser: Procedures that destroy the damaged vein; blood is rerouted through other veins, and the damaged vein is absorbed by the body.

Bypass: An artificial or transplanted vein is connected to the damaged vein to help improve blood flow.

Compression stockings: They provide firm support to improve blood flow back to the heart and prevent leg swelling; available for both men and women; custom ordered to size.

Hospitalization and antibiotic therapy: For severe venous ulcers.

Stripping: A surgical procedure to remove the damaged vein.

Valve repair: A surgical procedure to shorten the valves and improve valve function.

SHERRY'S NATURAL PRESCRIPTION

Dietary Recommendations

Foods to include:

- A high-fibre diet is essential to prevent constipation and straining. Eat plenty of fruits, vegetables, whole grains, legumes, nuts, and seeds. These foods are also high in antioxidants and good fats, both of which are helpful for circulation.

Foods to avoid:

- Saturated fats (animal fats) and trans fats (fast food and processed food) impede circulation, cause free radical damage, and trigger inflammation.
- Reduce sodium intake (soft drinks, chips, crackers, and deli meats) as it can increase fluid retention and swelling.

Lifestyle Suggestions

- Exercise regularly: Activities that involve the calf muscle will help pump blood back to the heart. Try walking, cycling, and swimming.
- Elevate your legs above the thighs when resting.
- Avoid standing or sitting in the same spot for a long time. Move around, flex your ankles, circle your feet, do calf raises, and shift your body weight.

- Lose excess weight, which will reduce pressure on your legs.

- Avoid excessive heat on your legs (sunbathing and hot baths), which causes the veins to dilate, thus worsening the problem.

- Don't cross your legs, as it hampers circulation and worsens symptoms.

- Avoid wearing high heels and tight shoes or clothing, as they impair circulation.

- Avoid constipation and straining on the toilet, as this can increase vein pressure.

- Don't smoke, as smoking damages the veins and blood vessels, increases blood pressure, and impairs circulation.

Top Recommended Supplements

Diosmin: A bioflavonoid that improves the tone and strength of the veins, reduces swelling, fights free radical damage, and stimulates lymphatic flow. Numerous studies have found diosmin safe and effective for improving vein disorders, including chronic venous insufficiency and varicose veins. It has a quick onset of action (one to two weeks). Dosage: 600 mg once daily of a product standardized to provide 95 percent diosmin and 5 percent hesperidin (the active constituents).

Horse chestnut seed extract: Promotes circulation, improves vein wall tone, and relieves pain and swelling. It offers modest benefits and may take six to eight weeks to begin working. Dosage: 300 mg twice daily; standardized to 50 mg of aescin.

Oligomeric proanthocyanidin complexes (OPCs): A group of flavonoids found in high levels in grape seed and pine bark that offers antioxidant activity, strengthens capillaries, improves circulation, and supports vein health. A few small studies have shown benefits. Dosage: 100–300 mg daily.

Complementary Supplements

Antioxidants: Help improve circulation and vein health. In addition to diosmin and OPCs, other antioxidants to consider include vitamins C and E and bilberry. Follow label instructions.

Butcher's broom: Improves the strength and tone of the veins, acts as a mild diuretic, and has mild anti-inflammatory effects. Dosage: 150 mg two to three times daily.

Gotu kola: A plant extract shown in preliminary research to reduce swelling, pain, fatigue, sensation of heaviness, and fluid leakage from the veins. Dosage: 60–120 mg daily.

FINAL THOUGHTS

To prevent and improve CVI, consider the following:

- Boost intake of fibre and antioxidant-rich foods; reduce your intake of saturated fats, processed foods, and sodium.
- Don't smoke.
- Exercise regularly, elevate your feet when resting, and avoid standing or sitting in the same spot.
- Wear compression stockings.
- Consider supplements of diosmin, horse chestnut seed, or OPCs.

COLD SORES

Cold sores, also known as fever blisters, are small lesions that appear on the lips or surrounding skin. They are primarily caused by infection with the herpes simplex type 1 virus (HSV-1), although they can result from herpes simplex type 2 virus (HSV-2), which is the virus that causes genital herpes. Approximately 80 percent of people carry the HSV-1 virus, and of those, 20 to 40 percent experience recurrent cold sores (two or more outbreaks per year).

Most people contract the HSV virus during childhood, although some people get it later in life.

After infection with the virus, it can remain dormant in the nerve cells of your skin for long periods of time and then periodically cause outbreaks, particularly when the immune system is weakened. There is no cure for the virus. However, there are a number of methods to reduce the risk of recurrence and speed healing of an outbreak.

SIGNS & SYMPTOMS

The initial infection may cause flu-like symptoms (fever and fatigue). An outbreak of cold sores causes

• Clusters of tiny, red, fluid-filled blisters

• Crusting once they burst

• Pain

Cold sores typically last for seven to ten days. However, they can become infected if picked, which delays healing.

WARNING SIGNS: Those who get recurrent cold sores typically experience prodromal symptoms before an outbreak—tingling, itching, or burning around the lips. These symptoms usually occur 24 to 48 hours prior to the eruption of a lesion.

RISK FACTORS

The virus is spread through contact with the fluid from the cold sore blisters or the saliva of an infected individual. Kissing, using the same eating utensils, sharing personal items (such as a razor), and receiving oral sex from someone who has HSV-1 can cause you to contract the virus. The lesions remain contagious until they have healed completely. Once you carry the virus, risk factors for an outbreak include

• Drying of the lips (exposure to sun and wind)

• Fatigue

• Fever

- Hormonal changes in women (menstruation or pregnancy)

- Illness

- Stress

- Trauma

Those with a weakened immune system (having cancer, AIDS, or an organ transplant) are prone to more frequent and severe bouts of cold sores. In these individuals, cold sores can become a serious health risk.

DOCTOR'S ORDERS

Cold sores generally clear up without treatment. Contact your doctor if the sores do not heal within two weeks, the symptoms are severe, you get frequent recurrences, or you experience pain or irritation in your eyes (this could indicate that the virus has infected your eyes, which is a serious condition).

Prescription antiviral drugs such as Valtrex and Zovirax may shorten the duration and severity of the infection, but are not approved for prevention. These drugs are expensive, associated with side effects (nausea, vomiting, and headache), and not recommended for children, pregnant women, or those with impaired kidney or liver function.

There are several over-the-counter products used to protect the skin, relieve pain, and speed healing. Abreva can help shorten the duration of an outbreak (by about 18 hours). Lipactin, which contains heparin and zinc, is used to soothe the skin but it does not shorten the duration of an outbreak. The Polysporin cold sore patch helps conceal the cold sore and promote healing. Some topical products like Zilactin contain anaesthetics, such as benzocaine, that help reduce the pain. Topical moisturizers can also be used to hydrate and protect the skin from drying out.

Aspirin, acetaminophen (Tylenol), or ibuprofen may be used to help reduce pain.

HOMEOPATHIC RECOMMENDATIONS

Natrum muriaticum: This remedy sometimes stops a cold sore outbreak if it is taken in the early, tingling stage.

Rhus toxicodendron: Herpes (cold sore virus) outbreaks in any location, especially around the lips, the corners of the mouth, or on and near the genitals and inner thighs, may respond to this remedy. Eruptions, which are red and swollen with burning pain and itching, are relieved by hot water or warm applications. The person feels a constant need to move around.

Combination recommendation: Herpezostin R68 by Reckeweg

SHERRY'S NATURAL PRESCRIPTION

There are several natural methods to speed healing of cold sores and prevent outbreaks.

Dietary Recommendations

Foods to include:

• Foods high in the amino acid lysine (legumes, fish, chicken, meat, apricots, figs, avocados, potatoes, eggs, and dairy) may help to reduce levels of arginine.

• Fruits, vegetables, and whole grains provide essential nutrients to support immune heath.

• Garlic contains compounds that have antiviral activity.

Foods to avoid:

• Foods that contain high amounts of arginine (chocolate, nuts, oysters, crab, oats, barley, wheat, and gelatin) allow the cold sore virus to replicate (thrive).

Lifestyle Suggestions

To avoid contracting or spreading the virus, don't share personal items such as drinking glasses, toothbrushes, razors, lipstick, or towels. If you have a cold sore, wash your hands before touching another person.

Those who suffer from recurrent cold sores can benefit from the following:

• Sunscreen: Apply to lips and face before going out in the sun and reapply regularly. Use a minimum of SPF 30.

• Moisturize: Use lip balm regularly to prevent the lips from becoming dry, chapped, or cracked.

• Relax: Work on reducing stress, which is a common trigger for cold sores. Try yoga, meditation, tai chi, or breathing exercises to promote relaxation.

• Sleep: Get adequate rest, which is essential for the immune system.

Once the blisters have appeared, try the following:

• Apply an ice pack, wrapped in a washcloth, for five minutes several times a day to ease pain.

• Dab the cold sore with witch hazel on a cotton ball. Witch hazel has antiviral activity against HSV-1 and can reduce inflammation and pain. Pharmacies keep this behind the counter, so you will have to ask for it.

• Do not pick or squeeze a cold sore blister or scab. This may cause it to spread, delay the healing process, and lead to infection.

Top Recommended Supplements

Lemon balm: An herb, also known as *Melissa officinalis*. Lemon balm has antiviral properties that can help speed healing and shorten the duration of an outbreak. Look for a cream containing 1 percent lemon balm extract. Apply two to four times daily for a week to 10 days.

C

Cold Sores

Lysine: An amino acid that inhibits growth of the cold sore virus and may help prevent recurrence. It may also reduce symptom severity and duration when an outbreak occurs. Dosage: 1,000 mg one to three times daily as a preventative. Creams containing lysine can help promote healing, but do not prevent outbreaks.

Propolis: A sticky resin that bees collect from trees. It has antiviral, antibacterial, anti-fungal, and anaesthetic properties. Studies done using a particular extract called propolis ACF (COLDSORE-FX) found that it can shorten the duration of an outbreak by about four days and also reduce pain. Dosage: Apply a small amount to the area four to six times daily until healed. It can be used at any stage of an outbreak (at first tingle or even when the sore erupts) to reduce pain and speed healing.

Complementary Supplement

Antioxidants: The antioxidants vitamins C and E may help to promote healing and strengthen the immune system's response to the virus. Vitamin E oil can also be applied directly to the affected area. In some studies this was found to reduce pain and accelerate healing.

Siberian ginseng (*Eleutherococcus sinticosus*): There is some evidence that it can help reduce the frequency and severity of outbreaks when taken regularly for prevention. Dosage: 2 g daily.

FINAL THOUGHTS

Cold sores are an unpleasant but largely preventable health concern. Here are the main points to keep in mind:

- To cut your risk of an outbreak, get adequate rest, reduce stress, avoid sharing utensils or personal items, and wear sunscreen and lip balm.
- Eat a healthy diet, including lysine-rich legumes and fish.
- Never pick or squeeze cold sores.
- Use a cold pack and witch hazel to relieve pain and prevent spreading, and a cream with lemon balm or propolis to promote healing.
- To prevent outbreaks, consider lysine supplements.

COMMON COLD

The common cold is an infection of the upper respiratory tract caused by a virus. There are over 200 viruses that cause colds; the most common is the rhinovirus. Colds are a major cause of doctor's appointments and lost work and school days. Children are most susceptible to contracting the virus and may experience as many as 10 colds a year. As we get older, we develop immunity to many viruses and are less likely to get colds.

Colds are highly contagious. The virus enters your body through your nose or mouth. For example, if you are beside someone who has the virus and coughs or sneezes and you inhale those virus droplets, then you can catch a cold. It can also be spread by hand-to-hand contact or by touching an object that has been contaminated with the virus and then rubbing your eyes, nose, or mouth.

A healthy functioning immune system is your best defence against a cold. If you catch a cold, there are a variety of lifestyle measures and supplements that can help speed healing and improve symptoms.

SIGNS & SYMPTOMS

Since there are many viruses that cause colds, symptoms and intensity vary, and include

• Cough

• Head and body ache

• Low-grade fever

• Nasal discharge (yellow/green)

• Sinus congestion and runny nose

• Sneezing

• Sore, scratchy throat

• Watery eyes

Note: Colds typically last for 7 to 14 days and improve without treatment. In some cases, though, a cold can lead to an ear infection, sinusitis, strep throat, bronchitis, pneumonia, or a flare-up of asthma.

IS IT A COLD OR FLU?

These infections are caused by different types of viruses. However, they do share some common symptoms such as aching, weakness, sore throat, and congestion. Here is where they differ: The flu causes a sudden onset of severe aching, pain, headache, and high fever (39–40°C). Colds develop more slowly, they don't usually cause fever, and they cause only mild aching and fatigue. The flu is a serious respiratory illness and can lead to bronchitis, pneumonia, and respiratory failure.

RISK FACTORS

- **Age:** Children are more susceptible because they have not developed resistance to viruses, plus children play together closely and are not careful about washing their hands and covering their mouths when they cough or sneeze.

- **Poor diet:** Nutritional deficiencies and excessive alcohol intake have all been linked to increased susceptibility.

- **Season:** Colds occur more frequently during the fall and winter because people spend more time indoors and are close together, which increases transmission; viruses survive better in low humidity, and cold temperatures make your nose drier and more susceptible to contracting a virus.

- **Smoking:** Damages nasal passages and makes it easier for viruses to enter.

- **Stress and lack of sleep:** Weaken the immune system and increase susceptibility.

DOCTOR'S ORDERS

Colds are not caused by bacteria, so antibiotics should not be used to treat a cold unless you develop a secondary bacterial infection such as strep throat or bronchitis.

Over-the-counter remedies, such as antihistamines, decongestants, and cough suppressants, may provide some symptom relief, but these products do not prevent or speed healing. As well, most of these products cause side effects. Antihistamines cause dry eyes/nose/mouth and drowsiness, and decongestants can raise blood pressure and cause dizziness and insomnia.

Tylenol (acetaminophen) can help reduce fever, aches, and pains, but it should be avoided by those with liver or kidney disease. Aspirin can also help these symptoms, but it should not be taken by children or teenagers because of the risk of Reye's syndrome. Those with kidney disease, ulcers, or risk of bleeding (taking blood thinners) should also avoid aspirin.

It is not necessary to see your doctor for a cold unless you or your child have a fever greater than 38°C along with aching, fatigue, sweating, and chills; if there is vomiting, ear pain, or coloured phlegm; or if symptoms persist longer than 10 days.

HOMEOPATHIC RECOMMENDATIONS

Aconite napellus: This remedy is excellent at the onset of a cold, denoted by symptoms that are intense and that come on suddenly. Exposure to cold and wind, stress, or traumatic experience may precipitate the illness. Symptoms include a dry, stuffy nose with a hot, thin discharge; tension in the chest; a scratchy throat; and choking cough. The person often feels thirsty, chilly, anxious, and agitated.

Kali bichromicum: This remedy is usually indicated for later stages of a cold with thick, stringy mucus that is difficult to clear from the nose and throat. The person typically experiences hoarse coughing with persistent phlegm.

Combination recommendation: Coryzalia by Boiron

SHERRY'S NATURAL PRESCRIPTION

Dietary Recommendations

Foods to include:

- Fruits and vegetables (especially garlic, onions, ginger, and horseradish) provide important nutrients and compounds that support immune function.

- Drink plenty of fluids (water, juice, herbal tea, and soup) to stay hydrated. Elderberry juice has antiviral activity. Green tea contains antioxidants that help support the immune system. There is some evidence that chicken soup can help reduce symptoms (congestion and sore throat) and speed healing.

- Herbal teas, such as Throat Coat, which contains marshmallow and licorice, has been shown to help relieve sore throat.

- Eat foods fortified with Wellmune, a natural ingredient that activates immune cells and enhances immune function without overstimulating the immune system. It is found in various juices, cookies, bars, and soups. It is safe for children as well as adults.

Foods to avoid:

- Excessive sugar intake can hamper immune function, so avoid eating candy and sweets.

- Cow's-milk dairy can worsen congestion in those with sensitivity.

- Alcohol suppresses immune function and should be avoided.

Lifestyle Suggestions

- Get extra rest to allow your body to recover.

- Manage stress—try breathing techniques, exercise, or meditation.

- For a sore throat, gargle with warm salt water and try lozenges that contain one or more of the following ingredients: slippery elm, marshmallow, vitamin C, zinc, eucalyptus, or menthol.

- For dry nose, try a nasal lubricant like Secaris or a saline nasal spray. Use a cool mist humidifier or vaporizer to add moisture to the air. Adding eucalyptus oil will help relieve nasal and sinus congestion and cough.

- Nasal irrigation, such as using a Neti pot or nasal wash, can help clear pollen and mucus from your nasal passages, relieve congestion and dryness, and improve breathing. Make a salt-water solution by mixing 1 tsp salt with 500 mL (16 ounces) purified lukewarm water. Lean forward over a sink and slowly pour the solution into one nostril and let it run out the other nostril. This can be repeated a few times daily. You can also use a nasal wash solution with essential oils such as menthol, eucalyptol, thymol, camphor, and wintergreen, which provide decongestant benefits.

To prevent acquiring or spreading a cold:

- Wash your hands frequently.

- Don't rub your eyes, nose, or mouth unless you have just washed your hands.

- Cover your mouth and nose when you sneeze or cough.

- Avoid exposure to those who have a cold.

- Don't share drinking glasses and utensils.

• Disinfect your kitchen, bathroom, and common living areas, especially when someone in the house has a cold.

• Exercise regularly, as exercise enhances immune function.

Top Recommended Supplements

American ginseng: Helps support immune function. Studies conducted with a particular extract of American ginseng (COLD-FX), standardized to polysaccharides, found that it can reduce the frequency, severity, and duration of colds by boosting the immune system. Dosage: 200–300 mg twice daily.

Echinacea: Some studies show it can reduce the severity and duration of cold symptoms. Look for *Echinacea purpurea*. Dosage: 300–600 mg capsules twice daily, or 2–4 mL tincture four to six times daily at the first sign of a cold for seven to ten days. Studies have not found this herb effective in children or as a cold preventative.

Vitamin C: Essential for immune health. Several studies have shown that vitamin C can help reduce the duration and severity of colds. Supplements may also play a role in prevention of colds, particularly in those with poor dietary intake or under stress and in athletes. Dosage: 500–2,000 mg daily throughout the cold season.

Zinc lozenges: Zinc is essential for immune function. Studies show that lozenges can help relieve symptoms (coughing, sore throat, and runny nose) and shorten the duration of a cold. Look for a product that provides 10–13.3 mg of zinc (gluconate or acetate). Take at the first sign of a cold. Dosage: One lozenge every few hours while awake, up to a maximum four to six lozenges daily.

Complementary Supplements

Aged garlic extract: Has antioxidant, anti-inflammatory, and immune-boosting properties. Taken regularly, it may help prevent colds by supporting immune function. Recent research also suggests it can reduce symptoms and duration in those who get sick. Dosage: 600–1,200 mg twice daily.

Probiotics: Support immune function and may help to prevent colds. Look for a product that provides at least 1 billion live cells and includes *Lactobacillus acidophilus* and *Bifido-bacterium*. Dosage: Take two to three times daily with meals. For infants and young children, consider BioGaia, available as a drop or chewable tablet. A study of infants in daycare given BioGaia found that it reduced fever, infections, and antibiotic use.

Propolis: A resin collected from trees. Some research suggests that it can help prevent and shorten the duration of a cold. Dosage: 500 mg twice daily.

FINAL THOUGHTS

To reduce your chances of catching a cold and speed the healing process when you do get a cold, consider the following:

• Eat a diet rich in fruits and vegetables; drink plenty of fluids.
• Exercise regularly and reduce stress.
• Wash your hands frequently and don't rub your eyes, nose, or mouth.
• For prevention, consider COLD-FX and vitamin C.
• To shorten the duration of a cold, try echinacea and zinc lozenges.

CONGESTIVE HEART FAILURE

Congestive heart failure (CHF), known simply as heart failure, occurs when your heart can't pump enough blood to meet your body's needs. CHF often results from other heart conditions, such as coronary artery disease or high blood pressure, which over time can damage and weaken the heart. When the heart can no longer pump blood efficiently through your body, blood and fluids back up into the circulatory system, causing swelling in your lungs, legs, feet, and ankles, and congestive symptoms such as shortness of breath.

Heart failure can develop suddenly due to damage caused by a heart attack, or it can develop gradually after years of having high blood pressure, coronary artery disease, or a defective heart valve. A number of lifestyle factors contribute to heart failure such as smoking, obesity, and diet. In some cases, though, the heart becomes weakened without explanation. This is called idiopathic dilated cardiomyopathy.

Heart failure is treatable with medication and lifestyle modifications. In many cases it is possible to prevent heart failure by controlling the risk factors that damage the heart. Maintaining a healthy diet, exercising regularly, not smoking, and reducing stress can help significantly. There are also a variety of supplements that can strengthen the function of the heart.

SIGNS & SYMPTOMS

- Difficulty concentrating or decreased alertness

- Fatigue and weakness

- Irregular or rapid heartbeat

- Lack of appetite and nausea

- Persistent cough or wheezing

- Reduced ability to exercise

- Shortness of breath when you exert yourself or lie down

- Sudden weight gain from fluid retention

- Swelling in your legs, ankles, feet, or abdomen

ACUTE HEART FAILURE

Acute heart failure occurs when something suddenly affects your heart's ability to function, such as a heart attack, a virus that attacks the heart muscle, severe infections, an allergic reaction, or a blood clot in the lungs. Signs and symptoms are similar to those of chronic heart failure, but are more severe and start suddenly. Acute heart failure can trigger a rapid heartbeat and abnormal rhythm. This requires immediate medical attention.

RISK FACTORS

- Age: Risk increases with advanced age (those over the age of 65 are at greatest risk).

- Gender: Men are at higher risk for heart failure.

- Ethnicity: Blacks are at greater risk to develop and die from CHF.

- Alcohol: Excessive intake weakens the heart muscle.

- Arrhythmia, an abnormal heartbeat, weakens the heart.

- Congenital heart defects put individuals at increased risk.

- Coronary artery disease: Plaque buildup causes the arteries to narrow, which limits the heart's supply of oxygen-rich blood.

- Diabetes increases the risk of high blood pressure and coronary artery disease.

- Heart attack damages the heart muscle.

- High blood pressure forces the heart to work harder.

- Kidney disease can cause high blood pressure and fluid retention, which contributes to heart failure.

- Obesity puts individuals at increased risk.

- Sleep apnea, an inability to breathe properly at night, results in low blood oxygen levels and increased risk of abnormal heart rhythms.

- Viral infections can damage the heart muscle.

DOCTOR'S ORDERS

Heart failure is a serious disease that requires medical care. Your doctor will recommend a combination of lifestyle measures and medications to help improve the strength of the heart and reduce symptoms of heart failure.

Commonly used medications include

Angiotensin-converting enzyme (ACE) inhibitors: Vasodilator drugs that widen or dilate blood vessels to lower blood pressure, improve blood flow, and decrease the workload of the heart. Examples include enalapril (Vasotec), lisinopril (Prinivil, Zestril), and ramipril (Altace). A major unpleasant side effect of these drugs is a chronic cough.

Angiotensin II (A-II) receptor blockers (ARBs): Work the same as the drugs above, but do not cause coughing. Examples include losartan (Cozaar) and valsartan (Diovan).

Beta blockers: Slow your heart rate and reduce blood pressure. Examples include carvedilol (Coreg), metoprolol (Lopressor), and propranolol (Inderal).

Digoxin (Lanoxin): Increases the strength of your heart muscle contractions and slows the heartbeat.

Diuretics: Commonly called water pills, diuretics make you urinate more frequently and keep fluid from collecting in your body. Examples include furosemide (Lasix) and spironolactone (Aldactone).

In some cases, surgery can be done to correct the underlying problem, such as replacing a faulty heart valve or doing bypass surgery on severely narrowed arteries. For those with severe heart failure that can't be helped by surgery or medications, a heart transplant may be necessary.

SHERRY'S NATURAL PRESCRIPTION

The key to managing or preventing heart failure is to get the risk factors under control, namely high blood pressure and coronary artery disease. Below are some recommendations to help improve heart function.

Dietary Recommendations

Foods to include:

- Cold-water fish contains omega-3 fatty acids that can help reduce blood pressure and cholesterol. Omega-3s are also found in chia seed and flaxseed.

- Drink green tea, which contains antioxidants that offer benefits for the heart.

- Eat small, frequent meals. Overeating is hard on the heart.

- Garlic and onions contain antioxidants that help lower blood pressure and cholesterol.

- Soy foods can help lower blood pressure. Incorporate soy milk, tofu, soy protein, and soy nuts into your diet.

- Whole grains, vegetables, fruits, beans, and legumes contain lots of fibre along with essential nutrients, which help lower blood pressure and cholesterol.

Foods to avoid:

- Alcohol can weaken heart function and interacts negatively with many heart medications. Avoid or limit alcohol to one drink per day.

- Caffeine can increase heart rate and affect heart rhythm.

- Saturated fat (red meat and dairy) and trans fats can increase cholesterol and the risk of coronary heart disease.

- Sodium (salt) can cause water retention and worsen heart failure. Limit sodium intake to 2,000 mg per day. Those with high blood pressure and other risk factors may be asked to limit sodium intake to 1,500 mg per day. Foods high in sodium include snack foods (chips, pretzels), deli meats, soft drinks, and fast foods. Don't add salt to your foods—season with herbs instead.

Note: Those with heart failure may need to limit fluid intake to prevent water retention. Speak with your doctor about this.

Lifestyle Suggestions

- Don't smoke, and avoid second-hand smoke. Tobacco damages blood vessels, reduces the oxygen in your blood, and makes your heart beat faster.

- Maintain a healthy body weight. Being overweight increases stress to the heart. Check your weight regularly as sudden weight gain can indicate worsening of symptoms.

- Get regular, moderate-intensity exercise, such as walking or swimming. Studies have shown that exercise can improve quality of life and function in those with CHF.

- Manage your stress. Stress increases heart rate and blood pressure, straining the heart. Try yoga, acupuncture, or meditation.

- Get adequate sleep at night (seven to nine hours). If you have shortness of breath during the night, prop up your pillow.

Top Recommended Supplements

Coenzyme Q10: An antioxidant that enhances energy production in the heart muscle. People with CHF have lower levels of Q10. Several studies have shown that supplements can significantly improve CHF symptoms and quality of life. Dosage: 100–300 mg daily.

Fish oils: Numerous studies have shown that the omega-3 fatty acids in fish oil can help lower blood pressure, reduce atherosclerosis, and protect against heart attack. There is also evidence that fish oil can reduce the risk of death in those with CHF. Dosage: 1–3 g of EPA plus DHA three times daily.

Hawthorn: Improves the heart's pumping ability and improves blood flow. Numerous studies have found that it can reduce symptoms of CHF and improve exercise capacity. Some research suggests that it may also help to prevent arrhythmias. Dosage: 300–600 mg three times daily.

L-carnitine: An amino acid naturally found in all cells. It helps the heart contract and produce energy more efficiently. Studies show that it improves heart function and can reduce the symptoms of CHF. Dosage: 500–1,000 mg two to three times daily.

L-taurine: An amino acid that helps increase the force and effectiveness of heart muscle contractions. Research has shown that taurine can reduce the symptoms of CHF. Dosage: 2 g three times daily.

Magnesium: Essential for heart health, proper muscle contractions, maintaining normal heart rhythm, and blood vessel health. Levels of magnesium are depleted by diuretics and digoxin, commonly used CHF drugs. Several studies suggest magnesium can promote modest reductions in blood pressure and improve CHF. Dosage: 100–300 mg daily as advised by your health care provider.

Complementary Supplements

Aged garlic extract: Helps lower blood pressure and cholesterol, reduces clotting, and prevents plaque formation in the arteries. Dosage: 600 mg twice daily.

Arginine: An amino acid required by the body to make nitric oxide, a substance that increases blood flow. There is some evidence that it can help improve symptoms and kidney function in those with CHF. Dosage: 5–15 g daily.

Potassium: Deficiency is common in those with CHF and is associated with risk factors and complications such as arrhythmias and blood vessel constriction. Some diuretics cause loss of potassium while others promote potassium retention, so check with your doctor before taking potassium.

Vitamin B1: Required for energy production in the cells of the heart. Taking diuretics depletes levels of vitamin B1, and some studies have shown that vitamin B1 supplements can help improve heart function and symptoms of CHF. Dosage: 100 mg daily as part of a B-complex.

FINAL THOUGHTS

To improve the management of CHF, consider the following:

- Boost intake of fibre, fish, fruits, vegetables, garlic, and green tea.
- Minimize intake of sodium, alcohol, caffeine, and saturated fat. Speak with your doctor about guidelines for fluid intake.
- Don't smoke.
- Get regular exercise and reduce your stress.
- Various supplements can help with CHF, but it is important to get advice from your health care provider and ensure that there are no interactions with prescribed medications.

CONSTIPATION

Constipation is a disorder of the lower gastrointestinal tract marked by a decrease in the frequency of stools, difficulty defecating, or the passage of dry, hard stools. Most people experience an occasional change in bowel habits; when it is persistent, it is referred to as chronic constipation.

During the digestive process, food passes from the stomach to the intestine where nutrients and water are absorbed into the body. The waste products of digestion create a stool, which travels through the intestines with muscle contractions. It normally takes 6 to 24 hours to pass a stool. Anything that slows the passage of stools through the intestines or increases the amount of water absorbed by the body—such as a lack of fibre, fluids, or physical activity; medication; or ignoring the urge to defecate—can lead to constipation.

Chronic constipation affects 31 percent of people between the ages of 19 and 65, and approximately 45 percent of people over age 65. This can be a debilitating and uncomfortable problem, but there are a number of lifestyle recommendations that can help.

SIGNS & SYMPTOMS

- Abdominal pain, bloating, and gas

- Bowel movements less than three times a week

- Passing hard stools

- Straining during a bowel movement

Chronic constipation can also cause bad breath, headache, fatigue, and hemorrhoids (due to straining), and worsen varicose veins.

Severe constipation may cause fecal impaction, a mass of hardened stool. This can be dangerous and may require removal by a doctor.

Note: See your doctor if you notice blood in your stool or have black stools, as this could signify a serious problem.

RISK FACTORS

- Age (more common in older adults)

- Diet (lack of fibre or fluids)

- Intolerance to cow's milk

- Health conditions: Irritable bowel, celiac disease, colon cancer, liver disease, and low thyroid

- Lack of activity (sedentary or bedridden)

- Medications: Sedatives, narcotics (codeine), chemotherapy, blood pressure drugs, Parkinson's drugs, and some antidepressants, antihistamines, and iron supplements

- Pregnancy (due to hormonal changes and pressure on the intestines)
- Stress (reduces intestinal motility)

DOCTOR'S ORDERS

Lifestyle approaches, such as increasing fibre and water intake and regular exercise, should be tried first. If this is not successful, your doctor may recommend drug therapy.

Stimulant laxatives irritate the colon wall to stimulate a bowel movement. Examples include bisacodyl (Dulcolax), senna (Senokot), castor oil, and cascara. These drugs work quickly (overnight), but may cause abdominal cramping and are recommended for short-term (a few days) use only. When taken regularly, they can cause dependence and other problems (see below).

Bulk-forming laxatives add bulk and water to the stools, which improves passage through the intestines. They are taken daily with plenty of fluids, and it may take a week to notice benefits. Side effects include temporary gas and bloating. Examples include bran, psyllium (Metamucil), methylcellulose (Citrucel), and inulin (Benefibre).

Stool softeners, such as docusate (Colace) and glycerin suppositories, cause water and fats to penetrate the stool, easing movement through the intestines. They may lead to tolerance and become ineffective with prolonged use. Mineral oil makes the stool slippery to facilitate passage; however, it should not be used regularly as it can reduce the absorption of fat-soluble vitamins (A, D, E, and K).

Enemas are reserved for severe cases. They should not be used regularly because they can cause electrolyte imbalances.

HOMEOPATHIC RECOMMENDATIONS

Graphites: This remedy is indicated when large stools look like little round balls. An achy feeling in the anus after the bowels have moved is commonly reported.

Lycopodium: A person who needs this remedy has frequent indigestion with gas and bloating, and many problems involving the bowels. Rubbing the abdomen or drinking something warm may help to relieve the constipation.

Combination recommendation: Laxative Combination R68 by Reckeweg

CAUTION: DO NOT OVERUSE LAXATIVES

Overuse of laxatives may cause dependence (lazy bowel syndrome), poor absorption of vitamins and nutrients (particularly potassium), dehydration, damage to the intestinal tract, and worsened constipation. Those who take laxatives for a long time may need to go off them slowly to allow the bowels to return to normal function.

SHERRY'S NATURAL PRESCRIPTION

Dietary Recommendations

Foods to include:

- High-fibre foods improve bowel regularity. Most foods contain a combination of both soluble and insoluble fibre, and both are important. Soluble fibre dissolves in water and forms a gel, adding volume to the stool and making it easier to pass. Good sources of soluble fibre include apples, avocados, bananas, plums, cereal grains (oats, barley, amaranth, kamut, and buckwheat), beans, nuts, and seeds (chia and flax). Insoluble fibre does not dissolve in water, but rather forms a soft pulp as it moves through the colon, aiding contractions of the colon. Insoluble fibre is found in wheat bran, many vegetables, and some fruits (apple and grape skin, berries, rhubarb, pineapple, and oranges). Several types of dietary fibre provide prebiotics, which are non-digestible food components that feed the beneficial bacteria (probiotics) in your gut. Good sources of prebiotics are inulin (chicory root and Jerusalem artichoke), soybeans, unrefined wheat and barley, and supplements as noted on the next page.

- Broccoli, spinach, and kale contain magnesium, which improves gut motility.

- Current guidelines recommend a daily fibre intake of 25 g and 38 g for women and men, respectively. (*Note:* Most Canadians consume less than half of the recommended amount of fibre.)

- Drink plenty of fluids. This is essential when increasing fibre intake. Fluids work with fibre to increase the bulk of the stool and ease passage. Water is best, but pure fruit and vegetable juices and herbal teas are also fine.

Foods to avoid:

- Refined and processed foods are high in sugar and contain little fibre.

- Cow's milk should be avoided by those with an intolerance as it can worsen constipation.

- Alcohol is dehydrating and should be minimized.

- Caffeine (coffee and tea) is also dehydrating; however, caffeine also promotes contractions in the bowel and many people find it helps initiate a bowel movement.

Lifestyle Suggestions

- Increase physical activity, as exercise helps stimulate intestinal and bowel contractions. Try walking, biking, or swimming.

- Set aside time to have a bowel movement each day, such as after breakfast.

- Don't resist the urge. The longer you delay going to the toilet once you feel the urge, the more water is absorbed from the stool and the harder it becomes.

- Acupuncture, massage, and reflexology may help by improving intestinal motility.

- Detoxification, such as a short-term cleanse or juice fast, along with fibre supplements, allows the body to focus on removal of waste. This is particularly helpful for chronic constipation. See Appendix C.

Top Recommended Supplements

Fibre supplements: Products containing psyllium husks, oat bran, guar gum, glucomannan, and fenugreek are effective and can be taken regularly. To minimize gas and bloating, start with a small amount (one tablespoonful daily) and gradually increase to allow your bowels to adjust. Take with plenty of water. Prebiotic fibre supplements help improve microflora balance and aid both constipation and diarrhea. An example is Sunfiber, a soluble dietary fibre made from hydrolyzed guar gum through a slow fermentation process, which leads to less gas, bloating, and discomfort.

Probiotics: Supplements containing these "friendly bacteria" help to restore the normal gut flora and have been shown to relieve constipation. Dosage: One to three capsules daily.

Complementary Supplements

Aloe vera juice: Aids bowel movements by working as a stimulant laxative and improving intestinal contractions. For short-term use only; may cause significant cramping. Dosage: 65 mL twice daily.

Magnesium: Aids intestinal function and helps stool retain water; may be deficient in those with constipation. Dosage: 200 mg twice daily. Higher dosages are used to relieve acute constipation.

Vitamin C: High dosages can help promote a bowel movement by stimulating contractions of the colon, but this should only be done to relieve an acute bout of constipation. Vitamin C may be combined with magnesium Dosage: 4 g. Buffered vitamin C is easier on the stomach while still providing benefits.

FINAL THOUGHTS

To prevent constipation and optimize bowel function:

• Consume 25 g or 38 g of fibre daily (for men and women, respectively). Best sources are whole grains, vegetables, fruits, and legumes.
• Drink lots of fluids, especially after exercising.
• Get regular physical activity to stimulate intestinal contractions.
• Consider fibre supplements to complement your diet.
• Probiotics can help improve intestinal health and function.

CROHN'S DISEASE AND COLITIS

Crohn's disease and colitis are categorized as inflammatory bowel diseases, or IBD. These diseases affect the digestive system and cause the intestinal tissue to become inflamed, develop sores, and bleed. Over 200,000 Canadians suffer from IBD. These diseases can be painful and debilitating and may lead to life-threatening complications, especially if untreated.

Crohn's disease and ulcerative colitis are very similar in that they both inflame the lining of your digestive tract and can cause severe bouts of watery or bloody diarrhea and abdominal pain. Where they differ is that Crohn's disease can occur anywhere in your digestive tract, often spreading deep into the layers of affected tissues, whereas ulcerative colitis usually affects only the innermost lining of your large intestine (colon) and rectum. Symptoms may come and go and those affected may also experience long periods of remission.

The actual cause of these diseases is unknown. Stress can aggravate symptoms and was once considered to be the underlying cause, but that is no longer the case. Many practitioners, especially those with knowledge of nutrition and preventative medicine, feel that diet may be responsible for triggering these diseases. Both diseases are rare in developing countries and among cultures that eat whole, unprocessed foods. As well, it wasn't until the mid-1900s that these diseases became a problem in North America. Our diets have drastically changed over the decades, and consumption of fast foods and processed and refined foods and ingestion of chemical food additives is now common. Food allergies may also play a part.

It is also possible that the inflammation may stem from the immune system's response to infection with a virus or bacterium. Since the diseases are more common among those with a family history, genetic mutations may also be to blame.

While there is no known medical cure for Crohn's disease or colitis, there are a variety of lifestyle approaches, supplements, and medications that can reduce the symptoms and even bring about long-term remission.

SIGNS & SYMPTOMS

The signs and symptoms of Crohn's disease and ulcerative colitis can vary widely, depending on the severity of inflammation and where it occurs, and include the following:

• Abdominal pain and cramping: Inflammation and ulceration causes the walls of the bowel to swell and develop scar tissue, which causes pain as food moves through your digestive tract.

• Blood in the stool: Caused by the inflammation and ulceration.

• Diarrhea and gas: The inflammation causes cells in the intestine to secrete large amounts of water and salt, leading to loose stools or diarrhea.

• Fatigue, nausea, and headache.

- Loss of appetite and weight loss: The pain and cramping can affect appetite, and the damage to the intestine can impair food and nutrient absorption.

- Nutrient deficiencies are common in those with IBD because of intestinal damage, impaired nutrient absorption, poor appetite, and drug-induced depletion.

- Sores, ulcers, fistulas, and perforation of the intestine.

- Aspirin use: Emerging evidence suggests that taking aspirin regularly may increase the risk of developing Crohn's disease. One recent study reported that those taking aspirin regularly for a year or more were around five times more likely to develop Crohn's disease.

Some people with these diseases experience inflammation in other areas of the body (joints, skin, and eyes).

RISK FACTORS

- Age: Those between the ages of 15 and 35 are at greatest risk.

- Diet: Eating a diet high in refined foods and fat and low in fibre increases the risk.

- Family history: Having a parent or sibling with the condition greatly increases the risk.

- Race: Caucasians, Jewish people, and those of Eastern European descent are four to five times more likely to develop Crohn's disease and colitis.

- Smoking significantly increases risk of Crohn's disease. Smokers who have Crohn's also experience more severe symptoms and face a higher rate of relapse, surgery, and need for drug therapy. It is thought that smoking lowers the intestines' defences, decreases blood flow to the intestines, and causes inflammation in the intestines.

DOCTOR'S ORDERS

The goal of medical treatment is to reduce inflammation and promote healing of the intestine. In some cases it is possible to achieve long-term remission. Dietary changes and supplements can be very helpful. Depending on your situation and the severity of the symptoms and intestinal damage, your doctor may prescribe drug therapy to control the inflammation. Commonly used drugs include sulfasalazine, mesalamine (Asacol), and corticosteroids, such as prednisone. There are also drugs that reduce inflammation by suppressing the immune system, such as azathioprine (Imuran) and infliximab (Remicade). These drugs are used for moderate to severe forms of the disease and carry the risk of serious side effects. Some drugs work well for some people, but not for others. It is important to discuss the benefits and risks with your doctor.

Antidiarrheal medications or laxatives may sometimes be necessary. Iron supplements are used for anemia, which occurs from chronic intestinal bleeding. For severe cases, surgery to remove the diseased portions of the bowel may be necessary, but this is always the last resort.

Crohn's Disease and Colitis

SHERRY'S NATURAL PRESCRIPTION

Dietary Recommendations

Diet plays a very important role in managing IBD. Ensuring adequate nutrient intake is critical since vitamin and mineral deficiencies are common.

Foods to include:

• Aloe vera juice has anti-inflammatory activity. One study of people with colitis found that 100 mL of aloe vera juice twice daily resulted in a complete remission or an improvement in symptoms in 47 percent of cases, compared with 14 percent of those given a placebo.

• Barley and wheat grass juice contain various vitamins, minerals, natural enzymes, and chlorophyll. There is some evidence that these juices can reduce intestinal inflammation and reduce symptoms of IBD.

• Soluble fibre can help improve symptoms of both constipation and diarrhea. Good sources include apples (pectin), bananas, berries, chia seed, oats, carrots, and potatoes. Gradually incorporate soluble fibre into your diet, and be cautious during periods of active disease.

• Yogurt with active cultures provides beneficial bacteria that can support intestinal health and aid digestion. It is also a good source of protein. Choose a natural, unsweetened yogurt.

• Green tea is an antioxidant that supports digestion and immune function and cuts the risk of disease.

• Dark chocolate: A recent study found daily consumption of 40 g of dark chocolate can improve gut microflora and metabolism by lowering levels of stress hormones.

• Drink plenty of fluids (water, broth, and juice) to prevent dehydration from chronic diarrhea. Herbal teas made from chamomile, slippery elm, and marshmallow can be very soothing to an inflamed gastrointestinal tract. These herbs also help facilitate digestion.

• Eat small, frequent meals, which is easier on digestion.

• Ensure adequate protein intake as protein deficiency is common in those with IBD. Eat lean poultry, fish, beans, and legumes. Fish contains beneficial omega-3 fatty acids (EPA and DHA), which can help reduce inflammation. The best sources of these fatty acids are salmon, herring, mackerel, albacore tuna, and sardines.

• Whole grains (whole oats, brown rice, and quinoa), vegetables, and fruits as tolerated provide energy and essential nutrients. During flare-ups, when the intestines are inflamed, raw vegetables and fruits can be irritating, so it is best to cook (steam) these foods.

Foods to avoid:

• Alcohol, caffeine, and spicy foods can irritate the intestines.

• Dairy and gluten/wheat are common triggers for those with IBD. Lactose intolerance is also common in those with IBD. Carrageenan, a compound used to stabilize milk proteins, has been shown to induce ulcerative colitis in animals. Cow's milk contains a bacterium (*Mycobacterium avium paratuberculosis*) that survives pasteurization and has been linked to Crohn's disease.

- Fast foods are typically high in saturated fat, refined starches, and preservatives, all of which can worsen symptoms. One study found that those who eat fast foods at least two times per week more than triple their risk of developing Crohn's disease.

- Refined flour (white bread and foods made with refined flour) is associated with worsening of symptoms.

- Saturated fats (e.g., butter, cream, cheese, meat) can worsen inflammation and irritate your intestine.

- Sugar has been shown in some research to worsen IBD, so limit intake from all sources (table sugar, candy, soft drinks).

Try an elimination diet to determine if food allergies are worsening your symptoms. See Appendix D for more information.

Lifestyle Suggestions

- Manage stress—stress can trigger flare-ups.

- Try acupuncture. There is some evidence that it can improve symptoms of Crohn's.

- Don't smoke—smoking can increase the risk of relapse.

- Get regular exercise to reduce stress and improve mood and energy levels.

Top Recommended Supplements

Fish oil: Contains omega-3 fatty acids, which have been shown to reduce inflammation and improve symptoms of IBD. One study also found that fish oil supplements reduced the risk of relapse and flare-up. Dosage: Take a daily dosage that provides at least 3–6 g of EPA/DHA.

Multivitamin and mineral complex: Nutrients most commonly deficient in those with IBD include vitamins A, B12, C, D, E, and K, folate, calcium, copper, magnesium, selenium, and zinc. Taking a quality multivitamin every day can help restore nutrient levels and improve overall health. Those with severe damage to the intestine may not be able to absorb vitamin B12; sublingual (under the tongue) tablets or injections can be taken in these cases. Additional antioxidants such as glutathione may provide benefits to reduce free radical damage caused by inflammation.

Probiotics: IBD can cause the normal bacteria flora of the intestine to be depleted, which can lead to digestive and bowel problems. Replacing the flora with probiotic supplements can help improve digestion and nutrient absorption and relieve constipation and diarrhea. Choose a probiotic that has been studied specifically for IBD, such as VSL#3 (8 strain probiotic). VSL#3 has shown benefits for adults and children with active ulcerative colitis and those in remission. There is also evidence that it can help those with IBD who develop pouchitis (inflammation of the lining of a pouch, an internal reservoir created following surgical removal of the colon).

Complementary Supplements

Boswellia: An herb with anti-inflammatory properties. Some research has shown that it can reduce symptoms of both Crohn's disease and colitis, similarly to prescription drugs. Dosage: 1,200 mg three times daily.

Curcumin (from the spice turmeric): Preliminary research shows it can help maintain remission in individuals with ulcerative colitis. Dosage: 1 g twice daily.

Digestive enzymes: People with IBD may be deficient in digestive enzymes, particularly those with severe intestinal damage. Supplements can help aid food digestion and nutrient absorption. Dosage: Take one or two capsules with each meal.

Glutamine: An amino acid that helps repair the intestinal lining. Dosage: 1,000 mg three times daily on an empty stomach.

Greens supplements: Contain barley and wheat grass, which can help soothe an inflamed intestine and provide essential nutrients. Recommended products include Greens+ and Kyo-Green. Dosage: Powders should be mixed with water or juice and taken daily.

Vitamin D: Deficiency is common in those with IBD and can lead to osteoporosis. Supplements can help maintain adequate vitamin D levels and support bone health. Dosage: 400 to 1,000 IU daily.

FINAL THOUGHTS

To manage the symptoms of Crohn's disease and colitis, consider the following:

- Avoid processed/refined/fast food, sugar, and dairy.
- Eat small, frequent meals of fish, brown rice, and vegetables (cooked).
- Drink barley, wheat grass, aloe vera juice, and plenty of water.
- Reduce stress, get regular exercise, and don't smoke.
- Fish oil, multivitamins, and probiotics (VSL#3) are highly recommended.

DEPRESSION

Depression is a disorder that affects your mood, thoughts, feelings, and behaviour. It is the most common psychiatric ailment in Western society. Depression affects approximately 1.7 million Canadians at any given time and is the second leading cause of long-term disability. It is much more than a case of the "blues." Depression can be serious and debilitating.

Although the exact cause of depression is not known, a variety of underlying factors may be involved, including the following:

Biological: Imbalance of neurotransmitters (chemical messengers in the brain—dopamine, serotonin, and norepinephrine) or hormone imbalance (as occurs with postpartum depression and menopause or with low thyroid function)

Environmental: Exposure to chemicals that disrupt brain chemistry (cigarette smoking, heavy metals, prescription and recreational drugs)

Nutritional: Deficiency of vitamins (B12), minerals (magnesium), or essential fatty acids; food allergies

Situational: Stress, trauma, injury, divorce, job loss, death of a loved one

Anyone suffering with depression should seek professional help to determine the underlying cause and an appropriate treatment.

SIGNS & SYMPTOMS

Major depression is diagnosed when a person has five or more of the following symptoms over a two-week period. At least one of the symptoms must be either a depressed mood or a loss of interest or pleasure.

• Agitation or sluggishness in movement and thought

• Depressed mood most of the day (feeling say, empty, or tearful)

• Difficulty concentrating, thinking, or making decisions

• Fatigue or loss of energy

• Feelings of worthlessness or excessive or inappropriate guilt

• Insomnia or increased sleep

• Loss of interest or pleasure in usual activities

• Recurrent thoughts of death or suicide

• Significant weight loss or weight gain; changes in appetite

RISK FACTORS

- Family history (previous depression or having a parent or grandparent with depression)

- Gender (twice as many women experience depression than men, likely due to hormonal changes—postpartum, menopause, and PMS)

- Having few friends or personal relationships

- Insomnia (due to the effect on hormones in the brain)

- Medical conditions (cancer, stroke, heart disease, diabetes, HIV/AIDS, headaches, anxiety, hypothyroidism, obesity, and other hormonal imbalances)

- Medications (sedatives, narcotics, corticosteroids, blood pressure and cholesterol-lowering drugs) and drug abuse (alcohol, nicotine, illicit drugs)

- Personality characteristics (low self-esteem; pessimism; attention, conduct, or learning disorders)

- Stress (loss of loved one, financial or relationship problems, trauma)

INSOMNIA AND DEPRESSION

There is a strong link between insomnia and depression. Studies estimate that 20 percent of people with insomnia suffer from major depression and 90 percent of people with depression have insomnia.

HOMEOPATHIC RECOMMENDATIONS

Aurum metallicum: This remedy can be helpful for serious people who are strongly focused on work and achievement, and who become depressed after a strong sense of failure. Discouragement, self-reproach, humiliation, and anger can lead to feelings of emptiness and worthlessness. This symptom picture is usually accompanied by nightmares and oversleeping that fluctuates with insomnia.

Staphysagria: This is used for feelings of hurt, shame, resentment, and suppressed emotions that can lead to depression. If under too much pressure, they can sometimes lose their natural inhibition and fly into rages or throw things. A person who needs this remedy may also have insomnia (feeling sleepy all day, but unable to sleep at night), toothaches, headaches, stomach aches, or bladder infections that are all stress related.

Combination recommendation: There is no effective combination remedy known; use Rescue Remedy by Bach for short periods when feeling overwhelmed.

DOCTOR'S ORDERS

Medical treatment typically involves prescription drugs and counselling. There are several classes of antidepressant drugs: tricyclic antidepressants (TCAs), monoamine oxidase inhibitors (MAOIs), selective serotonin reuptake inhibitors (SSRIs), serotonin and norepinephrine reuptake inhibitors (SNRIs), norepinephrine and dopamine reuptake inhibitors (NDRIs), and atypical drugs. TCAs include amitriptyline, clomipramine, and imipramine. MAOIs include moclobemide (Manerix). These two classes are less commonly used since the discovery of the newer classes. SSRIs include fluoxetine (Prozac), fluvoxamine (Luvox), citalopram (Celexa), paroxetine (Paxil), and sertraline (Zoloft). SNRIs include duloxetine (Cymbalta) and venlafaxine (Effexor XR). NDRIs include bupropion (Wellbutrin) and atypical drugs include mirtazapine (Remeron).

While antidepressant drugs may be necessary and do help some people, recent studies suggest that counselling (psychotherapy) is just as effective for mild to moderate depression. It may take several weeks to notice improvement with antidepressant drugs. All of these drug classes can cause a range of side effects. The most common side effects of SSRIs and SNRIs include nausea, weight gain/loss, headaches, anxiety, nervousness, insomnia or drowsiness, diarrhea or constipation, sweating, tremors, and sexual dysfunction (decreased sexual desire and delayed orgasm). Bupropion is less likely to cause sexual side effects, but it can cause significant agitation, dry mouth, insomnia, and seizures (particularly at higher dosages). Common side effects of mirtazapine include abnormal dreams, constipation, dizziness, dry mouth, and weight gain.

There are numerous drug interactions with all antidepressant drugs; consult with your pharmacist before taking any other prescription or natural products.

SHERRY'S NATURAL PRESCRIPTION

Dietary Recommendations

A healthy diet helps balance mood. Follow dietary recommendations outlined in Chapter 4. Eat small, frequent meals to maintain good energy and mood. Since food allergies can also trigger depression, refer to Appendix D for information on identifying possible allergies.

Foods to include:

• Vegetables, fruits, whole grains, nuts, and seeds are good sources of vitamins and minerals, which may be depleted in those with depression.

• Cold-water fish provide omega-3 fatty acids, which support brain health. Vegetarian sources of omega-3s include chia seed, flaxseed, and nuts.

• Turkey and salmon contain the amino acid tryptophan, which elevates serotonin production.

Foods to avoid:

• Sugar, soft drinks, and refined carbohydrates (white flour) can cause blood sugar fluctuations and trigger mood swings and irritability. Caffeine may also trigger mood swings and anxiety in some people; however, some recent research suggests it may play a protective role in depression. The antioxidants in coffee may protect the brain against free radical damage.

• Processed and fast foods often contain chemicals and preservatives that may upset brain chemistry.

• Alcohol is a nervous system depressant and should be minimized or avoided completely, especially by those taking medication.

Note: If you are taking MAOI drugs, avoid soy sauce, bologna, canned meats, fermented sausage, salami, ripened cheese, red wine, and yeast concentrates.

Lifestyle Suggestions

• Acupuncture: Studies have found it beneficial for depression. It may work by stimulating the production of neurotransmitters.

• Counselling: Therapy with a psychologist or psychiatrist can be very beneficial. Some research has found cognitive therapy equally effective as drug therapy.

• Exercise: Research has shown that exercise offers powerful benefits for relieving depression and stress and improving mood, well-being, and sleep. Aim for 30 minutes to one hour of activity daily—walking, cycling, swimming, yoga, or any activity you enjoy. Gradually build up intensity, as high intensity seems to be more effective to boost well-being.

• Massage and reflexology: Both help to relieve stress and tension and promote relaxation.

• Get adequate sleep: Quality sleep is essential for mental and physical health. If you are struggling with insomnia, refer to that section of this book for recommendations.

Top Recommended Supplements

Fish oil: Rich in omega-3 fatty acids, which are essential for the nervous system and support neurotransmitter function. Levels may be depleted in those with depression. Studies show benefits for depression, especially for those not getting adequate response to antidepressant drugs. Dosage: 1–2 g of EPA daily.

L-theanine: An amino acid present in green tea. Studies of a patented and pure form of L-theanine (Suntheanine) show it reduces stress and anxiety without causing drowsiness or addiction and also improves sleep quality. It works quickly to promote calming (30 minutes to one hour), and there are no known side effects. Dosage: 50–200 mg daily.

S-adenosylmethionine (SAMe): Supports the production of serotonin, dopamine, and norepinephrine; improves communication between nerve cells; and is an antioxidant (protects brain tissues against damage from free radicals). Numerous studies demonstrate benefits for improving depression with results comparable to conventional antidepressants. SAMe is well tolerated, has positive side effects (supports joint and liver health), and has a quick onset of action (two weeks). Not recommended for those with bipolar disorder (manic depression) as it can worsen the manic symptoms. Dosage: 400–1,600 mg daily on an empty stomach; start with a low dose and gradually increase if needed.

St. John's wort: Increases neurotransmitter levels. Numerous studies show it is effective for mild to moderate depression with effects comparable to prescription drugs. May take two to four weeks to notice benefits; side effects are rare and include stomach upset, fatigue, itching, sleep disturbance, skin rash, and sun sensitivity. St. John's wort interacts with many drugs, such as oral contraceptives, blood thinners, and other antidepressants; check with your pharmacist. Dosage: 300 mg three times daily.

Vitamin D: A deficiency has been reported in many people with depression, and supplements have been shown to improve mood in several studies. Dosage: 1,000–2,000 IU or even more as advised by your health care provider.

Complementary Supplements

B-complex: B-vitamins (such as B12 and folic acid) may be deficient in those with depression. Folic acid works with SAMe to boost neurotransmitter levels. Several studies have found benefits. Take 400–1,000 mcg folic acid, 1,000 mcg vitamin B12, along with 50–100 mg of other B-vitamins daily to support brain function.

5-hydroxytryptophan (5-HTP): A substance used by the body to create serotonin. Preliminary research shows benefits for depression. Side effects are rare and minor (upset stomach). Avoid use with other products that affect serotonin levels. Dosage: 100 mg three times daily.

Ginkgo biloba: Improves blood flow to the brain, improves memory and cognitive function, and may also improve serotonin response. Supplements may be particularly beneficial for the elderly. Dosage: 40–120 mg daily. *Note:* Ginkgo may enhance the effect of blood-thinning medications.

Tyrosine: An amino acid that helps depression. Dosage: 200–500 mg daily. Do not combine with prescription antidepressants.

FINAL THOUGHTS

If you or someone you know is suffering with depression, seek professional help and consider the following:

- Eat a healthy diet and avoid sugar, refined/processed foods, caffeine, and alcohol.
- Exercise regularly to reduce stress and improve mood and sleep.
- Try acupuncture, massage, and professional counselling.
- Consider SAMe or St. John's wort; both offer significant benefits for depression.
- Take fish oils, a B-complex, and vitamin D daily for overall brain function and improved mood, and consider Suntheanine to reduce stress and anxiety.

DIABETES

Diabetes is a chronic disease where the body does not make enough insulin or becomes insensitive (resistant) to the insulin that is produced. According to the Canadian Diabetes Association, over 9 million Canadians have diabetes or pre-diabetes (the precursor to diabetes). Unfortunately, this figure is expected to rise.

When we consume food, it is broken down into glucose, which causes a rise in blood glucose levels. Insulin is a hormone secreted by the pancreas in response to that rise in blood sugar. Insulin's role is to transport glucose from the bloodstream into the cells to be used for energy.

There are currently three main types of diabetes. Type 1 diabetes is responsible for approximately 10 percent of cases and occurs when the pancreas produces little or no insulin. The exact cause of type 1 diabetes is unknown, but it is thought that the immune system attacks and destroys the insulin-producing cells of the pancreas. Genetics may also play a role. Type 1 diabetes was previously known as juvenile diabetes or insulin-dependent diabetes because it typically appears during childhood or adolescence, and people who get this form require insulin injections to manage their blood sugar.

Type 2 diabetes is the most common form, accounting for about 90 percent of people with diabetes. This form occurs when the pancreas does not produce enough insulin or when your cells become resistant to the action of insulin. Obesity, inactivity, and poor diet (eating too many high-glycemic foods) are some of the causes of type 2 diabetes. Other risk factors are discussed on page 208. In the past, type 2 diabetes affected primarily adults. However, a growing number of children and adolescents are being diagnosed today. Pre-diabetes refers to a condition where your blood sugar levels are higher than normal but not yet considered diabetic. Not all people with pre-diabetes develop type 2 diabetes; lifestyle changes can play a significant role in preventing the progression to type 2 diabetes.

Diabetes can also occur during pregnancy, which is called gestational diabetes. It affects approximately 3.5 percent of all pregnancies and involves an increased risk of developing diabetes for both mother and child.

Recent research has identified another form of diabetes that affects the brain and may eventually be called type 3 diabetes. Numerous studies have found that diabetes significantly increases the risk of cognitive decline and dementia, including Alzheimer's disease. It is thought that hyperglycemia, insulin resistance, oxidative stress, and the production of inflammatory compounds is what leads to cognitive decline.

All forms of diabetes can have serious consequences if left untreated. While there is no cure for type 1 and type 2 diabetes, gestational diabetes and pre-diabetes are often reversible. With all forms of diabetes there is much that can be done from a lifestyle perspective to improve blood sugar control and prevent potentially life-threatening complications.

SIGNS & SYMPTOMS

Type 1 diabetes:

• Increased thirst and frequent urination (as excess sugar builds up in your bloodstream, fluid is pulled from your tissues, which can make you thirsty, so you may drink and urinate more than usual)

• Extreme hunger (your muscles and organs become energy depleted because insulin is not able to move glucose into your cells, which can trigger persistent hunger)

• Unusual weight loss (muscle and fat stores may shrink because they are not getting the necessary glucose)

• Extreme fatigue and irritability

Type 2 diabetes:

• Any of the type 1 symptoms

• Frequent infections

• Blurred vision (high blood sugar causes fluid to be pulled from all tissues, including the lenses of the eyes, which can affect vision)

• Cuts/bruises that are slow to heal

• Circulatory problems: Numbness or tingling in the hands or feet; difficulty getting or maintaining an erection

• Recurring skin, gum, or bladder infections

Note: Many people with type 2 diabetes have no obvious symptoms until they develop complications of the disease.

DIABETIC COMPLICATIONS

If left untreated, diabetes can lead to serious complications. Uncontrolled high blood sugar can cause damage to blood vessels throughout the body. Diabetes dramatically increases the risk of heart disease and stroke. In fact, about 75 percent of people who have diabetes die of some type of heart or blood vessel disease. Other complications include kidney and eye disease, nerve damage (diabetic foot and erectile dysfunction), and increased risk of infection.

RISK FACTORS

Type 1 diabetes:

• Genetics: Having a parent or sibling with type 1 diabetes

• Race: Type 1 diabetes is more common in Caucasians

• Possible factors that are still being explored include environment (viral illness) and diet (low intake of vitamin D and early exposure to cow's milk)

Type 2 diabetes:

• Age: The risk of type 2 diabetes increases with age, especially after age 40. Aging does not cause diabetes, but people tend to exercise less and gain weight with age.

• Gestational diabetes: Developing diabetes during pregnancy increases the risk of developing type 2 diabetes later in life. Giving birth to a baby that weighed more than 4 kg (9 lbs) is also associated with increased risk of developing diabetes.

• Heredity: Having a parent or sibling with either type of diabetes increases the risk.

• Impaired glucose tolerance or impaired fasting glucose increases the risk.

• Inactivity increases the risk of type 2 diabetes; conversely, physical activity improves insulin sensitivity and reduces the risk.

• Obesity (especially belly fat) greatly increases the risk of type 2 diabetes because carrying excess body fat reduces insulin sensitivity.

• Race: Those of Aboriginal, Hispanic, Asian, or African descent are at greater risk.

• Having high blood pressure, high cholesterol, or triglycerides, or being diagnosed with polycystic ovarian syndrome, acanthosis nigricans (a skin disorder that causes darkened patches of skin), or schizophrenia increases the risk.

Note: A growing body of research suggests that a high-glycemic-index diet (consuming quick-release carbohydrates that are high in the glycemic index) increases the risk of type 2 diabetes, although this is not an established risk factor. There is also significant evidence that following a low-glycemic diet can help improve blood glucose control and insulin sensitivity in those with either type 1 or type 2 diabetes.

Gestational diabetes:

• Age: Being over age 35

• History of polycystic ovarian syndrome (PCOS) or acanthosis nigricans

• Medication: Use of corticosteroids

• Previous diagnosis of gestational diabetes

• Race: Aboriginal, Hispanic, South Asian, Asian, or African descent

• Obesity: BMI of 30 kg/m^2 or higher

SKIN TAGS AND DIABETES

Recent research has found a link between skin tags and type 2 diabetes. Skin tags are associated with impaired carbohydrate metabolism, and their presence can indicate that a person is at risk of developing type 2 diabetes. Several studies suggest that having as few as three skin tags can increase the risk of diabetes. Studies have also shown that those with skin tags have higher cholesterol, blood sugar, and C-reactive protein than those without skin tags (all risk factors for diabetes and cardiovascular disease).

DOCTOR'S ORDERS

People with type 1 diabetes require insulin injections to manage blood sugar. In the past the only way to get insulin was through injection with a needle and syringe. Now there are insulin pen devices and pumps that are more convenient and less painful.

There are also several types of insulin that vary in their onset and duration of action. Your doctor will help devise a plan based on your needs.

Some people with type 2 diabetes can manage their blood sugar with diet and exercise alone, but in some cases medication or insulin is required. There are a variety of oral medications used for diabetes:

- Glyburide (Diabeta), gliclazide (Diamicron), and repaglinide (GlucoNorm) work by stimulating the pancreas to produce and release more insulin.
- Metformin works by reducing the amount of glucose produced by the liver and increasing your body's sensitivity to insulin.
- Drugs like rosiglitazone (Avandia) and pioglitazone (Actos) help insulin work better in the muscle and fat and also reduce glucose production in the liver.
- The newest class of oral medications, the DPP-4 inhibitors, such as sitagliptin (Januvia), work by preventing the breakdown of a naturally occurring compound in the body called glucagon-like peptide (GLP-1). GLP-1 reduces blood glucose levels in the body, so by interfering with its breakdown, these drugs allow it to remain active in the body longer, lowering blood glucose levels only when they are elevated.
- The newest class of injectable drugs are the GLP-1 receptor agonists, such as exenatide (Byetta) and liraglutide (Victoza). These drugs improve glycemic control by enhancing glucose-dependent insulin release from the pancreas, suppressing inappropriately elevated glucagon secretion, and slowing gastric emptying. These drugs are used primarily for managing type 2 diabetes.

All of these drugs have potential side effects and drug interactions, which should be reviewed by your doctor and pharmacist.

A number of factors can affect blood sugar levels, such as diet, activity level, illness, medication, alcohol, and stress. Careful monitoring is essential to ensure that your blood sugar levels are within the recommended range. Depending on your situation, your doctor may advise you to check your blood sugar once a day or more often. Fasting blood glucose levels should be between 4 and 7 mmol/L. The recommended range two hours after meals is between 5 and 10 mmol/L.

In addition to daily blood sugar monitoring, your doctor may recommend an A1C test, which measures your average blood sugar level for the past 120 days. This test indicates how well your diabetes treatment plan is working overall. The recommended A1C level for diabetics is 7 percent or less.

HYPOGLYCEMIA

Hypoglycemia, or low blood sugar, occurs when your blood sugar drops to less than 4 mmol/L. Symptoms include shakiness, lightheadedness, irritability, confusion, racing heart, and sweating. Hypoglycemia can result from not eating at regular intervals, intense physical activity, taking too much medication, or drinking alcohol. Blood glucose levels can drop quickly, and in severe cases can lead to loss of consciousness and seizures, so it is important to act quickly and eat or drink a fast-acting carbohydrate such as glucose tablets, honey, juice, or candy to raise blood sugar levels.

SHERRY'S NATURAL PRESCRIPTION

Dietary Recommendations

Foods to include:

- Cinnamon contains compounds that work synergistically with insulin, helping to reduce blood sugar levels. One study found benefits with just 1/2 tsp daily. Add cinnamon to your cereal, oatmeal, or breakfast shakes.

- Chromium is essential for blood glucose regulation. It is found in brewer's yeast, whole grains (especially wheat germ), onions, and garlic.

- For a natural and healthy sugar substitute, try stevia or xylitol.

- High-fibre, low-glycemic (slow-release) carbohydrates such as whole grains (quinoa, buckwheat, whole wheat, oats, brown rice, spelt), vegetables, fruits, seeds (chia, flax, and hemp), and legumes help to balance blood sugar.

- Protein (lean poultry, meat, and fish) and healthy fats (nuts, seeds, olive oil, and palm fruit oil) in each meal will slow carbohydrate digestion and promote better blood sugar control.

Note: To promote steady blood sugar levels, eat small, frequent meals (every two to three hours).

Foods to avoid:

- Alcohol can cause either high or low blood sugar depending on how much you drink and if you are eating while drinking. Limit alcohol intake to no more than two drinks daily.

- High-glycemic (quick-release) carbohydrates, such as white bread and baked goods, refined cereals, potatoes, white rice, and sugar (candy, cookies, soda), cause rapid and profound increases in blood sugar, creating a problem for diabetics. Studies have also found that those who eat high-glycemic diets are also at increased risk of developing type 2 diabetes.

- Saturated fat (animal products such as meat and dairy) can worsen blood glucose control.

Lifestyle Suggestions

- Lose excess weight: Being overweight can impair insulin sensitivity.

- Limit sugar intake to less than 10 percent of total caloric intake: Consuming more than this can negatively impact blood sugar and triglyceride levels.

- Get regular physical activity: Aim for 30 minutes to one hour of moderate-intensity activity each day, such as brisk walking, cycling, or swimming. Exercise helps with weight management and also improves blood glucose control and insulin sensitivity.

- Don't smoke: People with diabetes who smoke are at greater risk for heart, kidney, and eye disease, and nerve damage.

- Manage your stress: Stress triggers the release of hormones that impair insulin sensitivity. Try yoga, meditation, or other relaxation techniques.

- Practise good oral hygiene: Brush your teeth at least twice a day and floss daily to reduce the risk of gum infection. Visit your dentist regularly for professional cleaning.

- Take care of your feet: Diabetics are prone to nerve damage, which can make sores on the feet unnoticeable and delay wound healing. Inspect your feet daily for blisters or cuts. Apply moisturizer, particularly to your heels. See your doctor if you develop any sores that do not heal within a few days.

- Have regular physicals and eye exams to screen for potential complications.

Top Recommended Supplements

Alpha lipoic acid: A powerful antioxidant that can help improve insulin sensitivity and reduce the risk of diabetic complications such as neuropathy and nephropathy (kidney disease). Dosage: 600–1,200 mg daily.

Chromium: An essential trace mineral that plays a role in sugar metabolism. It helps improve insulin sensitivity and glucose tolerance. Some studies have found that diabetics are deficient in chromium and that supplements can help improve blood sugar management. Look for chromium picolinate as this is the most widely studied form of chromium. Dosage: 200–1,000 mcg daily.

Soluble fibre: Helps improve blood glucose control, reduces cholesterol and triglyceride levels, and supports weight management. Studies involving fibre supplements of fenugreek, psyllium, oat bran, guar, and glucomannan have shown benefits for diabetics by slowing carbohydrate digestion and absorption and aiding in weight management. Prebiotic fibre supplements, such as Sunfiber, can also help improve gut microflora balance and digestion. Sunfiber is made from hydrolyzed guar through a special fermentation process, leading to better tolerability (less gas and bloating). Take with plenty of water.

Complementary Supplements

B-vitamins: Essential for proper nerve function and energy metabolism. Take a B-complex or a multivitamin that contains at least 50 mg of the B-vitamins.

Chirositol: A nutrient derived from carob juice. Preliminary studies show it can help improve blood glucose metabolism, improve insulin sensitivity, and aid weight loss. This supplement may be particularly beneficial for those with pre-diabetes or type 2 diabetes, and those who are overweight. Dosage: 600–1,200 mg daily.

Fish oil: Helps improve glucose tolerance, reduces triglycerides and cholesterol levels, and may help improve diabetic complications (neuropathy and nephropathy). Dosage: Look for a product that provides at least 400 mg EPA and 200 mg DHA per dosage, and take three times daily.

Gymnema: Preliminary research shows that this herb can help stimulate insulin secretion and improve blood glucose control in those with both type 1 and type 2 diabetes. Dosage: 400 mg once or twice daily of a product standardized to 25 percent gymnemic acid.

Magnesium: Required for energy metabolism and nerve function. People with diabetes tend to have low magnesium levels, and a deficiency is associated with insulin resistance. Supplements can help improve insulin sensitivity and glucose control. Dosage: 200–600 mg daily.

Phase 2: White kidney bean extract that reduces starch digestion. Studies have shown that it can lower after-meal blood sugar levels. This supplement may be particularly helpful for those who are overweight and pre-diabetic. Dosage: 500–1,000 mg before starchy meals.

Vitamin D: Plays a role in insulin secretion. A deficiency can have a negative impact on insulin secretion and glucose tolerance. Some studies suggest that supplements can help improve blood sugar control and reduce neuropathy. Dosage: 400–2,000 IU daily.

Vitamin E: Helps to improve glucose tolerance and reduces glycosylation (binding of sugar to proteins in blood vessels). Many studies have found that it can prevent and reverse nerve damage and help protect against retinopathy and nephropathy. Dosage: 800 IU daily. Other antioxidants that have shown some benefits for improving blood glucose and reducing risk of complications include bilberry, coenzyme Q10, ginkgo biloba, green coffee extract, pycnogenol, and vitamin C.

FINAL THOUGHTS

To improve blood sugar control and reduce the risk of diabetic complications, consider the following:

- Eat small, frequent meals with low-glycemic, high-fibre carbohydrates, protein, and healthy fats. Add cinnamon to your diet.
- Avoid eating fast/processed/refined foods, alcohol, and saturated fat.
- Reduce your stress and aim for at least 30 minutes of activity daily.
- Maintain good oral and foot hygiene and see your doctor regularly for checkups and blood glucose testing.
- Consider supplements of alpha lipoic acid, chromium, and soluble fibre.

DIARRHEA

Diarrhea, which is loose, watery stools, is one of the most common digestive disorders. In fact, most people will experience diarrhea several times every year. Diarrhea is considered acute if it lasts just a few days or chronic if it persists for more than four weeks.

During digestion, the food we eat is broken down and nutrients are absorbed through the intestine. The waste material passes through the colon where most of the fluids are absorbed, creating a soft stool. The most common causes of acute diarrhea are dietary factors and infection. The body secretes extra fluid and intestinal contractions propel the toxins out of the body. When diarrhea occurs, the food and fluids you eat pass quickly through the colon so that the fluids are not adequately absorbed, causing soft, watery stools. Chronic diarrhea can occur due to digestive disorders or use of medications that affect bowel function.

Aside from being unpleasant and embarrassing, diarrhea can lead to serious complications, such as dehydration and nutrient deficiencies. In some cases it will clear up on its own, and in other cases treatment is necessary to get it under control and prevent complications.

SIGNS & SYMPTOMS

- Abdominal pain or cramps

- Bloating and gas

- Fever

- Frequent, loose, watery stools

Note: Diarrhea can lead to dehydration rapidly, especially in young children. When dehydration occurs, immediate medical attention is required. Signs of dehydration include excessive thirst, dry mouth or skin, little urination, severe weakness, dizziness or lightheadedness, or dark urine. Signs of dehydration in infants include dry mouth, crying without tears, unusual sleepiness, sunken eyes or cheeks, and skin that doesn't flatten if pinched and released. If this occurs, see your doctor immediately.

RISK FACTORS

- Diet: Fast foods, processed foods, preservatives, and artificial sweeteners such as sorbitol and mannitol

- Digestive disorders: Crohn's disease, colitis, celiac disease, and irritable bowel syndrome

- Infection with bacteria, viruses, or parasites, such as travellers' diarrhea or food poisoning

- Lactose intolerance

- Medication side effects: Antibiotics can destroy beneficial bacteria that normally are present in the gut, which can lead to diarrhea. Many other medications can cause diarrhea, in particular the non-steroidal anti-inflammatory drugs (NSAIDS), chemotherapy, colchicine, and drugs used to treat heart arrhythmias.

DOCTOR'S ORDERS

Acute diarrhea often clears up in a few days and rarely requires treatment. However, to prevent dehydration your doctor will advise you to increase fluid intake. There are special rehydration solutions, such as Gastrolyte and Pedialyte, available in pharmacies that contain electrolytes (sodium, potassium, and other minerals) that are necessary for health and to prevent dehydration. If you become depleted in these nutrients, it can lead to heart problems and other consequences.

If you develop diarrhea while taking an antibiotic, contact your doctor and stop the medication. Antibiotics destroy both the good and bad bacteria, which can disturb the balance of normal flora in your intestine, leading to overgrowth or potentially dangerous bacteria, such as *Clostridium difficile*, which can cause very serious diarrhea and requires medical treatment.

Diarrhea caused by a bacteria or parasite may require antimicrobial treatment.

If lactose intolerance is causing the diarrhea, you will be advised to avoid dairy products or to take lactase (an enzyme needed to digest lactose) when eating dairy.

Over-the-counter antidiarrheal medications, such as loperamide (Imodium) and bismuth subsalicylate (Pepto-Bismol), can help to slow diarrhea. However, these drugs should not be used if you have infectious diarrhea as they can prevent your body from eliminating the offending organism and can worsen the problem.

HOMEOPATHIC RECOMMENDATIONS

Phosphorus: This remedy is indicated for weak or empty feelings in the abdomen, followed by extreme liquid diarrhea.

Podophyllum peltatum: This can relieve diarrhea with severe cramping pain. The diarrhea occurs most often in the morning, and is often caused by overconsumption of fruits.

Sulphur: This remedy is indicated when there is extremely urgent diarrhea with burning felt in the digestive tract and an itchy, irritated anus and hemorrhoids.

SHERRY'S NATURAL PRESCRIPTION

Dietary Recommendations

Foods to include:

• Carob contains tannins that have an astringent or binding effect on the mucous membranes of the intestinal tract. Preliminary research in infants with diarrhea found that carob powder (at a dose of 1 g per kilogram of body weight per day) significantly improved resolution of diarrhea as compared to a placebo. Carob can also be used for treating adult diarrhea. It is available in health food stores and some grocery stores.

• Drink plenty of fluids (water, vegetable juice, broth). Teas containing chamomile, marshmallow, slippery elm, blackberry, blueberry, or red raspberry leaves can be helpful in alleviating diarrhea because these herbs contain tannins, which have astringent properties. Ginger tea can help reduce intestinal inflammation.

- During an acute attack, avoid solid foods and consume liquids. As you start to feel better, eat foods that are nutritious and easy to digest, such as bananas, brown rice, and potatoes. When your bowel movements have normalized, add more fibre-rich foods back into your diet.

- Fermented milk products (yogurt and kefir) help to restore beneficial bacteria in the gut and suppress growth of pathogenic bacteria. Look for a natural, unsweetened yogurt with live cultures, which have been shown to help prevent antibiotic-associated diarrhea, such as DanActive.

Foods to avoid:

- Caffeine, alcohol, and spicy foods (hot peppers) are stimulating to the digestive tract and can worsen diarrhea and upset stomach.

- Dairy products (other than fermented dairy), fats, and oils can worsen symptoms and should be avoided until the diarrhea has cleared.

- Sugar should be avoided if you have a bacterial infection. Fruit juices (especially apple and pear) are high in sugar and should be minimized until you have recovered.

Lifestyle Suggestions

- Get plenty of rest to allow your body to recover.

- See your doctor if diarrhea persists beyond five days or if you or your child develops dehydration.

- To reduce the risk of travellers' diarrhea, avoid tap water and ice cubes while on vacation and drink only bottled water and beverages; avoid raw fruits and vegetables unless you can peel them yourself; avoid raw or undercooked meats; use bottled water to brush your teeth; and keep your mouth closed while showering. Taking a probiotic (friendly bacteria) every day while away can also help reduce the risk of traveller's diarrhea. These beneficial bacteria (such as *Lactobacilli* and *Bifidobacteria*) normally live in the colon and inhibit the overgrowth of disease-causing bacteria.

Top Recommended Supplements

Multivitamin and mineral complex: Persistent diarrhea can lead to deficiencies of various vitamins and minerals, and taking a multivitamin can help prevent deficiencies. Certain nutrients (such as folic acid and zinc) can promote healing of the intestine. Speak to your pharmacist or health adviser for a recommendation as products vary depending on age, activity level, lifestyle, and gender.

· ·

CAUTION: If you have diarrhea, avoid taking large doses of vitamin C or magnesium (more than 500 mg or 100 mg, respectively), as these nutrients can cause loose stools.

· ·

Probiotics: Regular use of these beneficial bacteria can help prevent travellers' diarrhea and also help treat and prevent infectious diarrhea. Numerous clinical studies have shown that certain probiotics can reduce the severity and duration of diarrhea and help prevent it from occurring. Certain probiotics have been specifically studied for treating infectious diarrhea, such as BioGaia, which is safe for adults and children and available as drops and chewable tablets. Probiotics that have been studied for prevention of antibiotic-induced diarrhea include BioGaia and Bio-K. To prevent antibiotic-induced diarrhea, take your probiotic when you start your antibiotic and for at least two weeks after the antibiotic is finished. *Note:* While probiotics can help prevent and treat diarrhea, those with severe, dehydrating diarrhea should see their doctor.

Soluble fibre: Can help improve diarrhea by reducing water in the colon and firming the stool. Prebiotic fibre supplements, such as Sunfiber, help regulate the colon, aiding in both constipation and diarrhea. This type of fibre also helps improve gut microflora balance and aids digestion. Take with plenty of water.

Complementary Supplements

Brewer's yeast: Some research has shown that this supplement can help relieve infectious diarrhea, particularly when caused by *Clostridium difficile* (associated with antibiotic use). Dosage: Three capsules three times daily.

Goldenseal: Has antibiotic properties and contains a chemical called berberine, which prevents infectious bacteria from attaching to the gut and blocks the action of toxins produced by bacteria. Dosage: 250–500 mg three times daily, or 1 mL of tincture three times daily.

Lactase: This enzyme helps the body digest/breakdown lactose. Lactase supplements can help those who get diarrhea as a result of lactose intolerance. The typical dosage is 6,000–9,000 IU taken at the beginning of each meal.

FINAL THOUGHTS

To manage diarrhea, consider the following:

- Drink lots of fluids (especially water and herbal teas).
- Avoid dairy, fats, oils, spicy food, sugar, caffeine, and alcohol.
- Get adequate rest.
- Take a probiotic, multivitamin and mineral complex, and rehydration solution.
- See your doctor if diarrhea persists beyond five days or if you develop dehydration.

DIVERTICULAR DISEASE

Diverticulosis is a common condition where small, bulging pouches (diverticula) develop in the gastrointestinal tract. Diverticula usually develop when weak places in your colon give way under pressure, causing the formation of pouches, which can protrude through the colon wall. These pouches rarely cause problems, so people often don't realize that they have them. However, if the diverticula become infected (diverticulitis), this can cause abdominal pain, fever, nausea, and change in bowel habits.

Diverticula most commonly develop in the large intestine; however, they can form anywhere in your digestive system, including your esophagus, stomach, and small intestine.

It is possible to prevent diverticular disease by eating a high-fibre diet and avoiding constipation.

SIGNS & SYMPTOMS

Most people with diverticulosis do not have any symptoms. If diverticulitis occurs, it can cause

• Abdominal pain (mild to severe and sudden onset)

• Constipation or diarrhea

• Fever, nausea, vomiting

• Rectal bleeding

Note: Complications of diverticulitis include blockage in the colon and abscess or fistula formation. If a pouch ruptures, the waste material can spill into the abdominal cavity, leading to peritonitis, which is a serious medical problem that needs immediate attention.

RISK FACTORS

• Age: Diverticular disease is most common in those over age 40. About 10 percent of those over age 40 and 50 percent of those over age 60 are affected.

• Poor diet: Lack of fibre

• Lack of exercise

• Obesity

• Smoking

....

THE FIBRE FACTOR

Diverticular disease is very rare in countries where people eat a high-fibre diet, but it is very common in Canada, the United States, and Europe, where people eat more refined carbohydrates and less fibre. Prior to the 1900s, when refining of grains started, diverticular disease was rare in North America. A high-fibre diet can reduce your risk of diverticular disease and also help prevent flare-ups in those who already have it.

....

DOCTOR'S ORDERS

The treatment of diverticulitis depends on the severity of the symptoms. For those with mild symptoms, dietary changes and antibiotics for the infection may be all that is needed. During a flare-up, your doctor will advise a temporary low-fibre diet to allow the colon to heal. Once the symptoms subside, you can gradually increase the fibre in your diet.

Surgery is a last resort, but may be necessary for those with bowel obstruction or severely damaged intestine.

SHERRY'S NATURAL PRESCRIPTION

Dietary Recommendations

Nutrition plays an important role in the prevention and management of diverticular disease.

Foods to include:

- Drink plenty of fluids (water, juice, herbal tea) to aid the effect of fibre.

- Eat healthy fats (fish, olive oil, chia seed, and flaxseed), which can help reduce inflammation.

- Eat small, frequent meals to facilitate digestion and elimination.

- Fermented milk products (yogurt and kefir) can help reduce the risk of infection by supporting growth of beneficial bacteria in the gut.

- High-fibre foods, such as fresh fruits and vegetables and whole grains (oats, whole wheat, brown rice, and chia and flaxseed), keep stools soft, reducing the pressure on your colon, and preventing constipation. Aim for 25–30 g of fibre daily. Increase your intake gradually to avoid bloating and gas. Minimize fibre intake during an acute bout of diverticulitis. Let the colon rest and heal before resuming a high-fibre diet.

Foods to avoid:

- Fast foods and processed foods contain chemicals that can damage intestinal health.

- Minimize saturated fat (red meat).

- Refined grains (white flour/bread/rice/pasta) contain little to no fibre.

In the past, those with diverticular disease were told to avoid nuts or seeds, but there is no evidence that these foods trigger flare-ups, so they can be enjoyed as part of a healthy diet.

Lifestyle Suggestions

• Get regular physical activity. Aim for 30 minutes to one hour each day. Studies have found that jogging can help protect against diverticular disease.

• Maintain a healthy body weight.

• Don't smoke.

• Respond to bowel urges. Avoid holding it in as that can create dry, hard stools that are hard to pass, increasing colon pressure.

Top Recommended Supplements

Fibre: Helps prevent constipation and improve bowel function. Supplements play an important role in preventing and managing diverticular disease. Choose a product high in soluble fibre that mixes well with water, such as Sunfiber, which studies have shown can improve both constipation and diarrhea. Sunfiber is also a prebiotic fibre, meaning it can improve levels of beneficial bacteria in the gut. This type of fibre is also less likely to cause gas and bloating. Another supplemental form of soluble fibre to consider is glucomannan, which is derived from konjac root. Dosage: Varies with the product. Aim for 25–38 g of fibre daily from foods and supplements. Take with plenty of water. Avoid fibre supplements during an acute bout of diverticulitis.

Probiotics: Beneficial bacteria that support gut health. Supplements may help to re-establish the normal flora, which is often altered in those with diverticular disease, reduce intestinal inflammation, help to reduce the risk of gut infection, and also aid digestion and nutrient absorption. Probiotics that have been studied for diverticular disease include *Lactobacillus acidophilus, Lactobacillus plantarum, Lactobacillus casei, Bifidobacteria,* and *Saccharomyces boulardii.*

Complementary Supplements

Fish oil: Helps reduce inflammation. Dosage: 1–3 g daily.

Glutamine: An amino acid that supports good intestinal health. Dosage: 400 mg three to four times daily.

FINAL THOUGHTS

To prevent diverticular disease, consider the following:

• Boost your fibre intake by eating whole grains and avoiding refined foods.
• Include healthy fats (fish, chia seed, and flaxseed) and fermented milk products (yogurt and kefir) in your diet.
• Drink plenty of fluids.
• Get regular exercise.
• Consider fibre supplements and probiotics to complement your diet.

EAR INFECTIONS

Ear infections are the most common childhood illness, and the reason for more children's visits to the doctor than any other illness. Seventy-five percent of children have had at least one ear infection by one year of age. Ear infections, known medically as otitis media, are a non-contagious infection of the middle ear, just behind the eardrum.

Ear infections often develop from a viral infection, such as a cold. If the middle ear becomes inflamed from the infection, fluid builds up behind the eardrum, creating a breeding ground for infection. These infections can also occur when there is swelling or problems with the eustachian tubes (the tubes that connect the middle ear to the inner nose). These tubes equalize pressure inside and outside the ear. In children, the eustachian tubes are narrower and shorter, making it easier for fluid to get trapped in the middle ear during an infection.

In most cases, ear infections will clear up without treatment. More serious infections, particularly in infants and toddlers and those caused by bacteria, may require medical treatment. A healthy diet and lifestyle can help support proper immune function and reduce the risk of developing ear infections.

SIGNS & SYMPTOMS

Pain in the ear is the most common symptom of an ear infection. Children often don't recognize that their ears are the source of their discomfort, so it is important to look for other signs and symptoms, such as

- Balance difficulties

- Crying and irritability

- Ear drainage (look for a thick, yellow fluid, but do not be alarmed)

- Fatigue/malaise

- Fever

- Hearing problems

- Trouble sleeping

- Tugging at ears (though this is not a telltale sign)

RISK FACTORS

- Age: Children under three years of age are most at risk for developing an ear infection. Young children are at greater risk because their eustachian tubes are not fully developed (they are shorter and more horizontal), making fluid drainage more difficult.

- Ethnicity: Inuit and First Nations are at increased risk.

- Exposure to smoke and air pollution increases risk.

- Group child care increases the spread of germs and risk of infections.

- Oral or facial abnormalities, such as cleft palate.

- Not being breastfed.

- Pacifier use can increase the risk of recurrent ear infections by about 25 percent. The risk is related to frequency of use. Several factors may be responsible for this: Pacifiers may act as receptacles for viruses, and the sucking pressure may bring bacteria up from the throat and infect the ears.

- Premature birth.

- Season: Ear infections are more common during the fall and winter (cold and flu season).

- Swollen adenoids can block the eustachian tubes.

- Teething and feeding position: Babies who drink from a bottle while lying down tend to get more ear infections than those who feed upright.

- Weakened immune system: Colds or flus can increase a child's risk of getting an ear infection.

SWIMMER'S EAR

Swimmers often suffer from painful plugged ears when water becomes trapped in the outer ear and ear canal. When this happens, the skin inside the ear becomes watery, reducing the natural acidity that fights incoming pathogens and infection may result. Swimmer's ear usually clears up on its own, but requires a trip to the doctor if there is pain. To help prevent swimmer's ear, try an ear solution called Buro-sol (available over the counter) after you bathe or shower. This product is an astringent. It helps dry up water in the ear and inhibits bacterial growth, which is responsible for the pain, itching, and inflammation of the ear.

DOCTOR'S ORDERS

About 80 percent of all ear infections are viral and clear up on their own without antibiotic treatment. For infants older than six months who are otherwise healthy and have mild symptoms, it is recommended to just keep an eye on your child for 72 hours. If symptoms persist beyond this period, a visit to the doctor is recommended. If the doctor sees pus and suspects bacterial infection, then a course of antibiotics may be required to avoid complications. Antibiotics should only be used when necessary because of the risk of side effects (diarrhea) and antibiotic resistance. Analgesics such as Tylenol or Advil can be used to relieve pain.

For severe cases where a child has recurrent ear infections, surgery may be recommended to place small tubes inside the ears to drain fluid and relieve pressure. The concern is that hearing loss from chronic ear infections may delay language and speech development. A specialist will place a small plastic tube in a surgical hole made in the eardrum. The tubes allow air to enter the middle ear and fluid to drain out of it properly. They are also thought to relieve pressure and pain. Children are under general anaesthesia during surgery and usually recover quickly with little pain. There are maintenance issues and minor complications that may result from ear tubes, so it is important to discuss all factors with your doctor before proceeding with surgery.

HOMEOPATHIC RECOMMENDATIONS BY BRYCE WYLDE

Chamomilla: A sudden intolerable outburst of pain suggests a need for this remedy. Children may seem angry and beside themselves, and often become violent. They need to be carried constantly and walked around or rocked. Ear pain and other symptoms are worse from heat and wind, and the cheeks (often only one) may be hot and red.

Pulsatilla: This remedy is often indicated for ear infections that accompany a cold. Symptoms include a stuffy nose and yellow or greenish mucus. The ear is hot and swollen, and the person feels that something is pressing out of it. Pain is usually a pulsing sensation that gets worse at night.

Combination recommendation: Earache relief drops by Similasan

EAR TUBES VS. WATCHFUL WAITING

A large study published in the *New England Journal of Medicine* (July 2007), found that early treatment with ear tubes did not affect developmental outcomes when comparing treated and untreated children. Children involved in this long-term study were followed from approximately age 3 to age 11. Some were treated with tubes and some were not. Over the years, the researchers tested the children for reading, writing, spelling, behavioural issues, social skills, and intelligence, and found that there was no significant difference between the two groups. As a result of this groundbreaking study, guidelines regarding the treatment of chronic ear infections with tubes were re-evaluated and changed to encourage a watchful, waiting approach to treatment.

SHERRY'S NATURAL PRESCRIPTION

Dietary Recommendations

Food allergies can trigger ear infections. Consider an elimination diet (Appendix D) to determine if food allergies are an underlying cause.

Foods to include:

- Brightly coloured vegetables, fruits (especially berries), and whole grains contain essential vitamins and minerals that support the immune system.

- Chewing gum that contains xylitol (a natural sugar found in some fruits) can help reduce the risk of ear infections. Studies have shown that xylitol interferes with the growth of some bacteria that cause ear infections.

- Fish and flaxseed contain essential fatty acids that help to reduce inflammation.

- Yogurt with active cultures contains beneficial bacteria (probiotics) that help to reduce the risk of infections. One product that has been studied is DanActive, a yogurt drink that contains *Lactobacillus casei*. In a study of 638 children, those given this probiotic drink had a 19 percent decrease in common infections, including ear infections, compared to those who did not consume the probiotic. (*European Journal of Clinical Nutrition,* May 2010)

Foods to avoid:

- Dairy products may increase the risk of infection in those with sensitivities or allergies to cow's milk.

- Sugar suppresses immune function. Minimize soft drinks, candy, and sweets.

Lifestyle Suggestions

- Avoid second-hand smoke, as it weakens immunity.

- Breastfeeding supports lifelong healthy immunity. Exclusive breastfeeding until at least three months of age reduces the incidence of ear infections, and this effect persists four to twelve months after breastfeeding ceases. Always breastfeed (or bottle feed) with the baby slightly vertical; never put a child to sleep with a bottle.

- Discourage children from submerging their heads in water for prolonged periods, especially in lakes that are polluted. Use earplugs for swimming and bathing for children who are prone to infections.

- Minimize use of a pacifier.

- Ensure that your child gets adequate sleep; lack of sleep can hamper immune function.

- If your child exhibits signs of an ear infection, keep a close eye and check his or her temperature. See a doctor if the temperature is above 39°C or there is severe pain.

- Regular exercise boosts immune function.

- Wash hands regularly to avoid infections, and encourage your children to wash their hands and avoid rubbing their eyes, nose, or mouth.

Top Recommended Supplements

Probiotics: Beneficial bacteria that play an important role in supporting immune health and preventing infections. One probiotic that has been studied specifically in infants and children is *Lactobacillus reuteri* (BioGaia). A study of infants in a daycare setting given BioGaia showed that the infants experienced significantly fewer infections (including ear infections) and doctors' visits, less use of antibiotics, and fewer absent days. Dosage: five drops or one chewable tablet daily.

Xylitol: A natural sugar found in various fruits. Chewing gum with xylitol has been shown in several studies to significantly reduce the risk of ear infections. In order for it to be an effective preventative, the xylitol gum must be used five times daily. Look for CulturedCare, a probiotic gum that contains xylitol.

Complementary Supplements

Echinacea: Can help to reduce the severity and duration of cold symptoms, which may help to prevent ear infections from developing, although this has not been specifically studied. Dosage: 1–2 mL (depending on age) of echinacea liquid taken three times per day or more.

Echinacea should be started as soon as symptoms appear and continued until a few days after they are gone.

Garlic: Contains potent sulphur compounds that boost immune function. Studies have shown that aged garlic extract has activity against the major bacteria that cause ear infections. Dosage: For adults, take two to six capsules daily; liquid form is available for infants and children dosed according to age and tolerance as advised by a health care provider.

Vitamin C: Helps support immune function and reduces the severity of cold symptoms. Dosage: Adults should take 500–1,000 mg daily; children should take 250–500 mg three times daily.

FINAL THOUGHTS

To help reduce the risk of ear infections, consider the following:

- Encourage a healthy diet, including lots of vegetables, fruits, whole grains, fish, flaxseed, and yogurt. Minimize sugar intake.
- Keep children away from cigarette smoke and pollution.
- Discourage children from submerging their heads underwater for prolonged periods.
- Encourage regular hand washing, especially for children in daycare facilities.
- Consider BioGaia and xylitol gum for prevention.

ECZEMA

Also known as dermatitis, eczema is an inflammatory skin condition marked by extremely itchy, red, scaly, and irritated skin. Eczema affects about 7 million Canadians and is the most common skin problem in children under the age of 12. In fact, up to 25 percent of Canadian children get eczema. While many will outgrow the condition, in some it can persist throughout their lives. There are several forms of eczema; the most common ones include the following:

Atopic dermatitis: Atopic dermatitis is the most common form of eczema, affecting about 10 percent of all Canadians. It usually begins in infancy and varies in severity during childhood and adolescence. It is thought to be caused by a combination of dry, irritable skin and a malfunction in the body's immune system.

Contact dermatitis: This is caused by exposure to an irritant or allergen, such as laundry soap, dyes, cosmetics and skin products, cleaning products, or plants (poison ivy).

Neurodermatitis: This form develops in areas where something, such as tight clothing, rubs or scratches your skin and causes irritation.

Seborrheic dermatitis: Seborrheic dermatitis is a red rash with yellowish and oily scales, which is known as cradle cap when it affects infants. It may also affect adults and can be triggered by stress or other health conditions such as Parkinson's disease.

Stasis dermatitis: This may be caused by varicose veins and chronic venous insufficiency, which cause a buildup of fluid beneath the skin of the legs. This fluid buildup interferes with your blood's ability to nourish your skin and places extra pressure against the skin.

While eczema can be uncomfortable to deal with, it is not contagious and can be managed well with a variety of conventional and natural methods.

SIGNS & SYMPTOMS

Eczema can appear on various parts of the body. Symptoms vary in severity and include the following:

- Dryness

- Itching

- Redness

- Skin lesions (small red bumps; crusty, scaly patches)

- Swelling

In severe cases, fluid-filled vesicles, ulcers, or cracks may occur. Open sores and ulcers can become infected if picked or scratched. If the skin becomes red and warm to the touch, it may be infected and require immediate medical attention.

RISK FACTORS

- Age: While eczema can occur at any age, it is most common in infants and young children.

- Diet (deficiency of essential fatty acids; exposure to food allergens)

- Digestive problems (leaky gut syndrome and celiac disease)

- Exposure to skin irritants (chemicals, detergents, latex, cosmetics, and pollution)

- Genetics: Having a parent with eczema, asthma, and allergies increase risk. About 80 percent of children born to parents who both have had or do have eczema will also have the condition.

- Having hay fever, allergies, asthma, or a family history of these conditions

- Stress (physical or emotional)

- Climate changes (especially cold, dry weather), stress and illness, or infections can trigger flare-ups.

DOCTOR'S ORDERS

Doctors often prescribe steroid creams, such as hydrocortisone, clobetasol (Dermovate), or mometasone (Elocom), to reduce the itching and inflammation. These products are typically not used long-term, as they may cause side effects such as thinning of skin, stretch marks, discolorations, and problems with absorption of the steroid into the bloodstream. Antihistamines are given for those with severe itching. Pimecrolimus (Elidel) is a drug that affects the immune system and helps reduce flare-ups. This is also not recommended for long-term use. Phototherapy with ultraviolet light can offer benefits for adults with severe atopic dermatitis.

HOMEOPATHIC RECOMMENDATIONS

Mezereum: This remedy is indicated when there are intense and itchy eruptions that start as blisters, then ooze and form thick crusts. Scratching leads quickly to thickened skin. The person who requires Mezereum is usually very anxious and has a strong craving for fat.

Sulphur: This remedy is very useful for those who have repeatedly used cortisone on eczema without success. Intensely burning, itching, inflamed eruptions that are worse from warmth and bathing suggest a need for this remedy. Affected areas are red, with scaling or crusted skin.

Combination recommendation: Calendula Gel by Boiron

SHERRY'S NATURAL PRESCRIPTION

Dietary Recommendations

Foods to include:

• Nuts, seeds (flaxseed, pumpkin, and hemp), cold-water fish, and olive oil contain essential fatty acids, which can help reduce inflammation. Pumpkin and sunflower seeds also contain zinc, which is important for skin health.

• Fruits and vegetables contain valuable nutrients that support skin health.

• Drink lots of purified water to help flush toxins out of the body.

Foods to avoid:

• Spices, dairy, caffeine, alcohol, and preservatives may trigger flare-ups.

Note: Food allergies are common in those with eczema, in particular, eggs, milk, peanuts, soy, wheat, and food additives (preservatives and dyes). Consider an elimination diet (see Appendix D) to determine if food allergens are the source of your skin problems.

Lifestyle Suggestions

If you have contact dermatitis, avoid exposure to known irritants. For all forms of eczema, the following tips can help reduce flare-ups:

• Use only hypoallergenic skin products, soaps, and detergents and rinse well with water.

• Take short baths or showers (five to ten minutes) with warm (not hot) water. Bathing in oatmeal can help reduce itching. Gently pat your skin dry; do not rub hard.

• Moisturize your skin after bathing and throughout the day. Look for creams that are thick and emollient and contain one or more of the following: chamomile, vitamins A, E, and C, calendula, licorice, lavender, and sea buckthorn. Avoid products containing perfumes, dyes, or chemical irritants.

• Witch hazel in astringent that helps dry up weeping eczema and reduces itching and inflammation. Apply topically with gauze pads.

• Wear soft, natural fabrics, such as cotton, hemp, or silk.

• Don't scratch or rub your skin. If you are itchy, apply moisturizer.

• Use a humidifier or vaporizer in your home to add moisture to the air.

Top Recommended Supplements

Fish oils: Contain omega-3 fatty acids (EPA) that reduce inflammation. Several studies have shown significant benefits with high dosages (10 g per day). Lower dosages (2–3 g daily) may also offer benefits.

Gamma-linolenic acid (GLA): An omega-6 fatty acid that may be lacking in those with eczema. Some studies have found benefits with GLA supplements (primrose, borage, and black currant oil) to reduce itching and improve eczema. Dosage range: 500–1,000 mg daily. It may take one to two months to notice benefits.

E

Eczema

Complementary Supplements

Celadrin: A mixture of fatty acids that reduces inflammation. Available in creams and capsules. Dosage: Three to six capsules daily; apply topical cream several times daily.

Probiotics: Beneficial bacteria with immune-regulating properties; help improve digestion and reduce allergic reactions. Probiotics may help in the prevention and management of eczema. Preliminary research has found benefits with *Lactobacillus GG*.

FINAL THOUGHTS

Eczema is a manageable condition. To reduce flare-ups, consider the following:

- Avoid exposure or ingestion of known allergens or triggers.
- Use only hypoallergenic household and skin products.
- Bathe briefly; moisturize regularly with products made for sensitive skin.
- Consider supplements of fish oil, GLA, or Celadrin.
- Probiotics may be helpful for those with digestive problems and to reduce allergic responses.

ENDOMETRIOSIS

Endometriosis is a condition where cells that make up the lining of the uterus grow outside the uterus, most commonly on the fallopian tubes, ovaries, or tissue lining the pelvis. This tissue behaves similarly to that within the uterus. It thickens, breaks down, and bleeds each month with the menstrual cycle. However, because there is nowhere for this blood to exit the body, it becomes trapped, irritates surrounding tissue, and may cause scar tissue to form, which is painful.

Endometriosis affects about 10 to 20 percent of women of childbearing age. The actual cause is unknown; however, it is known that endometriosis is an estrogen-dependent condition and estrogen is necessary to induce or maintain endometriosis. Women who have endometriosis experience a remission of symptoms during pregnancy and complete resolution with menopause.

One theory as to the cause is that menstrual blood containing endometrial cells flows back through the fallopian tubes, and cells start to grow outside the uterus. Many women have some retrograde menstrual flow, yet the immune system is able to clear the debris and prevent implantation and growth of cells. In some women, though, this endometrial tissue implants and grows. It is thought that a compromised immune system or environmental toxins (xenoestrogens) may be at play. Since endometriosis often occurs in those with a family history, it is possible that there could be a genetic flaw.

While endometriosis can be painful, it doesn't increase the risk of uterine cancer or ovarian cancer, and there are a number of lifestyle approaches and natural remedies that can be very helpful.

SIGNS & SYMPTOMS

One-third of women with endometriosis have no symptoms. When symptoms do occur, they include the following:

- Heavy or irregular menstruation

- Infertility or miscarriage

- Pain with bladder or bowel function, or abdominal pain

- Painful intercourse

- Pelvic pain, especially during menstruation

ENDOMETRIOSIS AND PREGNANCY

Approximately 30 to 50 percent of women who have difficulty becoming pregnant have endometriosis. Endometriosis can produce adhesions that can trap the egg near the ovary and prevent it from travelling through the fallopian tube to the uterus. Despite this, many women with endometriosis are still able to conceive, but it often takes them longer. During pregnancy, most women have no signs or symptoms of endometriosis.

E

Endometriosis

- Age: Women of childbearing age are at greatest risk

- Family history: Having a mother or sister with the condition can increase risk by up to tenfold

- Never having given birth

- Retrograde menstrual flow

- High estrogen levels (exposure to xenoestrogens)

- Immune system dysfunction

- History of pelvic infection

DOCTOR'S ORDERS

Doctors may prescribe anti-inflammatory medications such as ibuprofen (Advil and Motrin) to ease pain and swelling. Oral contraceptives and drugs that stop ovulation and menstruation are sometimes used to lower estrogen levels and control heavy bleeding. For women having difficulty conceiving, laparoscopic laser techniques can be done to shrink and remove lesions.

Hysterectomy should be considered only as a last resort for those with severe symptoms that have not benefited from other conventional and natural approaches. Having this radical surgery does not guarantee an end to the symptoms and is associated with various risks and complications.

SHERRY'S NATURAL PRESCRIPTION

The natural approach to endometriosis focuses on supporting liver function (the liver breaks down estrogen), optimizing intestinal health (normal flora aid in estrogen metabolism), and balancing immune function.

Dietary Recommendations

Foods to include:

- Increase intake of whole grains, fresh vegetables, and fruits. These foods are high in fibre and help balance levels of friendly bacteria in the intestine. Choose organic as much as possible.

- Eat liver-supporting foods such as beets, carrots, onions, garlic, leafy greens, artichokes, apples, and lemons.

- Broccoli, cauliflower, Brussels sprouts, and cabbage contain indole-3-carbinol, which helps the liver break down estrogen.

- Flaxseed, soy, beans, and legumes contain phytoestrogens, which may help reduce the impact of other hormones.

- Yogurt with active cultures increases the amount of friendly bacteria in the intestine and aids digestion and immune function.

Foods to avoid:

- Alcohol, caffeine, refined foods, food additives, sugar, and saturated fats may affect hormone balance, impair immune function, and worsen symptoms.

- Red meat and non-organic produce may contain hormones, pesticides, and chemicals that act as estrogen-mimickers. To avoid these chemicals and hormones choose organic meat and produce.

Lifestyle Suggestions

- Have regular pelvic examinations and report any changes in symptoms to your doctor.

- Get regular exercise. This is a natural pain reliever and boosts mood. Vigorous exercise has been found to reduce the risk of endometriosis. Try walking, cycling, or aerobics. Kegel exercises (contracting and releasing the pelvic muscles) may help release pelvic tension.

- Reduce stress, because stress can trigger flare-ups and worsen symptoms. Try yoga, Pilates, stretching, or breathing techniques.

- Acupuncture and massage may help relieve pelvic congestion and pain.

- A castor oil pack may help with abdominal pain and swelling. Apply oil directly to abdomen, cover with a clean soft cloth and plastic wrap. Place a heating pad on top and let sit for 30 to 60 minutes.

- Do not use tampons. They block menstrual flow and may increase the likelihood of retrograde blood flow. Use unbleached, unscented cotton pads instead.

- Minimize exposure to environmental estrogens or xenoestrogens (phthalates, parabens, and dioxins), which are present in pesticides, plastics, and certain skin care products and cosmetics.

Top Recommended Supplements

There has been little research on supplements and natural therapies to improve endometriosis. However, there is a role for using supplements to help symptoms by normalizing estrogen levels, improving detoxification, and reducing inflammation.

Calcium D-glucarate: Helps the liver detoxify and eliminate excess hormones (particularly estrogen). Dosage: 300–500 mg daily.

Chasteberry: Balances the estrogen-to-progesterone ratio and may help normalize ovulation. Dosage: 150–300 mg daily.

Indole-3-carbinol: A compound found naturally in cruciferous vegetables that aids in detoxification of estrogen, protects liver function, and may protect against hormonal cancers. Dosage: 400 mg daily.

Milk thistle: Supports liver function and aids in detoxification of estrogen. Dosage: 20–100 mg daily.

Complementary Supplements

Calcium and magnesium: Both aid in hormone metabolism and may help reduce menstrual pain. Dosages: 500 mg of calcium and 200 mg of magnesium three times daily.

Gamma linolenic acid: Found in evening primrose, borage, and black currant oil. It may help reduce pain and inflammation. Dosage: 1–3 g daily.

Fish oils: Contains omega-3 fatty acids, which may help with pain and inflammation. Dosage: 1 g three times daily.

Iron: Required for those with heavy bleeding and anemia. Dosage varies. Take only under advice from your health care provider.

Vitamin C: An antioxidant that supports immune function and protects against cell and tissue damage. It also improves healing of tissues damaged by lesions and scarring; it may also help control heavy bleeding by strengthening capillary walls. Dosage: 1,000 mg daily.

FINAL THOUGHTS

To improve endometriosis and prevent worsening, consider the following:

- Eat organic vegetables, fruits, whole grains, legumes, flaxseed, and yogurt.
- Minimize consumption of red meat, alcohol, caffeine, and refined foods.
- Get regular exercise and reduce stress.
- Avoid exposure to environmental estrogens.
- Top recommended supplements are indole-3-carbinol, calcium D-glucarate, chasteberry, and milk thistle.

ERECTILE DYSFUNCTION (IMPOTENCE)

Erectile dysfunction (ED), also known as impotence, is the inability to achieve or maintain an erection that is adequate for sexual performance. This is the most common sexual problem among men—almost every man will experience an episode of ED at one point in his life. ED is estimated to affect nearly half of Canadian men between the ages of 40 and 70. It is more common in men over age 50. For most men it occurs occasionally, but for some ED occurs frequently.

A series of factors are involved in developing an erection. Sexual arousal causes nerves in the brain and spine to signal arteries in the penis to swell up with blood. The spongy tissues in the penis expand and it becomes erect. Any interference with this process, whether physical or psychological, can prevent an erection.

As men age, there are changes in erectile function. It may take longer to develop an erection and it may not be as rigid, and more direct stimulation may be required. Orgasm may become less intense and the volume of ejaculate reduced.

There are many options today for men experiencing erectile dysfunction, from drug therapy to lifestyle measures and supplements.

SIGNS & SYMPTOMS

• Inability to obtain a full erection

• Inability to maintain an erection for sexual performance

RISK FACTORS

• Diabetes: High blood sugar damages blood vessels in the penis. About 80 percent of men with diabetes develop erectile dysfunction, and it occurs at an earlier age.

• Diseases of the nerves, blood vessels, heart, prostate, and kidneys

• Hormonal imbalances: Low testosterone, growth hormone, thyroid, or DHEA levels

• Surgery or trauma that causes nerve damage (spinal cord injury, prostate surgery)

• Drugs: Antidepressants, beta-blockers, antihistamines, tranquilizers, and anticancer drugs

• Alcohol, marijuana, cocaine, and other illicit drugs

• Smoking causes damage to blood vessels and nerves in the penis.

• Psychological factors: Stress, anxiety, depression, and lack of sleep

DOCTOR'S ORDERS

Medications such as sildenafil (Viagara), tadalafil (Cialis), and vardenafil (Levitra) work by enhancing the effects of nitric oxide, a chemical that relaxes muscles in the penis, leading to increased blood flow. Arousal and stimulation is still required for an erection, but the drug assists the physical aspect. Do not use these drugs if you have had a heart attack, stroke, or other serious heart problems, or if you are taking drugs for angina (nitroglycerine).

Yohimbe is a plant-based drug that dilates blood vessels and increases circulation. It has been shown in several studies to improve ED. Yohimbe was previously available over the counter, but is now available by prescription only due to numerous side effects such as nervousness, irritability, insomnia, and increased blood pressure. It should be avoided by those with heart or kidney disease.

Other medical options include injectable drugs, implants, hormone therapy, vacuum devices, surgery to repair blood vessels or nerves, and counselling.

HOMEOPATHIC RECOMMENDATIONS

Caladium: This may help those with a high libido but physical erectile dysfunction.

Lycopodium: People who need this remedy may have problems with erections because of worry, and may also experience memory loss.

Selenium metallicum: If the erectile dysfunction starts after a fever or exhausting illness, if the person feels weak but sexual interest is still present, or if there is hair loss (head, body hair, or eyebrows), there may be a need for this remedy.

SHERRY'S NATURAL PRESCRIPTION

Dietary Recommendations

Foods to include:

• Fibre-rich foods help promote blood sugar balance.

• Zinc helps support testosterone production; the best food sources are pumpkin seeds, soybeans, oysters, and wheat germ.

• Vitamin E dilates blood vessels and improves blood flow; the best food sources include nuts and seeds, whole grains, palm fruit oil, and leafy green vegetables.

Foods to avoid:

• Foods high in saturated and trans fats can be damaging to the blood vessels and reduce circulation (red meat, dairy, and processed and fast foods).

• Minimize refined flour and sugar as these foods cause blood sugar fluctuations, which can be damaging to the blood vessels.

• Minimize soy foods as they may reduce testosterone levels.

• Avoid alcohol before sex.

Lifestyle Suggestions

• Exercise: Regular activity is essential to improve blood flow and circulation, reduce stress, and increase energy levels. Activities such as walking, squats, and lunges are particularly good for increasing blood flow to the pelvic area.

• Don't smoke. Smoking damages blood vessels and nerves.

- Maintain a healthy body weight. Obesity leads to diabetes and heart disease, both of which can impact sexual function.

- Get adequate sleep at night and be aware that a lack of sleep can affect performance.

- Reduce stress whether through exercise, breathing techniques, or visualization. Find what works to promote relaxation and practise it regularly.

- Acupuncture and hypnosis may help improve erectile function.

- Communicate with your partner and your doctor.

Top Recommended Supplements

Arginine: An amino acid used to make nitrous oxide, a substance that dilates blood vessels and increases blood flow. Preliminary research suggests benefits for improving ED. One study combined arginine with pine bark extract with positive effects. Dosage: 1,000 mg three to five times daily.

Korean ginseng: Also called panax ginseng, Korean ginseng increases energy and the ability to maintain an erection; several studies have found it effective for improving erectile function. Dosage: 900 mg two to three times daily.

Tongkat ali: Also known as *Eurycoma longifolia*. Several clinical studies on a patented form of this plant called Physta show that it can increase testosterone and DHEA levels, improve sexual performance and satisfaction, and boost energy levels. Dosage: 200–600 mg daily.

Complementary Supplements

Antioxidants: Vitamins C and E and flavonoids (grape seed and pine bark) help improve blood flow and reduce oxidative damage to the blood vessels. Follow label directions.

Carnitine: An amino acid that has been shown to improve erectile function. Two studies found that it boosted the effectiveness of Viagra. Dosage: 2–4 g daily.

Ginkgo biloba: Opens blood vessels and increases blood flow to the penis. It is particularly helpful for ED caused by antidepressant drugs or vascular problems (diabetes). Dosage: 120–200 mg daily.

Maca: Rich in the amino acid arginine, which increases blood flow to the penis, and histidine, which helps support orgasm and ejaculation. Preliminary research has found it helpful, particularly for improving desire. Dosage: 1,500–3,000 mg three times daily.

FINAL THOUGHTS

To prevent or improve ED, consider the following:

- Exercise regularly; eat a high-fibre diet with lots of whole grains, nuts, and seeds; and reduce stress.
- Maintain a healthy body weight.
- Don't smoke, and minimize alcohol.
- The most-researched supplements for ED are Korean ginseng, arginine, and tongkat ali (Physta).
- Ginkgo biloba may be helpful for ED caused by antidepressant use or those who have diabetes.

FIBROCYSTIC BREASTS

Fibrocystic breasts are described as benign (non-cancerous) changes that occur in the breast tissue, making them lumpy and fibrous. This condition is also known as cyclic mastalgia. It was once known as fibrocystic breast disease, but the term "disease" is no longer used because research has shown that this condition is a variation of normal breasts, not a disease, yet it can cause significant pain and discomfort.

Fibrocystic breasts affect as many as 60 percent of women typically between the ages of 30 and 50. During the menstruating years, fluctuating monthly hormonal cycles can lead to the accumulation of fluid, cells, and cellular debris within the breast. It is believed that excess levels of the hormones estrogen and prolactin cause breast cysts to become chronically inflamed and surrounded by fibrous tissue, which can harden and thicken the cysts, creating the lumpy breasts. Other hormones, such as growth factor, insulin, and thyroid hormone, are also implicated.

While this condition can be painful, the lumps are benign and do not increase your risk of breast cancer. If you do discover a lump in your breast tissue, it is important to consult with your doctor.

There are a number of lifestyle modifications and natural treatments that can help reduce the symptoms of fibrocystic breasts and promote good breast health.

SIGNS & SYMPTOMS

- Breast pain and tenderness

- Changes in nipple sensation (itching) and nipple discharge (non-bloody)

- Dense and bumpy/lumpy consistency in the breast tissue

- Feeling of fullness in the breasts

- Swelling in the breasts before the menstrual period

Note: Symptoms may range from mild to severe, and typically peak just before each menstrual period and improve immediately after the menstrual period.

FIBROCYSTIC BREASTS AND BREAST CANCER

Fibrocystic lumps are benign and don't increase your breast cancer risk, but they can make diagnosing breast cancer more difficult because of the dense, fibrous tissue and lumps. Fibrocystic lumps move freely when touched and they get worse with the menstrual cycle. In contrast, a cancerous growth in the breast is often not tender or freely movable when touched. See your doctor if you notice a lump in your breast. To rule out breast cancer, a needle aspiration of the cyst or a mammogram can be done.

- Age: Women between the ages of 30 and 50 are at greatest risk

- Diet: High intake of saturated fat and caffeine

- Family history of fibrocystic breasts or breast cancer

- Irregular menstrual cycles

- Hormones: Having an imbalance of estrogen to progesterone (estrogen dominance), which can be caused by exposure to xenoestrogens (estrogen-like chemicals in food and the environment, such as pesticides and plastics) or taking estrogen replacement therapy

- Low thyroid function (hypothyroidism)

- Not having children

- Poor lymphatic drainage

DOCTOR'S ORDERS

There are a few drugs that can be given to manage the symptoms of fibrocystic breasts, but they are not always effective and there are potential side effects. Oral contraceptives are sometimes prescribed to help stabilize hormone levels. Side effects include increased risk of stroke, gallbladder disease, and breast cancer, to name a few. The drug danazol (Danocrine) is used for severe cases. It is a synthetic testosterone-like drug that works by decreasing the amount of estrogen made by the ovaries; side effects include hot flashes, vaginal dryness, increased body hair, and acne. Anti-inflammatory drugs such as ibuprofen (Advil and Motrin) may be used to manage the pain, but these drugs can cause stomach pain, bleeding, and ulcers.

There is some research that topically applied progesterone cream can be helpful for the management of fibrocystic breasts. In Canada, this is available by prescription through a compounding pharmacy. To determine whether your progesterone levels are low, a blood or saliva test can be done. See Appendix E for more information.

SHERRY'S NATURAL PRESCRIPTION

Dietary Recommendations

Foods to include:

- Boost fibre intake (whole grains, vegetables, and fruits) as fibre helps the body eliminate excess hormones and toxins, which worsen fibrocystic breasts. Onions, garlic, beets, artichokes, and lemon help support liver function and the elimination of hormones.

- Choose organic foods as much as possible to avoid harmful chemicals.

- Cruciferous vegetables (broccoli, cauliflower, Brussels sprouts, and cabbage) contain substances that help the body detoxify estrogen.

- Drink plenty of water. Try dandelion tea, which may help reduce breast pain and supports detoxification.

- Fish, chia seed, and flaxseeds contain beneficial fatty acids that can help reduce inflammation. Flaxseed also contains lignans, which act as a phytoestrogen and help block the effects of estrogen.

- Sea vegetables (kelp and nori) contain iodine, which may be deficient in those with fibrocystic breasts. Iodine deficiency can increase tissue sensitivity to estrogen stimulation.

- Soy products contain phytoestrogens, which can help balance hormone levels and counter the effects of excess estrogen stimulation. Soy also contains amino acids, which aid in detoxification.

- Use oils containing beneficial fats such as olive, flaxseed, and sunflower oil.

Foods to avoid:

- Minimize caffeine as it can worsen symptoms. Aside from coffee, it is also in black tea (and, to a lesser extent, green tea), cola, chocolate, and some over-the-counter medications.

- Reduce saturated fat (found in red meat and high-fat dairy products) as studies have shown that it can worsen fibrocystic breasts.

Lifestyle Suggestions

- Examine your breasts monthly.

- Exercise regularly to improve circulation and help the body detoxify.

- Work on losing excess weight. Women who are obese have higher levels of estrogen because this hormone can be stored in fat tissue.

- Reduce stress, which can cause hormonal changes that may worsen symptoms. Try yoga, tai chi, or breathing techniques.

- Get your hormones checked. Ask your doctor to check your thyroid as low thyroid function can worsen symptoms of fibrocystic breasts. Urine and saliva tests can be done to check for estrogen dominance. See Appendix E for more information.

- Massage can help improve circulation and lymphatic drainage.

- Wear a proper-fitting bra. If it is too tight, it can cut off circulation and worsen symptoms.

- Apply castor oil packs to the breasts. Soak flannel cloth in castor oil, wring out, and apply to breasts. Cover with a heating pad or hot water bottle and leave on for 30 minutes. This will help relieve pain and improve circulation.

Top Recommended Supplements

Chasteberry (vitex): Helps to balance hormone levels of estrogen, progesterone, and prolactin. Studies have shown that it can help reduce breast tenderness and swelling. Dosage: 150–300 mg daily of a product standardized to contain at least 0.5 percent agnuside. Do not take if you are on oral contraceptives or if you are pregnant.

GLA: Found in flaxseed, primrose, and borage oil, which contain beneficial fatty acids that may help reduce pain and inflammation associated with fibrocystic breasts. Dosage: 1 g two to three times daily.

Indole-3-carbinol: A compound found naturally in cruciferous vegetables that aids in detoxification of estrogen, inhibits free radical damage, protects liver function, and inhibits tumour growth. Dosage: 400 mg daily.

Complementary Supplements

Fish oils: Contain beneficial omega-3 fatty acids, which have anti-inflammatory effects, help reduce breast pain, and also help the body absorb iodine. Iodine deficiency is associated with fibrocystic breast changes. Dosage: 1 g three times daily.

Ginkgo biloba: Helps improve circulation, and preliminary research found it helped reduce cyclic breast tenderness. Dosage: 80 mg twice daily.

Magnesium: Helps reduce pain and inflammation of fibrocystic breast changes, particularly symptoms associated with the menstrual cycle. Dosage: 100–200 mg twice daily with meals.

Vitamin B6: Helps the liver process estrogen. Studies have shown that it can reduce breast pain and swelling associated with the menstrual cycle. Dosage: 50–100 mg daily as part of a B-complex.

Vitamin E: Helps reduce pain, tenderness, and swelling. Some (but not all) studies have found benefits. Dosage: 400–800 IU daily.

FINAL THOUGHTS

To prevent and manage fibrocystic breasts naturally, consider the following:

- Examine your breasts monthly and report any changes to your doctor.
- Reduce exposure to xenoestrogens (plastics, pesticides, non-organic meat and dairy). Eat more fibre, sea and cruciferous vegetables, and soy products.
- Reduce stress and get regular exercise.
- Try castor oil packs to relieve pain and promote better circulation.
- Consider supplements of chasteberry, GLA, and indole-3-carbinol.

F

Fibrocystic Breasts

FIBROIDS (UTERINE)

Uterine fibroids are non-cancerous tumours or growths of the uterus. They are also known as myomas, fibromyomas, or leiomyomas. Despite their name, fibroids are not fibrous; they are composed of connective tissue and muscle. They can appear in groups and grow either inside or outside of the uterus. Fibroids are the most common, non-cancerous tumours occurring in women of childbearing age. It is estimated that over 50 percent of women have fibroids, but many are unaware. They can be smaller than a pea or grow larger than a football. In very rare cases fibroids can develop into cancer; however, most often they are not harmful, but may cause pain and discomfort when they become large and put pressure on the abdomen and bladder.

Fibroids typically appear during the childbearing years, particularly between the ages of 30 and 40, and then shrink during menopause. While the actual cause of fibroids is uncertain, it is known that their growth is stimulated by estrogen, and genetic alterations likely play a role. Fibroids are becoming increasingly common today, which has been attributed to high amounts of xenoestrogens (estrogen-like compounds) in our food supply and environment.

ENVIRONMENTAL ESTROGENS

Xenoestrogens are substances that have estrogen-like activity in the body. They are present in foods (fish, meat, and dairy) and in the environment (plastics, pesticides, and skin care products). Research suggests that xenoestrogens may play a role in uterine fibroids, certain cancers, and premature sexual maturity in young girls.

SIGNS & SYMPTOMS

Many women do not realize they have fibroids until it is discovered as a result of a pelvic examination or prenatal ultrasound. For those who develop large fibroid tumours, signs and symptoms vary depending on location, and may include the following:

• Anemia (due to heavy bleeding)

• Back ache or leg pains

• Constipation

• Heavy menstrual bleeding and prolonged periods

• Infertility and miscarriages

• Pain during intercourse

• Pelvic pressure or pain

• Urinary frequency or incontinence

- Age: Most common between the ages of 30 and 40

- Estrogen excess (promotes growth of fibroids)

- Family history (fibroids contain genetic alterations)

- Insulin-like growth factor (may stimulate fibroid growth)

- Obese women are at a slightly increased risk

- Race (fibroids are three to five times more common among Black women)

Studies have found a link between consumption of red meat and ham with the presence of fibroids. Heavy metal contamination and hypothyroidism have also been associated with greater risk of fibroids.

Pregnancy and childbirth appear to have a protective effect against fibroids. Research suggests that use of birth control pills may actually be protective against developing fibroids except among those who start taking the pill between the ages of 13 and 16.

DOCTOR'S ORDERS

In most cases, doctors recommend watchful waiting for fibroids. Since fibroids tend to grow slowly and then shrink after menopause, surgical procedures are recommended only if the fibroids are large and cause heavy bleeding and pain, or if they are impairing fertility. Surgical options include myomectomy (an incision into the abdomen and removal of fibroids), hysterectomy (removal of the uterus), and uterine artery embolization (a procedure that cuts off blood supply to the uterus to cause the fibroid to shrink). Medications to reduce pain and inflammation such as anti-inflammatory drugs may be prescribed. Medications are also used to reduce estrogen levels and shrink fibroids; however, there are many side effects with these drugs. Progesterone cream is popularly used for fibroid treatment; however, in some women it can cause fibroids to grow, so it should be used only under a physician's supervision.

SHERRY'S NATURAL PRESCRIPTION

A holistic approach to treating fibroids is aimed at reducing levels of circulating estrogens and supporting liver function (the liver detoxifies estrogen). This can be achieved through dietary, lifestyle, and supplemental approaches.

Dietary Recommendations

Foods to include:

- Fibre-rich foods such as fruits, vegetables, and whole grains will help extract excessive estrogen stores from the body.

- Cruciferous vegetables such as broccoli, cauliflower, and Brussels sprouts are particularly helpful, as they contain compounds that help the liver detoxify estrogen.

- Choose organic foods whenever possible to reduce ingestion of xenoestrogens from pesticides.

- Foods containing phytoestrogens (plant-based estrogens), such as soy foods, flaxseed, buckwheat, oats, and beans help balance estrogen levels.

- Artichokes, beets, carrots, dandelion greens, garlic, and onions contain compounds that support liver function and detoxification of hormones.

- Drink more green tea, as it contains polyphenols that block the negative effects of estrogen and help protect against estrogen-related cancers.

- Those with heavy bleeding may require additional iron to prevent anemia. The best food sources of iron include clams, oysters, organ meats, beef, pork, poultry, and fish. Iron is also present in eggs, dried beans, fortified cereals, and dark green leafy vegetables.

Foods to avoid:

- Meat, dairy, and fish (especially farmed salmon) may contain dioxins and other xenoestrogens that can stimulate fibroid growth and worsen symptoms.

- Minimize sugar and caffeine, which can trigger pain and inflammation.

Lifestyle Suggestions

- Reduce stress, as it can cause hormonal changes that may worsen fibroid symptoms. Try yoga, tai chi, or breathing techniques.

- Regular exercise of moderate-intensity activity for one hour daily reduces stress and will help to maintain a healthy body weight.

- Acupuncture helps relieve pelvic pain and swelling.

- Apply castor oil to your pelvic area, and cover with plastic and a hot towel. Leave in place for one hour and do this three times per week.

Top Recommended Supplements

Calcium D-glucarate: Assists in the elimination of estrogen. Dosage: 400–500 mg daily.

Chasteberry: Helps to normalize hormone levels. Dosage: 160–240 mg daily.

Indole-3-carbinol: Helps with the detoxification or breakdown of estrogen. Dosage: 200–400 mg daily.

Complementary Supplements

Dandelion root and milk thistle: Help support liver detoxification. Dosage varies, so follow label directions or the advice of your health care provider.

Pancreatic enzymes: May help reduce unusual cell and tissue growths. Dosage: One capsule between meals three times daily.

Red raspberry tea: An astringent that helps reduce uterine inflammation and prevents fibroid growth. Dosage: 500–1,000 mL daily.

FINAL THOUGHTS

Fibroids are a common condition that affect women of childbearing years. To prevent and manage fibroids naturally, consider the following:

- Reduce exposure to xenoestrogens (plastics, pesticides, non-organic meat and dairy).
- Boost fibre intake; eat more cruciferous vegetables.
- Reduce stress and get regular exercise.
- Acupuncture can help relieve pain and promote relaxation.
- Consider supplements of indole-3-carbinol, calcium D-glucarate, and chasteberry.

FIBROMYALGIA

Fibromyalgia (FM) is a common disorder that has only recently received recognition by the medical community. The word "fibromyalgia" comes from the Latin terms for fibrous tissue (fibro), muscle (myo), and pain (algia). It is marked by widespread pain, fatigue, and tender points. It is estimated that 2 percent of Canadians have this condition.

The exact cause of FM is unknown. However, researchers have identified several factors that contribute to the development of FM:

- Allergies or chemical sensitivities
- Alterations in muscle metabolism: Reduced blood flow to muscles can cause fatigue and pain
- Chemical imbalance in the brain: Alterations in the neurotransmitters serotonin and norepinephrine
- Elevated levels of a chemical called substance P, which is involved in our sensation of pain signals
- Infection: Viruses (Epstein-Barr, HHV-6, and cytomegalovirus) and fungal infections by *Candida albicans* have been implicated
- Nutritional deficiencies in magnesium and antioxidants
- Sleep disturbances: Disturbed sleep patterns may be a cause rather than just a symptom
- Stress may play a role in the development of FM and it can also trigger flare-ups in those already diagnosed
- Trauma or injury, particularly in the upper spinal region

While there is no cure for FM, there are a number of lifestyle approaches that can help improve symptoms and quality of life.

SIGNS & SYMPTOMS

For many people, symptoms of FM develop slowly over time while for others it can occur suddenly after a stressful life event such as surgery, trauma, or infection. Symptoms of FM vary among individuals and can be affected by weather, stress, and physical activity.

- Anxiety
- Chest pain
- Depression
- Difficulty concentrating
- Dizziness
- Dry eyes, skin, and mouth
- Fatigue and sleep disturbance

- Headaches

- Irritable bowel or bladder

- Numbness or tingling in the hands and feet

- Pain (most commonly in the neck, shoulders, hips, lower back, and thighs)

- Painful menstrual periods

- Swollen lymph nodes

RISK FACTORS

- Autoimmune disease: Those with arthritis, lupus, and other autoimmune diseases

- Disturbed sleep: Those with nighttime muscle cramps, restless legs, or sleep apnea

- Family history: Those with a family member with FM

- Gender: Women are at greater risk

DOCTOR'S ORDERS

There is no cure for FM. Prescription drugs are given to reduce symptoms, often with limited success. Those commonly prescribed include muscle relaxants (Flexeril), anti-inflammatory drugs (ibuprofen), and pain relievers (acetaminophen or codeine). In some people, antidepressants help to improve sleep, depression, and anxiety, but use of these drugs is limited by undesirable side effects.

SHERRY'S NATURAL PRESCRIPTION

A comprehensive program that includes lifestyle strategies, nutrition, and supplements to reduce symptoms and improve well-being offers the greatest benefit for FM sufferers.

Dietary Recommendations

Foods to include:

- Focus on fresh fruits, vegetables, whole grains, lean protein (tofu, fish, beans, poultry, nuts, and seeds), and healthy fats (olive oil and palm fruit oil) to ensure your body gets essential nutrients and energy.

- Eat plenty of magnesium-rich foods such as green vegetables, soybeans, almonds, and cashews.

Foods to avoid:

- Caffeine interferes with sleep, causes anxiety, reduces mineral absorption, and can worsen several FM symptoms. Minimize caffeine from all sources, including coffee and soft drinks.

- Sugar reduces immune function, interferes with sleep, causes mood swings, and encourages growth of yeast, which has been linked to FM.

• Minimize or avoid processed/fast/fried foods, which are high in saturated fats and can trigger inflammation.

Note: Since food allergies have been implicated in FM, it is important to identify possible allergens. Refer to Appendix D for more information.

Lifestyle Suggestions

• Reduce stress, which can trigger or aggravate the symptoms of FM. Try breathing exercises, meditation, or yoga.

• Massage therapy can help improve a number of FM symptoms including muscle soreness, and it can also help improve range of motion, reduce stress, and improve sleep.

• Several studies have shown that regular low-intensity exercise can improve FM. Exercise improves mood, reduces pain, and improves overall well-being.

• Chiropractic improves spinal alignment and nerve flow, and can reduce pain and improve sleep. Craniosacral therapy can also be beneficial.

• Acupuncture can help reduce pain and promote relaxation.

• Sleep is essential; lack of sleep can intensify pain, anxiety, and responses to stress. Refer to the insomnia section of this book for tips on getting a better night's rest.

• Laughter improves mood and well-being; watch funny movies, read humorous books, and spend time with funny people.

Top Recommended Supplements

Melatonin: A hormone that regulates our sleep cycles. Supplements shorten the time needed to fall asleep, reduce night wakening, improve sleep quality, and reduce tender points. Dosage: 3 mg one hour before bed.

S-adenosylmethionine (SAMe): Supports production of neurotransmitters (serotonin), antioxidants, hormones, and joint compounds. Studies for FM have shown that it can reduce pain, fatigue, and stiffness and improve mood. SAMe is very safe and better tolerated than antidepressant drugs. Do not combine with antidepressants or products that modify serotonin levels unless advised by your doctor. Dosage: 800 mg daily. Choose a product that is enteric coated and take on an empty stomach. SAMe can also be given by injection by a doctor.

5-hydroxytryptophan (5-HTP): Elevates serotonin levels and alleviates depression; may also reduce tender points and anxiety, and improve sleep quality. Do not combine with prescription antidepressants or products that modify serotonin levels. Dosage: 100 mg three times daily. 5-HTP is not as well studied as SAMe, but it is less expensive and is a good second choice.

Complementary Supplements

Acetyl-L-carnitine: Preliminary research suggests it may help improve musculoskeletal pain, depression, and general health in those with FM. Dosage: 1,500 mg daily.

Capsaicin: A component of cayenne pepper that helps relieve pain and works by depleting substance P, thus reducing the sensation of pain. Look for Zostrix or Menthacin, which are available in a pharmacy without a prescription. Apply to painful areas; wash hands after application, as it can burn the eyes.

Celadrin: Reduces pain and swelling and improves joint mobility. Dosage: 1,500 mg daily. Celadrin is also available in a cream, which can be applied to sore joints and muscles.

Magnesium: Reduces inflammation and promotes muscle relaxation. Dosage: 200 mg three times daily; may provide additional benefits when taken with malic acid (1,200–2,400 mg), which reduces pain.

Ribose: A sugar compound involved in the production of cellular energy. Preliminary research suggests that it can help improve energy and sleep and reduce pain in those with FM. Dosage: 5 g three times daily.

Vitamin E: Antioxidants may be depleted in those with FM. Preliminary research found that vitamin E improved symptoms of FM. Dosage: 400 IU daily.

FINAL THOUGHTS

FM is a chronic and painful condition that is not curable but can be greatly improved with lifestyle strategies and supplements. Key points to keep in mind:

- Nourish your body with a healthy diet and eliminate foods that trigger inflammation.
- Exercise regularly to reduce stress and pain and improve sleep and mood.
- Consider massage, chiropractic, or acupuncture to reduce symptoms.
- Top supplements include SAMe or 5-HTP and melatonin.
- Consider supportive supplements of acetyl-L-carnitine, Celadrin, magnesium, and ribose.

F

Fibromyalgia

FLU

The flu, which is short for influenza, is a viral infection that affects the upper respiratory tract (nose, throat, bronchial tubes, and lungs). Every year, approximately 10 to 25 percent of Canadians are infected with the flu. While it can be unpleasant, most people recover within a week to 10 days. However, an estimated 4,000 to 8,000 Canadians, mostly seniors, die every year from pneumonia related to flu or from other serious complications of flu.

The flu is caused by three strains (types) of viruses: influenza A, B, and C. Type A is responsible for the deadly influenza pandemics (worldwide epidemics) that strike every 10 to 40 years. Type B can lead to smaller, more localized outbreaks that generally occur every 3 to 15 years. And either types A or B can cause the flu that circulates almost every winter. Type C is less common and causes only mild symptoms.

In Canada, flu season typically runs from November to April. During these months, when the weather is colder outside, we spend more time indoors, closer to one another and sharing germs. This is how the flu is spread—by close contact with someone who has the virus. The virus travels through the air in droplets when someone with the infection coughs, sneezes, or talks. You can inhale the droplets directly, or you can pick up the germs from an object (doorknob, telephone, or keyboard) and then transfer them to your eyes, nose, or mouth.

There is no cure for the flu, but there are measures that can be taken to reduce your risk of infection, and to speed healing and reduce complications if you are infected.

IS IT THE FLU?

Flu and cold are caused by different viruses. Colds are caused by rhinoviruses and differ from flu in that they have a slower onset, symptoms are milder, and they typically don't cause high fever or muscle or joint aching.

SIGNS & SYMPTOMS

Once you are in contact with the virus, it takes about 48 hours for symptoms to develop.

- Chills and sweats

- Headache

- Loss of appetite

- Nasal congestion

- Nausea and vomiting (more common in children)

- Sore throat, dry cough

- Sudden onset of fever, muscle and joint aching, weakness, and fatigue

Young children, the elderly, and those with a weakened immune system are at risk of developing complications such as ear infections, sinusitis, bronchitis, and pneumonia.

RISK FACTORS

Anyone can get the flu, but the following groups of people are at greatest risk of infection and developing complications from the flu:

- Adults and children with chronic heart and lung disease

- Health care workers

- People living in a nursing home or chronic care facility

- People with chronic conditions such as diabetes, anemia, cancer, immune suppression, HIV, or kidney disease

- Those younger than 2 years of age or over 65

DOCTOR'S ORDERS

For most people, the best way to manage the flu is to rest, drink fluids, and allow the infection to run its course. Those who are at risk of complications (infants, the elderly, and those listed above) should consult with their doctor. There are antiviral drugs (such as Tamiflu) that can be given within the first 48 hours to reduce the length of illness and help prevent complications.

Anyone with signs and symptoms of pneumonia should seek medical attention. These include a severe cough (with phlegm), a high fever, and a sharp pain in the lungs when you breathe deeply. If you have bacterial pneumonia, you'll need treatment with antibiotics.

Over-the-counter products such as Tylenol and Motrin can be used to help reduce pain and fever. While they may help ease the symptoms, they do not shorten the duration of infection and can cause side effects. Tylenol can be hard on the liver, and Motrin can cause stomach pain, bleeding, and ulcers. Children under age 16 should not be given aspirin because of the risk of Reye's syndrome, a rare but potentially fatal disease.

Health Canada recommends yearly flu vaccination for those at risk. Vaccines don't offer 100 percent protection, but they do help reduce the risk of infection and complications if you get sick. Children under six months and those who are allergic to eggs should not receive the vaccine.

There is great debate about the long-term safety of vaccination and possible consequences, such as allergic reactions and increased risk of Guillain-Barré syndrome, an autoimmune disease that attacks the nervous system and results in weakness and abnormal sensations. It is important to review the benefits and risks with your health care provider.

HOMEOPATHIC RECOMMENDATIONS

Gelsemium: Symptoms of fatigue and aching that come on gradually, increasing over several days, may indicate a need for this remedy. The face feels heavy, with droopy eyes. A headache may begin at the back of the neck and skull, and the person may feel chills and heat running up and down the spine. Anxiety, trembling, dizziness, perspiration, and moderate fever are other indications for *Gelsemium*.

Oscillococcinum: Oscillococcinum is the Boiron brand of a remedy widely used in Canada, the U.S., and Europe for treating flu symptoms. Lots of good research has shown that it has strong antiviral effects. Use this at the first sign of flu symptoms that include fever, chills, body aches and pains, and headaches.

Combination recommendation: PascoLeucyn by Pascoe

SHERRY'S NATURAL PRESCRIPTION

Dietary Recommendations

Foods to include:

• Citrus fruits and berries contain vitamin C, which helps support immune function.

• Drink plenty of fluids, especially during the first few days of infection, to prevent dehydration and weakness. Choose water, juice, herbal teas, and broth. Elderberry juice contains compounds that have antiviral activity and can speed healing.

• Eat light meals of nutritious foods such as soups and stews with vegetables and beans, brown rice, fish, and poultry.

• Garlic, ginger, and onions contain antioxidants that support immune function.

• Green tea contains antioxidants that help support the immune system.

• Eat foods fortified with Wellmune, a natural ingredient that activates immune cells and enhances immune function without overstimulating the immune system. It is found in various juices, cookies, bars, and soups. It is safe for children as well as adults.

Foods to avoid:

• Dairy products can worsen mucus (phlegm) in those with cow's milk sensitivity.

• Minimize sugar (candy, soft drinks, and sweets) as it can hamper immune function.

Lifestyle Suggestions

• Get adequate rest as this is essential to help your body recover. Not getting enough rest on a regular basis can weaken your immune system and make you more susceptible to the flu and other infections.

• Minimize stress, which can hamper immune function. Try meditation, yoga, or breathing techniques.

• Get regular exercise to support proper immune function. Studies have shown that those who exercise regularly have less severe symptoms and recover quicker than those who don't exercise. During an episode of the flu you will not have the energy to exercise and should rest.

• Wash your hands frequently (especially after touching your eyes, nose, or mouth and after coughing or sneezing) to prevent spreading germs to others.

Top Recommended Supplements

Echinacea: Contains compounds that are thought to stimulate the immune system. Studies have shown that supplements can reduce flu symptoms and duration of infection. There are many forms of echinacea. A mixture containing all the parts of *E. purpurea* above the ground (flowers, leaves, and stems) has the best supporting evidence for effectiveness in treating flu. Dosage: 3–5 mL of tincture or 300 mg of extract three times daily. Take at the first onset of symptoms and continue for 7 to 14 days. Preliminary research on a product called Flu Shield, which contains *Echinacea angustifolia*, found that taking this product regularly reduced the incidence of infections.

North American ginseng: Helps support immune function. Studies conducted with a particular extract of American ginseng (COLD-FX), standardized to polysaccharides, show that it can reduce the frequency, severity, and duration of colds and flu by boosting the immune system. Dosage: 200–300 mg twice daily.

Complementary Supplements

Aged garlic extract: Has antiviral properties and enhances immune function. Preliminary studies suggest that regular use can reduce the risk of cold and flu. Dosage: 600 mg daily.

Elderberry: Can stimulate the immune system and inhibit viral growth. Studies of a product containing elderberry, echinacea, and bee propolis found that it reduced symptoms and sped up recovery from influenza. Dosage: Follow label instructions.

Panax ginseng: Also known as Korean ginseng, this supplement strengthens immune function. A few studies have shown that it can reduce the risk of cold and flu. Dosage: 200 mg daily of an extract standardized to contain 4–7 percent ginsenosides.

Vitamin C: Some research suggests that supplements can play a protective role and also shorten duration of illness. Dosage: 100–2,000 mg daily.

Vitamin D: A vitamin D deficiency is associated with increased risk of flu, and some research suggests that supplements can play a protective role. Dosage: 1,000–2,000 IU daily or as advised by your practitioner.

FINAL THOUGHTS

To improve healing from the flu, consider the following:

• Drink plenty of fluids, such as water, elderberry juice, and herbal teas.
• Eat citrus, berries, garlic, onions, and ginger.
• Minimize consumption of sugar and dairy products during an infection.
• Get lots of sleep and rest to allow your body to recover.
• Consider echinacea to speed recovery and aged garlic extract for prevention.

GALLSTONES

Gallstones are solid deposits of cholesterol or mineral salts that form in your gall-bladder or nearby bile ducts. It is estimated that about 20 percent of Canadians have gallstones by the age of 60. In many cases they do not cause a problem or symptoms. However, some people with gallstones develop a gallbladder attack, which causes abdominal pain, bloating, and nausea.

The gallbladder is a pouch-shaped digestive organ that is located near the liver and is responsible for storing and concentrating bile, a greenish-brown fluid composed of bile salts, fatty compounds, cholesterol, and other chemicals produced by the liver. When you eat, food enters the small intestine and the gallbladder contracts and releases bile into the common bile duct. The common bile duct carries bile to the upper part of your small intestine (duodenum), where it helps break down fat from your food. Aside from aiding digestion, bile is also involved in the absorption of fat-soluble nutrients, the retention of water in the colon to promote bowel movements, the excretion of bilirubin (the residue from the breakdown of red blood cells), and the elimination of drugs and chemicals from the body. If the bile becomes chemically unbalanced, it can form into particles that eventually grow into stones, which can lead to inflammation and infection of the gallbladder, known as cholecystitis.

There are two main types of gallstones: cholesterol and pigment gallstones. Cholesterol gallstones, as the name implies, are composed mainly of cholesterol. They are yellow in colour and may also contain calcium and bilirubin. About 90 percent of gallstones are cholesterol stones. They can be caused by too much cholesterol in the bile (which is not related to high blood cholesterol) or infrequent or incomplete emptying of the gallbladder (which causes the bile to become more concentrated). Pigment gallstones are dark brown or black stones that form when your bile contains too much bilirubin. This may result from having cirrhosis, biliary tract infection, or sickle cell anemia.

Problematic gallstones are treatable with medications or surgery. Lifestyle measures can go a long way to help prevent gallstones and also to help eliminate them.

SIGNS & SYMPTOMS

Gallstones vary greatly in shape and size. They can be as small as a grain of salt or as large as a golf ball. They can be smooth and round or irregular with jagged edges. Some people get just one, and others have several or even hundreds of them. About 90 percent of people have no symptoms. Others may experience the following:

- Fever when the stones get trapped in the neck of the gallbladder

- Indigestion (gas and bloating)

- Nausea and vomiting

- Upper abdominal pain and aching

Untreated gallstones can lead to serious, even fatal, complications, such as the following:

- Blockage of the bile duct: Occurs when a small stone escapes the gallbladder and enter the ducts leading from your gallbladder, liver, or pancreas to your small intestine (common bile duct). Symptoms include yellowing of the whites of the eyes and skin (jaundice), dark urine, and pain in the upper abdomen. If the pancreas becomes inflamed, it can cause intense, constant pain in your upper abdomen that may radiate to your back or chest. The pain is usually worse when you lie down and better when you sit up. You may also have nausea, vomiting, and fever.

- Gallbladder cancer: Gallstones may cause your gallbladder to release bile more slowly, which increases inflammation and the amount of time cells are exposed to cancer-causing substances in the bile. This type of cancer is quite rare.

RISK FACTORS

- Age: Risk increases with age. About 25 to 30 percent of women and 10 to 15 percent of men develop gallstones by age 70.

- Diets high in saturated fat and cholesterol and low in fibre can significantly increase the risk of gallstones.

- Ethnicity: The incidence of gallstones is higher in certain racial groups. For example, in Canada, 70 to 80 percent of the Aboriginal population is affected by this disease. Mexicans are also at greater risk.

- Family history of gallstones puts individuals at greater risk.

- Gender: Women between the ages of 20 and 60 are three times more likely to have gallstones than men. This is attributed to estrogen, which causes more cholesterol to be excreted in the bile.

- Medical conditions such as cirrhosis, biliary tract infection, diabetes, and sickle cell anemia increase the risk of pigment gallstones.

- Obesity raises cholesterol levels in the bile and also reduces the frequency of gallbladder emptying.

- Multiple pregnancies and the use of oral contraceptives or estrogen therapy increase the risk.

- Yo-yo dieting: Rapid weight loss can upset bile chemistry, and skipping meals or eating too little fat can reduce gallbladder contractions and emptying and increase the risk of gallstones.

DOCTOR'S ORDERS

Most gallstones do not cause any symptoms. Treatment is required only if you are experiencing serious symptoms. The most common treatment for gallstones causing symptoms is removal of the gallbladder (cholecystectomy). This can be done by laparoscopic surgery where a small tube is inserted into the abdomen and tiny instruments are used to remove the gallbladder. This is preferred, as the incisions are small and recovery is quick (a few days). For severe cases, open surgery through a large abdominal incision is necessary. Recovery from this procedure can take weeks.

For those with small stones, sound-wave therapy can help break up stones. Medications, such as ursodiol, are then used to dissolve the stone fragments.

G

Gallstones

SHERRY'S NATURAL PRESCRIPTION

Dietary changes, exercise, and supplements can be helpful in preventing gallstones and to prevent them from growing and causing inflammation and infection. However, if you are experiencing severe pain, fever, or any of the above listed symptoms of a blockage of the bile duct, it is critical to see your doctor.

Dietary Recommendations

Foods to include:

• Beets, artichokes, and dandelion greens help to improve the flow of bile.

• Coffee is actually protective. Caffeine increases bile flow and stimulates gallbladder contractions. In one study of 46,000 men, those drinking two or three cups of regular coffee per day had a 40 percent lower risk of gallstones compared with men who did not drink coffee.

• Eat small, frequent meals.

• Diets high in fibre are associated with a lower risk of gallstones. Eat more wheat and oat bran, milled flaxseed, legumes, vegetables, and fruits.

• Include lean protein (fish and poultry) and healthy fats (olive, palm fruit, and flaxseed oil).

Foods to avoid:

• Diets high in sugar are linked to increased risk of gallstones. Minimize high-sugar foods such as candy, soft drinks, pastries, and other sweets.

• Eating lots of saturated fat and cholesterol increases the risk of gallstones. Minimize red meat, high-fat dairy, eggs, and deep-fried and processed foods.

Lifestyle Suggestions

• Maintain a healthy body weight. If you are overweight, follow a healthy diet (not a fad diet) and boost activity levels to promote slow, gradual weight loss. Rapid weight loss can actually increase your risk of gallstones.

• Get regular physical activity every day.

Top Recommended Supplements

Lecithin: Contains phosphatidylcholine (PC), which helps protect against gallstone formation. Some preliminary studies suggest that 300–2,000 mg per day of PC may help dissolve gallstones.

Milk thistle: May help prevent gallstones from occurring. The active component, silymarin, helps to reduce cholesterol levels in bile and improve bile flow. Dosage: 420 mg daily.

Peppermint oil: Aids digestion; some research has shown that it can help dissolve gallstones. Dosage: One capsule three times daily. Choose an enteric-coated capsule to prevent upset stomach.

Complementary Supplements

Betaine HCl: An acidic form of betaine, a vitamin-like substance. People with gallstones may have insufficient stomach acid and may benefit from supplementing with betaine HCl. Dosage: Follow label directions.

Vitamin C: Needed to convert cholesterol to bile acids. A low intake of vitamin C is associated with increased risk of gallstones. Dosage: 500 mg daily.

The herbs artichoke leaf, dandelion root, and turmeric are often used to treat gallstones. It is thought that they work by improving bile flow and stimulating the gallbladder to contract and expel the stone. The research to support the benefits of these herbs is weak and there are certain side effects, so it is important to consult with your health care provider.

FINAL THOUGHTS

To reduce the risk of gallstones, consider the following:

- Eat small, frequent meals that contain high-fibre grains, vegetables, and fruits along with lean protein and healthy fats.
- Coffee in moderation (two to three cups per day) is helpful for prevention.
- Get regular physical activity.
- Maintain a healthy body weight, but avoid fad diets and rapid weight loss.
- Consider supplements of lecithin, peppermint oil, and milk thistle.

GLAUCOMA

Glaucoma refers to a group of eye diseases that cause damage to the optic nerve and elevated pressure inside the eye, or intraocular pressure (IOP). One of the most common causes of blindness, glaucoma affects over 400,000 Canadians.

The optic nerve is a bundle of nerve fibres at the back of the eye that carries images from the back of the eyeball (retina) to the brain. As the optic nerve deteriorates, blind spots develop in the visual field, usually starting with the peripheral (side) vision. If left untreated, glaucoma may lead to blindness in both eyes.

Elevated IOP is one of the primary causes of optic nerve damage; however, not everyone with elevated IOP develops glaucoma, and glaucoma can develop in those with normal IOP. IOP is regulated by the production and drainage of aqueous humour, a fluid naturally and continuously produced in the front of the eye. In a healthy eye, fluid is produced and drained at equal rates. If too much fluid is produced or not enough is drained, then IOP increases.

The two main types of glaucoma are open-angle and angle-closure. Open-angle glaucoma is the most common form and occurs when the eye fluids drain too slowly, causing a fluid backup and increased IOP. Damage to the optic nerve occurs slowly and is painless, so visual loss may occur without symptoms. Angle-closure glaucoma develops when the drainage canals within the eye become blocked and IOP increases. This can result from a narrow drainage angle that you are born with or as a result of aging. If you have a narrow drainage angle and your pupils dilate, this can cause a sudden increase in IOP, along with severe pain and headache. Vision loss can occur rapidly and requires immediate medical attention.

Other forms of glaucoma include low-tension glaucoma in which IOP is normal, yet the optic nerve becomes damaged. The cause of this type of glaucoma is unknown. Childhood glaucoma is an inherited form of the disease that is similar to open-angle glaucoma. There may not be any symptoms initially, but it leads to blindness if left untreated. Congenital glaucoma appears soon after birth and causes noticeable signs, including tearing, light sensitivity, and cloudiness of the cornea. With secondary glaucoma, IOP increases due to a structural problem within the eye, such as eye injury or other medical conditions.

SIGNS & SYMPTOMS

Many people with glaucoma are unaware of it until a serious loss of vision occurs. Signs and symptoms vary depending on the type of glaucoma.

Open-angle glaucoma:

• Loss of peripheral vision

• Progressive visual loss

• Tunnel vision

Acute angle-closure glaucoma:

• Blurred vision, halos around lights

• Headache

• Intense eye pain

• Nausea and vomiting

• Red, watery eyes

• Age: Those over the age of 40 are at increased risk.

• Family history (genetic defects may be inherited)

• Increased intraocular (internal eye) pressure

• Injuries (trauma to the eye, eye tumours, or inflammatory eye disease)

• Medical conditions: Having diabetes, insulin resistance, high blood pressure, heart disease, hypothyroidism, or nearsightedness increases your risk.

• Medications (chronic use of corticosteroids)

• Race: Blacks are at much greater risk; Mexicans and Asians are also at increased risk.

G

Glaucoma

DOCTOR'S ORDERS

There is no cure for glaucoma and the damage to the optic nerve cannot be reversed. In the early stages, if there is no damage to the optic nerve, your doctor may just recommend more frequent exams to monitor any changes. Those with elevated IOP and nerve damage often require treatment for life. There are a number of therapies that lower IOP and prevent further damage, such as eye drops, oral medications, laser therapy, and surgery. Eye drops provide the mainstay of therapy. Here is a brief overview of the most commonly used products:

• **Alpha-agonists:** Reduce the production and increase drainage of aqueous humour. An example is brimonidine (Alphagan). Possible side effects include fatigue, dizziness, dry mouth, and red, itchy, or swollen eyes.

• **Beta blockers:** Reduce the production of aqueous humour. Examples include timolol (Timoptic) and betaxolol (Betoptic). Possible side effects include slowed pulse, hair loss, lower blood pressure, impotence, fatigue, depression, and memory loss. These drugs are not typically used in those with asthma, bronchitis, emphysema, or diabetes.

• **Carbonic anhydrase inhibitors:** Reduce the production of aqueous humour. Examples include dorzolamide (Trusopt) and brinzolamide (Azopt). Possible side effects include frequent urination and a tingling sensation in the fingers and toes.

- **Cholinergic drugs:** Increase the outflow of aqueous humour. Examples include pilocarpine (Isopto Carpine) and carbachol (Isopto Carbachol). Possible side effects are pain around or inside the eyes, blurred vision, nearsightedness, nasal congestion, sweating, increased salivation, and upset stomach.
- **Prostaglandin-like compounds:** Increase the outflow of aqueous humour. Examples include latanoprost (Xalatan) and bimatoprost (Lumigan). Possible side effects include stinging and redness of the eyes, darkening of the iris, changes in the pigment of the eyelid skin, and blurred vision from swelling of the retina.

Since the disease can progress without symptoms, regular checkups are critical.

SHERRY'S NATURAL PRESCRIPTION

Dietary Recommendations

Foods to include:
- Vegetables that contain vitamin C and carotenoids (antioxidants), such as carrots, bell peppers, broccoli, kale, collard greens, and tomatoes, are important for eye health.

- Berries and cherries contain plant pigments (anthocyanidins) that prevent free radical damage to the eye and protect blood vessels.

- Fish contain omega-3 fatty acids that may reduce the risk of glaucoma.

Foods to avoid:
- Regular coffee consumption (more than one cup per day) can increase IOP.

- Food allergies may be implicated in glaucoma. Refer to Appendix D.

- Alcohol impairs liver function, which can affect the removal of toxins. Studies also suggest that consuming more than one alcoholic drink a day can raise IOP.

....

CAFFEINE AND GLAUCOMA

Caffeine has been shown in studies to elevate intraocular pressure. If you have glaucoma, minimize your consumption of coffee, soda, tea, and other caffeinated beverages.

....

Lifestyle Suggestions
- Drink fluids in small amounts over the course of a day. Drinking a lot in a short time may increase eye pressure.

- Exercising at least three times per week has been found to reduce IOP in those with open-angle glaucoma. Avoid exercises that require you to lower your head (in certain yoga poses, for example), as this can increase IOP.

- Reduce stress, which can trigger an attack in those with angle-closure glaucoma. Try breathing exercises, acupuncture, massage, or meditation.

G

Glaucoma

- Wear sunglasses when outdoors and safety glasses or goggles for sports or when using tools or working with chemicals.

- Get frequent eye examinations as advised by your doctor.

Top Recommended Supplements

Note: Supplements may be used in conjunction with prescribed therapies under doctor's supervision. Do not stop taking any prescribed medication unless advised by your doctor.

Ginkgo biloba: One study found that ginkgo can improve vision in those with glaucoma. It may work by opening up blood vessels and enhancing circulation and reducing free radical damage. Dosage: 40 mg three times daily.

Vitamin C: Important for production of collagen, which supports the health and integrity of blood vessels in the eyes and elsewhere. Vitamin C levels may be lower in those with glaucoma. Several studies have shown that it can help to lower IOP. Dosage: 2 g or more daily. To reduce the risk of upset stomach, consider buffered vitamin C, such as calcium ascorbate.

Complementary Supplements

Alpha lipoic acid: May help improve vision. Dosage: 150 mg daily.

Bilberry: Helps improve blood flow and blood vessel health. One study found that a combination of bilberry and pine bark extract boosted the efficacy of a common glaucoma eye drop. Dosage: 160 mg twice daily.

G

Glaucoma

FINAL THOUGHTS

To prevent worsening of glaucoma and preserve your vision:

- Get regular eye exams and follow your doctor's orders.
- Exercise regularly, reduce stress, and eat a healthy diet.
- Wear appropriate eye protection.
- Eat more vegetables, berries, and fish; avoid caffeine and alcohol.
- Consider supplements of vitamin C and ginkgo biloba.

GOUT

Gout is a form of arthritis that occurs when uric acid accumulates in a joint, leading to a sudden onset of intense pain and inflammation. While this problem is not life-threatening, it can be debilitating.

Uric acid is a substance created by the breakdown of foods containing high amounts of purines, a component of protein found in organ meat, seafood, and fish. Gout was once known as the "disease of kings" because of its association with consumption of rich foods and alcohol. Uric acid is normally eliminated in the urine. However, some people produce high amounts or are not able to eliminate it properly, leading to a buildup in the blood and the formation of uric acid crystals in the joints.

There are two main forms of gout: acute and chronic. Acute gout usually involves one joint, most often the big toe or a joint in a lower limb. An attack can begin suddenly and is often triggered by eating too much purine-rich foods, alcohol, or trauma. The attack usually subsides in a few days, however most people who have an acute attack will have a recurrence within a year. Over time the attacks may become more frequent, last longer, and involve more joints. If the gout is not treated, an attack can persist and lead to chronic gout. Deposits of urate crystals can form around the joint (called tophi), which can lead to chronic inflammation and damage to the joint and soft tissues. This is referred to as tophaceous gout.

Gout has become increasingly common in our society over the past few decades. In Canada it affects about 2 percent of both men over the age of 30 and women over the age of 50. It is thought that changes in diet and lifestyle are contributing to the rising incidence of gout. There are a number of dietary and lifestyle interventions that can help in both the management and prevention of gout.

SIGNS & SYMPTOMS

Gout attacks often occur suddenly, affecting the big toe, heel, or ankle and then later progressing to the knees, wrists, elbows, and fingers. Symptoms include the following:

- Back pain
- Fever
- Intense pain
- Joint swelling
- Red and warm joints
- Upset stomach

RISK FACTORS

- Age: Those over 40 are at greater risk.
- Alcohol consumption (rye, beer, and wine): More than two drinks per day for men or one drink per day for women increases risk.

- Carrying excess weight
- Eating foods high in purines (see next page)
- Family history
- Gender: Men are affected more frequently.
- Lead exposure
- Medications (antibiotics, aspirin, chemotherapy, diuretics, niacin)
- Medical conditions such as high blood pressure, high cholesterol or triglycerides, kidney disease, and diabetes
- Stress (trauma, surgery, emotional stress)

DOCTOR'S ORDERS

For an acute attack, non-steroidal anti-inflammatory drugs (NSAIDs) such as ibuprofen, naproxen, or indomethacin are often prescribed. They reduce pain and inflammation and work within 12 to 24 hours, but may cause side effects, including upset stomach, bleeding stomach, and ringing in the ears. They can also be hard on the liver and kidneys. Use only when absolutely necessary—the lowest dose for the shortest period of time.

One of the oldest remedies for a gout attack is colchicine, which is derived from the herb autumn crocus. It can also be used for prevention, but is limited by unpleasant side effects, such as severe diarrhea and upset stomach.

The primary drug used for prevention is allopurinol. It reduces the production of uric acid and is generally well tolerated. Skin rash is the most common side effect. There are a number of drug interactions with allopurinol, so check with your pharmacist before taking new medications.

SHERRY'S NATURAL PRESCRIPTION

An acute gout attack will most likely require medical treatment. However, certain lifestyle changes and nutritional supplements may help ease symptoms of an attack and prevent recurrences.

Dietary Recommendations

Foods to include:

- Cherries (fresh, canned, or juice) help to reduce uric acid levels and inflammation. Preliminary research suggests eating 20 cherries (about one cup) a day can cut the risk of a recurring gout attack in half. Raspberries, blueberries, blackberries, and celery also seem to help, although there is less research backing their benefits.
- Flaxseed provides essential fatty acids, which help reduce inflammation.
- Foods high in vitamin C (red peppers, tangerines, mandarins, oranges, and red cabbage) reduce uric acid.
- Choose lean proteins such as tofu, eggs, nuts, and seeds and low-fat dairy. Limit intake of meat, fish, and poultry to one serving (4–6 ounces, or 113–170 g) daily.
- Pineapple is high in bromelain, a digestive enzyme that may help reduce inflammation.

G

Gout

- Drink plenty of water (2–3 L per day) to help flush uric acid through the kidneys. However, if you have heart or kidney disease and are on fluid restriction, consult your doctor before changing fluid intake.

- Coffee is fine in moderation. Some studies have actually found an association between drinking coffee and lower levels of uric acid. If you don't currently drink coffee, there isn't enough evidence to suggest that starting to drink coffee will be preventative.

- Whole grains and flaxseed are high in fibre and help with elimination of uric acid. Studies have found that those who eat a high-fibre diet have lower uric acid levels. A high-fibre diet also reduces other risk factors for gout, including diabetes and high cholesterol.

Foods to avoid:

- Organ meats (heart), sardines, herring, mackerel, mussels, and sweetbreads contain very high amounts of purines, which can substantially increase uric acid levels.

- Minimize (once weekly) anchovies, veal, bacon, liver, kidneys, goose, scallops, salmon, crab, lobster, turkey, and haddock, which contain high amounts of purines.

- Limit consumption (four times weekly) of legumes (dried beans, peas, and soybeans), asparagus, gravy, mushrooms, oysters, tongue, spinach, and tuna.

- Refined flour (white bread, pasta) and sugar should be minimized as these foods can raise uric acid levels and are also unhealthy.

- Reduce consumption of alcohol, especially beer, as it interferes with uric acid elimination.

Note: Purines are found in all protein foods and should not be eliminated completely. Avoid foods highest in purines during an acute attack, and gradually resume eating these foods once symptoms disappear.

Lifestyle Suggestions

- Acupuncture helps to relieve pain and inflammation and promote relaxation.

- Exercise: Activities such as swimming, cycling, and stretching can help improve blood flow, reduce pain, and promote relaxation. Avoid high-impact activities, such as running, which are hard on the joints.

- Go easy on the joints—be careful not to bruise or hurt your joints as this can bring on an attack.

- Massage: Gentle massage helps promote relaxation and encourages removal of toxins. Avoid rubbing the joints affected by gout.

- Reduce stress through massage, meditation, or breathing exercises, which can help prevent a recurrence of gout.

- Weight loss: Slow, gradual weight loss may reduce attacks. Avoid rapid weight loss or fasting as this can raise uric acid levels and aggravate gout.

Top Recommended Supplements

Vitamin C: Reduces uric acid levels and may help with both managing an acute attack and preventing an attack. Take 500 mg daily for prevention. Higher amounts (4 g and higher) have been used to relieve an attack, but this should be done only under the supervision of a health care professional.

Complementary Supplements

Bromelain: An enzyme that helps reduce inflammation during an attack. Dosage varies by product potency; check label directions.

Celadrin: Reduces joint pain and inflammation and also helps improve joint mobility. Dosage: 1,500 mg daily.

Fish oil: Omega-3 fatty acids help reduce inflammation and improve joint health. Dosage: 1 g three times daily.

Quercetin: A flavonoid that in preliminary studies was found to help prevent gout attacks. Dosage: 150–250 mg three times daily.

FINAL THOUGHTS

Gout is a painful condition that can often be prevented and certainly improved by dietary and lifestyle modifications. To reduce your risk of an attack, consider the following:

- Minimize intake of high-purine foods and alcohol.
- Eat gout-fighting foods such as cherries, berries, and pineapple; drink plenty of water.
- Try acupuncture and massage to reduce stress and pain.
- Engage in regular, light exercise such as swimming, cycling, and stretching.
- Consider supplements of vitamin C, fish oil, and Celadrin.

GUM DISEASE

Gum disease, also known as gingivitis, is a very serious yet often overlooked health problem. Initially it causes red, swollen, and bleeding gums. If left untreated, gum disease can lead to periodontitis, a serious infection that destroys the soft tissue and bone that support your teeth, leading to tooth loss. Chronic periodontitis is very serious as it can lead to other health problems such as high blood sugar and increased risk of heart attack and stroke. In pregnant women it can affect the health of the unborn child and lead to premature birth.

There are many factors that affect gum health such as smoking, heredity, and immune function. However, the most common cause of gum disease is poor oral hygiene. The disease starts with the formation of plaque on the teeth when starches and sugars in food interact with bacteria in the mouth, creating a sticky film on the teeth. Brushing and flossing help to reduce plaque formation, but it re-forms quickly and any that is missed and stays on the teeth longer than 24 hours can harden under the gum line into tartar. Tartar acts as a reservoir for bacteria. It cannot be eliminated by brushing or flossing; only professional cleaning can eliminate this substance.

Plaque and tartar irritate the gums, causing inflammation. In time this inflammation causes pockets to develop between the gums and teeth that fill with more plaque, tartar, and bacteria. Over time the pockets become deeper and more bacteria accumulate under the gum tissue, leading to loss of bone and tissue and even tooth loss.

With proper oral hygiene, regular dental cleaning, and a healthy diet and lifestyle, gum disease can be prevented and even reversed.

CHECK YOUR GUMS

Healthy gums are firm and pale pink. If your gums are puffy and red and bleed easily, see your dentist. The sooner you seek care, the better your chances of reversing damage and preventing more serious problems.

SIGNS & SYMPTOMS

- Breath odour or bad taste in the mouth

- Gum recession

- Loose teeth or a change in how the teeth fit together

- New spaces between teeth

- Pus between teeth and gums

- Swollen, red gums

- Tenderness and bleeding of the gums

- Diabetes increases the risk of gum infection, and gum disease impairs the body's ability to use insulin.

- Drugs: Antihistamines reduce saliva production; phenytoin (an anticonvulsant) causes gum inflammation; immune suppressants (organ transplant drugs) may increase the risk of infection.

- Dry mouth

- Family history of gum disease

- Hormonal changes during pregnancy and menopause

- Poor diet and nutritional deficiencies (vitamin C, B-vitamins, and calcium)

- Poor oral hygiene (not brushing or flossing regularly)

- Smoking or chewing tobacco hampers immune function and promotes bacterial growth

- Stress may increase risk of gum disease, likely because it may trigger an increase in behaviours such as smoking and poor oral hygiene and it compromises the immune system.

- Suppressed immune system (HIV/AIDS or those undergoing cancer treatments)

DOCTOR'S ORDERS

Practising good oral hygiene is the best defence against gum disease. If you have early-stage gum disease, your dentist may ask you to come in more frequently. Professional cleaning and scaling can remove tartar and bacteria that can't be accomplished with brushing or flossing. Root planing can be done to smooth the root surface and discourage further accumulation of tartar. Antibiotic mouth rinses may be prescribed to control infection.

For advanced periodontitis, you may be referred to a gum specialist called a periodontist, who can offer various treatments such as flap surgery (to reduce pockets), soft tissue or bone grafts, and tissue-regeneration procedures. Antibiotics are sometimes used in conjunction with scaling and root planing to treat advanced cases.

HOMEOPATHIC RECOMMENDATIONS

Calendula: When there is dental inflammation, infection, or an abscess, this remedy can help when applied to injured gums and areas around the teeth. Calendula can help reduce the chance of infection and help the tissues heal after being cut or bruised.

SHERRY'S NATURAL PRESCRIPTION

Dietary Recommendations

Foods to include:

• Cranberries and cranberry juice contain antioxidants that prevent bacteria from adhering to teeth and gums. Choose products that are sugar-free or sweetened with xylitol.

• Fish and flaxseed contain fatty acids, which help reduce gum inflammation and may help reduce bone destruction.

• Fruits and vegetables contain vital nutrients that support immune function and gum health. Citrus, berries, peppers, and cantaloupe are good sources of vitamin C, which is used in the synthesis of collagen.

• Garlic supports immune function and helps fight infection.

• Green tea contains compounds that fight infection and inflammation. Preliminary research on a chewable candy with green tea found it helped improve gingivitis.

• Xylitol is a natural sugar added to gum, candy, and toothpaste that helps prevent cavities and may help prevent gum disease. There is a gum that contains both xylitol and a probiotic (BLIS K12) called CulturedCare that can help prevent the overgrowth of harmful bacteria that cause bad breath and gingivitis, and it also helps promote good oral health. A chewing gum that contains pycnogenol has also shown benefits in reducing bleeding gums and plaque formation.

Foods to avoid:

• Refined, starchy carbohydrates (white bread/rice/pasta) and sugars (candy, sweets) stick to the teeth and lead to plaque and tartar formation. Even dried fruit such as raisins and prunes stick easily to teeth. Always brush your teeth after eating these foods.

Lifestyle Suggestions

• Brush your teeth after meals and at bedtime and floss daily.

• Visit your dentist yearly or more often if recommended to have your teeth professionally cleaned.

• Don't smoke, and avoid second-hand smoke.

• Support immune system function by getting adequate sleep and reducing stress levels.

• Try an oral rinse that contains thyme, chamomile, echinacea, myrrh, tea tree oil, or eucalyptus as these natural ingredients have shown some benefits for gum disease. Folic acid has also shown benefits as a rinse and in supplement form (see next page).

USING PROPER TECHNIQUE

First it is important to choose the right toothbrush. Dentists recommend soft bristles because hard bristles can injure the gums. Angled toothbrushes allow you to reach every tooth easily. Replace your brush every three to four months or when the bristles are worn down. Electric toothbrushes are very effective and may be helpful, especially for those with arthritis or problems with dexterity. To properly brush your teeth, use short, back-and-forth, then up-and-down strokes on the outer surfaces and vertical strokes on the inner surfaces. Use gentle pressure; the tips of the brush do the cleaning, so it isn't necessary to use force. You should spend about three to five minutes brushing your teeth. To properly floss, use about 18 inches of floss, hold the floss taut and bent around each tooth, and gently scrape up and down each side of each tooth. Each stroke should go slightly below the gum line.

Top Recommended Supplements

Coenzyme Q10: A powerful antioxidant that has been studied for gum health. It helps reduce gum pockets and speeds healing after dental surgery. Dosage: 50–100 mg daily.

Folic acid: Studies suggest it can reduce gum inflammation and bleeding. Use a solution of 0.1 percent of folic acid as a mouth rinse, 1 tsp (5 mL) twice daily. Benefits have also been seen when folic acid was taken in supplement form. Dosage: 4 mg daily.

Vitamin C: Essential for gum health; protects the gums from cell damage, hastens healing, and strengthens the immune system to fight off the bacterial infection that causes gum disease. Studies have found that those who are deficient in vitamin C are at increased risk of gum disease and supplementing can help to reduce symptoms. Vitamin C with flavonoids may offer additional benefits for reducing inflammation. Dosage: 250–1,000 mg daily, depending on dietary intake and other factors.

Complementary Supplements

Calcium: Essential for healthy bone and teeth. Research suggests that it can improve symptoms of periodontal disease (bleeding gums and loose teeth). It may be particularly helpful in those who are deficient in calcium. Dosage: 500 mg two or three times daily with meals.

Fish oils: Reduce inflammation and may reduce bone loss. Dosage: 1–3 g daily.

Vitamin E: Antioxidant properties help protect against free radicals produced by white blood cells attracted to diseased gums. Dosage: 400 IU daily.

FINAL THOUGHTS

To improve gum health and reduce the symptoms of gum disease, consider the following:

- Brush your teeth after meals and floss daily, and get your teeth professionally cleaned at least once a year.
- Add cranberries, fish, and green tea to your diet. Minimize refined starches and sugars.
- Try CulturedCare probiotic gum.
- Don't smoke, and avoid second-hand smoke.
- Consider supplements of coenzyme Q10, folic acid, and vitamin C.

HAIR LOSS

The human body sheds approximately 100 of its 100,000 to 150,000 strands of hair every day, and new ones grow to take their place. As we age, this renewal process may slow where more hairs are lost than grown.

Male pattern baldness is an inherited condition called androgenetic alopecia and it may begin as early as age 20. Male hair loss is distinguished by a receding hairline and thinning on the crown. The rate of hair loss may be slow, gradual, or fast. By age 50, about 50 percent of men will experience thinning and hair loss. For 40 to 50 percent of women, hair may begin to thin after age 50 (typically after menopause). This is called female pattern baldness. Women tend to see their hair thin throughout the head, but most visibly on the crown. Significant hair loss for women before age 50 is rare and usually triggered by hormonal fluctuations, stress, or a secondary health concern.

Other kinds of hair loss include the following:

Alopecia areata: This form of hair loss is characterized by patchy baldness or bald spots. It affects both men and women equally, both adults and children, but it is rare, affecting less than 2 percent of the population. Hair loss due to alopecia areata is usually triggered by an immune system disorder. Once addressed, the hair usually grows back.

Anagen effluvium: This condition occurs when hair in the growth phase falls out prematurely. Prescription medications used for the treatment of cancer are the most common cause of this condition. Chemotherapy patients may lose up to 90 percent of their hair as a result of anagen effluvium.

Telogen effluvium: A natural part of the hair growth cycle includes a resting phase called telogen, which involves 10 percent of hair at any given time. Telogen effluvium occurs when up to 30 percent of hairs on the head are in the resting phase at any given time. This condition may be caused by physical or emotional stress, and hair growth will return to normal as stress is eased.

The health of your hair is a reflection of the overall state of your health, so it is important to address hair loss from a multipronged approach that includes both the use of standard medical treatments to slow hair loss and nutritional and lifestyle changes to address and improve health.

SIGNS & SYMPTOMS

- Bald patches

- Scalp irritation

- Sudden, excessive, or increased hair loss

- Visible thinning of the hair around the top and sides of the head

If hair loss is accompanied by other symptoms such as fatigue, cold hands and feet, dry skin and hair, and menstrual fluctuations, it may be the warning signs of hypothyroidism or an underactive thyroid. See your doctor immediately for further tests.

- Age: Hair loss is more common with increased age.

- Burns, injuries, and skin infections such as ringworm

- Drugs used to treat gout, arthritis, depression, heart problems, and high blood pressure, and birth control pills

- Genetics

- Hair treatments: Chemicals used for dying, bleaching, straightening, or perming can damage and break hair if they are used incorrectly; hairstyles that pull hair tightly can cause hair loss, which is known as traction alopecia.

- Hormonal changes such as pregnancy and menopause

- Immune disorders (lupus, diabetes, thyroid disease)

- Nutritional deficiencies: Inadequate protein, iron, or essential fatty acids

- Severe gastrointestinal disorders that cause malabsorption of nutrients, such as celiac disease, Crohn's, or colitis

- Stress: Emotional stress, fever, surgery, flu

- Weight problems and extreme dieting

PUT A LEASH ON DHT

DHT stands for dihydrotestosterone, a hormone formed when the enzyme 5-alpha-reductase breaks down testosterone. DHT is the primary underlying cause of male pattern baldness. DHT shortens the hair growth cycle, causing the hair follicles to shrink and stop production of hair, leading to hair loss. DHT not only affects men but also women, particularly after menopause when levels of estrogen decrease. Some drugs used to treat baldness work by inhibiting the action of 5-alpha-reductase, thus reducing the formation of DHT. High-fat diets can also boost DHT levels.

DOCTOR'S ORDERS

If you experience sudden or excessive hair loss or bald patches, see your doctor to rule out nutritional deficiencies, thyroid concerns, and other health problems.

Hair loss due to aging and genetics must be treated as early as possible to stabilize hair loss and stimulate regrowth.

The most highly recommended topical solution is minoxidil (Rogaine). Minoxidil is a vasodilator (a drug that causes the blood vessels in the body to become wider) and was originally introduced as a blood pressure–lowering drug. When it was found to have an added benefit of hair regrowth, it was reformulated as a topical 2 percent solution and is now sold over the counter. Minoxidil is applied to the scalp twice daily. It has been shown to benefit approximately 40 percent of people who use it for hair loss as early as two months after the initial application. Studies show hair weight and hair counts increase with the 2-percent solution, and more so with the 5-percent solution where hair weight increased by 45 percent. Minoxidil must be used on a daily basis for life to ensure hair growth. It may cause irritation and itchiness. Discontinue use if symptoms persist.

Another recommended treatment for hair loss is finasteride (Propecia), an oral prescription medication taken once daily for life. Finasteride is only for men. It has been shown to stop hair loss in 83 percent of cases and to stimulate regrowth in 66 percent of cases. Finasteride works by inhibiting DHT.

SHERRY'S NATURAL PRESCRIPTION

Dietary Recommendations

Proper nutrition is important to supply nutrients to the hair follicles in the scalp.

Foods to include:

• Ensure adequate protein intake as protein is necessary for hair growth. Choose lean sources of protein (fish, poultry, lean cuts of meat, beans, nuts, seeds, and soy). Meat, poultry, and fish also contain iron, which is required for proper hair growth.

• Fish, chia seed, and flaxseed contain essential fatty acids necessary for proper hair growth.

• Nuts and seeds; almonds contain magnesium, which is important for hair growth.

• The outer skin of plants such as potatoes, cucumbers, green and red peppers, and sprouts can strengthen hair because they are rich in the mineral silica.

• Whole grains, vegetables, and fruits are good sources of essential nutrients and fibre.

Foods to avoid:

• Caffeine and alcohol can deplete the body of nutrients and also raise adrenal levels, which can trigger hair loss.

• Foods high in sugar can raise cortisol levels (a stress hormone) and cause the body to produce more androgens, promoting hair loss.

• High intake of salt has been linked to hair loss. Foods high in salt include processed and snack foods, deli meats, and the salt shaker.

• Reduce or eliminate pro-inflammatory foods: saturated fat (fatty meats and dairy) and trans fats (processed foods and fried foods). Saturated fat reduces the amount of sex hormone binding globulin (SHBG), a substance that normally binds to testosterone. With less SHBG, more testosterone can be converted into DHT, which promotes hair loss.

Lifestyle Suggestions

• Regular exercise and healthy sleep habits will increase circulatory and overall health, promoting healthy hair.

• Reduce the frequency of washing and drying your hair. Use a gentle shampoo and conditioner. Some research has found that essential oils can benefit those with alopecia areata. In one study, daily application of a combination of thyme, rosemary, lavender, and cedarwood in a base of grape seed and jojoba oils yielded significant improvement in hair growth after seven months of use.

• Avoid using hot water and hair dryers or curling irons whenever possible.

- Avoid exposing hair to chlorinated pool water and other chemicals (perms and dyes).

- Do not overbrush your hair. Limit grooming and always be gentle when brushing or combing hair. Keep braids and ponytails loose.

- Give yourself a weekly deep conditioning treatment and scalp massage to protect the hair shaft and stimulate new hair follicle growth.

- Wear a wide-brimmed hat when outdoors to protect your scalp and hair from the sun's damaging rays.

- Don't smoke. According to one report, smokers were four times more likely to have grey hair than non-smokers and were more prone to hair loss.

Top Recommended Supplements

B-vitamins: Essential for proper hair growth. A deficiency of the B-vitamins biotin and PABA can cause hair loss. Supplements of biotin may strengthen hair, stimulate new hair growth, slow hair loss, and prevent greying, particularly in those who are deficient in this nutrient. PABA (para-aminobenzoic acid) may protect hair roots and help prevent hair loss. It can also reverse greying in cases where the cause is a deficiency of PABA or other B-vitamins. Dosage: Take a B-complex vitamin daily.

Essential fatty acids: A deficiency can cause hair loss; supplements can help improve the health of scalp and hair. Take a blend of fish and evening primrose or borage oil. Dosage: 2–3 g daily.

Orthosilicic acid: Enhances collagen formation and makes hair stronger and thicker. One study found that it improved brittleness of hair and nails. Taking silicon supplements will not yield the same results as silicon is poorly absorbed. Orthosilicic acid is the bioavailable (usable) form of silicon and is available in Canada under the name BioSil. Dosage: 6–10 drops daily in juice (to mask the bad taste). Drink immediately.

Complementary Supplements

Grape seed extract: A potent antioxidant that has been shown in preliminary research to stimulate hair growth. Dosage: 50–100 mg daily.

Minerals: Iron, selenium, and zinc are essential for hair growth; a deficiency can cause hair loss. Dosage: Take as part of a daily multivitamin/mineral complex.

Saw palmetto: Used primarily for the treatment of enlarged prostate. It blocks the production of DHT and thus may be helpful for treating hair loss due to high DHT levels, although this has not been tested in humans yet. Consult with your health care provider before supplementing with saw palmetto.

FINAL THOUCHTS

To improve the health of your hair and prevent hair loss, consider the following:

- Eat lots of vegetables, fruits, whole grains, fish, nuts, seeds, and lean protein.
- Reduce or minimize saturated fat, caffeine, sugar, and salt.
- Get regular exercise and don't smoke.
- Avoid using harsh chemicals and heat on your hair. Do a scalp massage with essential oils weekly.
- Consider supplements of B-vitamins, essential fatty acids, and orthosilicic acid.

HEART DISEASE (CARDIOVASCULAR DISEASE)

Heart disease, also known as cardiovascular disease, refers to diseases of the blood vessels and heart. While cancer is highly feared, heart disease is actually the leading cause of death worldwide and among Canadians, accounting for about one-third of all deaths.

There are several forms of heart disease, including coronary artery disease (CAD), hypertension, congestive heart failure, congenital heart disease (a defect that you are born with), arrhythmia (irregular heartbeat), cardiomyopathy (enlargement of the heart), heart block, valve disorders, and pericarditis (infection of the membrane surrounding the heart).

This chapter focuses specifically on CAD, also known as atherosclerosis or hardening of the arteries. The coronary arteries supply your heart with blood, oxygen, and nutrients. CAD is thought to start when the inner lining of the arteries become damaged. The blood vessel wall reacts to this injury by depositing cholesterol, calcium, and other substances on the inner lining of the artery. The result is a progressive thickening of the blood vessel wall, which reduces the supply of oxygen-rich blood to the heart, leading to chest pain (angina). If the coronary arteries become completely blocked and the flow of blood is cut off, a heart attack (myocardial infarction) occurs, which results in damage to the heart muscle.

High blood pressure, high levels of cholesterol and triglycerides in the blood, and smoking can all contribute to the development of plaque. Chronic inflammation is a recently recognized factor that contributes to CAD. Inflammation causes damage to the arterial walls and further narrows the passageways.

This process does not happen overnight. Damage may begin as early as childhood. Years of smoking, stress, high blood pressure and cholesterol, uncontrolled blood sugar (diabetes), and poor diet take a toll on your heart and contribute to the development of heart disease. The good news is that there are many ways to keep your heart healthy, reduce your risk of heart disease, and improve heart health if you already have heart disease.

CHOLESTEROL: THE GOOD AND THE BAD

Cholesterol is a fatty substance manufactured in the liver and also obtained from consuming saturated and trans fats. There are two forms of cholesterol: LDL and HDL. LDL (low-density lipoprotein) is called "bad" cholesterol because it can build up in the artery walls of the brain and heart, narrowing the passageways for blood flow. HDL (high-density lipoprotein) is called "good" cholesterol because it picks up the LDL deposited in the arteries and transports it to the liver to be broken down and eliminated.

SIGNS & SYMPTOMS

- Chest pain and tightness (often triggered by physical or emotional stress); women may notice pain in the back, arm, neck, or abdomen
- Fatigue with exertion
- Shortness of breath
- Swelling in your feet and ankles

RISK FACTORS

- Age
- Diabetes
- Family history of heart disease
- Gender: Men are at greater risk of coronary artery disease than women. However, the risk for women increases after menopause.
- High blood pressure
- High cholesterol: High LDL (bad cholesterol) and low HDL (good cholesterol)
- History of stroke or a TIA (transient ischemic attack)
- Inactivity (sedentary lifestyle)
- Obesity
- Poor diet (high in saturated and trans fats; low in fibre); excess alcohol consumption
- Smoking
- Stress

MULTIPLYING YOUR RISK

Most people with heart disease have more than one risk factor, and the more risk factors you have, the greater your likelihood of heart disease and death. For example, obesity often leads to diabetes, high blood pressure, and cholesterol. This cluster of problems is called metabolic syndrome, which greatly increases the risk of heart disease.

In recent years, research has identified other factors that may increase your risk of heart disease. They include:

- C-reactive protein (CRP), a marker of inflammation, which is a factor in the development of atherosclerosis. High CRP levels are correlated with an increased risk of heart attack and stroke.

H

Heart Disease (Cardiovascular Disease)

- Fibrinogen, a protein in your blood that is involved in blood clotting. High levels of fibrinogen may promote excessive clumping of platelets, which can cause a clot, leading to a heart attack or stroke.

- Homocysteine, an amino acid made by the body during normal metabolism. Studies suggest that elevated homocysteine increases the risk of heart disease by damaging the lining of the arteries and promoting clots. Homocysteine metabolism is controlled by vitamins B6, B12, and folic acid, and a deficiency of these nutrients can increase levels. However, studies have not found that lowering homocysteine reduces heart disease risk.

- Lipoprotein (a), a substance that forms when a low-density lipoprotein (LDL) cholesterol particle attaches to a specific protein. The protein that carries lipoprotein (a) may disrupt your body's ability to dissolve blood clots, and high levels of this substance may increase the risk of cardiovascular disease.

DOCTOR'S ORDERS

Lifestyle approaches (diet, exercise, and not smoking) are essential for the management of heart disease. If these approaches aren't effective, then your doctor will likely prescribe a medication depending on your needs. There are drugs to lower cholesterol or blood pressure, which are mentioned in those sections of this book. Low-dose daily aspirin (ASA, 81 mg daily) is often recommended to thin the blood and reduce the risk of clotting, which can lead to heart attack and stroke. New guidelines issued by the Canadian Cardiovascular Society now recommend ASA for all people who have had a heart attack, stroke, or peripheral artery disease. ASA is no longer recommended for primary prevention for people who have not had a heart attack or stroke or other vascular disease.

For those with angina, nitroglycerin tablets, spray, or patches may be used to open up the coronary arteries and improve blood flow.

There are also various procedures, such as angioplasty and coronary artery bypass surgery, which can be done to improve blood flow.

SHERRY'S NATURAL PRESCRIPTION

Dietary Recommendations

Foods to include:

- Green tea contains antioxidants that offer benefits for the heart.

- Fish, chia seed, and flaxseed contain beneficial omega-3 fatty acids that reduce inflammation and LDL cholesterol, prevent blood clotting, and reduce the risk of heart disease. Try to eat two to three servings per week of fresh cold-water fish such as salmon, trout, herring, mackerel, and tuna. Reduce consumption of toxins by choosing wild (not farmed) fish.

- Fruits and vegetables contain an array of antioxidants, including flavonoids, which have been associated with a lower risk of heart disease. These compounds help reduce inflammation, promote relaxation of blood vessels, lower cholesterol levels, and reduce blood clot formation. Some of the best food sources include apples, berries, grapes, citrus, onions, tea, and cocoa.

- Garlic helps reduce cholesterol and thin the blood, and has antioxidant properties. Try to eat one fresh clove daily.

- Moderate alcohol consumption (one drink daily for women and two for men) has been shown to have heart-protective effects. Alcohol increases protective HDL cholesterol and also helps to thin the blood. Higher amounts can be hard on the liver and increase blood pressure and the risk of heart disease.

- Nuts (almonds and walnuts) help lower cholesterol levels. Nuts contain fibre and nutrients such as vitamin E, alpha-linolenic acid, magnesium, potassium, and arginine, which are important for heart health. Although nuts are high in calories, some studies have found that increasing nut consumption by several hundred calories per day does not cause weight gain.

- Oat bran is rich in a soluble fibre called beta glucan, which has been shown to lower cholesterol levels. A typical dose of oat bran is 5–10 g taken with each meal. Beta glucan is also available in supplement form. The recommended intake is 10–15 g of beta glucan per day.

- Olive oil is a monounsaturated fat that can help reduce blood clots and lower LDL cholesterol. Add it to your salads and recipes in place of other vegetable oils. Olive oil is best to add to foods after they are cooked or used in salad dressings. It is not heat stable and not recommended for cooking.

- Palm fruit oil is rich in poly- and monounsaturated fatty acids and antioxidants like beta carotene and tocotrienols (a potent form of vitamin E). Research conducted on the tocotrienols in Malaysian palm fruit oil have shown that it can help raise HDL cholesterol and lower LDL cholesterol. Palm fruit oil is heat stable, thus ideally suited for cooking. Many food companies have replaced the hydrogenated oils (trans fats) in their products with palm fruit oil. Pure (virgin) coconut oil has similar properties and benefits.

- Phytosterols (plant sterols) are plant compounds that are effective in lowering LDL cholesterol levels. They are thought to work by attaching to cholesterol in the digestive tract and carrying it out of the body. They also remove cholesterol from substances made in the liver. They are naturally present in small amounts in fruits, vegetables, nuts, seeds, and legumes. Manufacturers are now adding plant sterols to a variety of foods, such as orange juice (Minute Maid Heart Wise with CoroWise plant sterols), margarine (Becel pro.activ), and yogurt (Danacol).

- Soluble fibre—which is found in oats, flaxseed, chia seed, beans, psyllium, and fruits—helps lower cholesterol levels. Insoluble fibre—which is found in whole grains, vegetables, and fruits—does not lower cholesterol, but studies have shown that it helps protect against heart disease. Current Canadian guidelines recommend adults consume 21–38 g of fibre daily. Fruits and vegetables also contain vital antioxidants, and studies have shown that those who consume antioxidant-rich diets have lower rates of heart disease. Appendix B lists low-glycemic foods.

- Soy products (tofu, soybeans, miso, and soy protein powder) can help lower cholesterol and triglycerides. Substituting as little as 30 g (1 ounce) per day of soy protein for animal protein can significantly lower cholesterol.

- Tomatoes contain an antioxidant called lycopene, which has been shown to help reduce LDL cholesterol and slow the progression of atherosclerosis. Aim for 10 servings of tomato products weekly or consider a supplement.

- Yogurt and fermented milk products have been shown to lower cholesterol levels.

Foods to avoid:

- Foods high in cholesterol, such as organ meats, egg yolks, shrimp, squid, fatty meats, and whole milk products, may have a small effect on raising blood cholesterol levels in those with high blood cholesterol or type 2 diabetes. However, studies have shown that in healthy people with no history of heart disease, diabetes, or high blood cholesterol, eating an average of one egg per day does not increase the long-term risk of heart disease. If your cholesterol levels are normal you may eat up to one egg per day (or seven eggs per week). If you have diabetes or high blood cholesterol, limit your whole eggs to no more than four per week.

- Foods high in sugar and refined starches (white flour) can raise triglyceride and insulin levels, which increases the risk of heart disease.

- Salt causes water retention and increases the pressure inside your arteries. Reducing salt intake reduces blood pressure in most people. Aim for no more than 2,300 mg daily. Avoid adding salt to foods and minimize eating processed and fast foods such as deli meats, snacks (chips, pretzels), french fries, and burgers.

- Saturated fat, which is present in animal foods (beef, pork, and dairy), can raise cholesterol levels and is associated with increased heart disease risk. Vegetable and plant oils also contain some saturated fat, but much less than animal products. Limit daily consumption of saturated fat to 10 percent of total calories. Read food labels carefully. Dairy products labelled "low fat" can be misleading. For example, 25 percent of calories in 2 percent milk come from fat. The 2 percent refers to the fraction of volume filled by fat, not the percentage of calories coming from fat.

- Trans fatty acids are found in hydrogenated oils, which are present in some margarines, snack foods (chips and microwave popcorn), and deep-fried foods (french fries). These fats can raise cholesterol levels and increase the risk of heart disease. Look for non-hydrogenated margarines. Many snack food companies are now making products that are free of trans fatty acids.

Lifestyle Suggestions

- Don't smoke, and avoid second-hand smoke, as this increases many risk factors for heart disease. Smoking lowers the good HDL cholesterol, increases blood pressure, and causes serious damage to blood vessels. It is never too late to quit. Within one year of quitting, your risk of heart disease is half that of a smoker's. After 15 years, your risk is similar to that of someone who has never smoked.

- Lose excess weight. Losing even 5 to 10 percent of excess weight can lower cholesterol and blood pressure.

- Exercise regularly. Moderate-intensity activities, such as brisk walking, biking, or swimming, can reduce cholesterol and blood pressure and help with weight management. Aim for one hour daily.

- Reduce stress levels. Stress causes the liver to increase the production of cholesterol, which is used to make stress hormones. Try meditation, exercise, or yoga to promote calming and relaxation.

- Manage your blood sugar levels. If you have diabetes or are at risk for diabetes, work on improving your blood sugar levels with exercise and a low-glycemic diet (see Appendix B).

- See your doctor regularly for checkups and to monitor your blood pressure, cholesterol, and blood sugar. Discuss the results with your doctor.

Top Recommended Supplements

Aged garlic extract: Helps lower total and LDL cholesterol and triglycerides, reduces blood clotting, and prevents atherosclerosis. Dosage: 600 mg or more daily.

Coenzyme Q10: An antioxidant that has been widely studied and found to lower blood pressure and cholesterol and strengthen the function of the heart. Dosage: 100 mg twice daily.

Fish oils: Fish oil contains the beneficial omega-3 fatty acids, eicosapentaenoic acid (EPA) and docosahexaenoic acid (DHA). Numerous studies show fish oil can significantly lower triglycerides, modestly raise HDL cholesterol, and reduce inflammation and blood clotting. Dosage: Minimum of 1 g of EPA and DHA daily; usual dose for those with heart disease is 3 g daily, although higher amounts have been used in some studies.

Niacin (vitamin B3): Numerous studies have shown that niacin can lower LDL cholesterol, triglycerides, and lipoprotein-A levels and raise HDL cholesterol. Dosage: 1–4 g daily. Niacin can cause liver inflammation at higher dosages (more than 500 mg daily) and requires physician monitoring.

Stanols and sterols: Plant substances that have been shown in many studies to lower LDL cholesterol. They are thought to work by attaching to cholesterol in the digestive tract and carrying it out of the body. They also remove cholesterol from substances made in the liver. A sterol ester, called beta-sitosterol, has been shown to decrease cholesterol absorption by about 50 percent. Dosage: Varies depending on the product and potency.

Complementary Supplements

Flavonoids: Antioxidant compounds that can help lower cholesterol and blood pressure. There is some evidence that they can help reduce atherosclerosis. Those that have been researched include Sytrinol (citrus and palm fruit extract), MegaNatural BP (grape seed extract), and Pycnogenol (pine bark extract). Follow label directions.

Soluble fibre: Helps to lower cholesterol. Those that have been studied include glucomannan (PGX), partially hydrolyzed guar gum (Sunfiber) beta glucan, and psyllium (Metamucil). Dosage varies depending on the product and amount of fibre per serving. Add gradually to the diet to avoid gas and bloating. Dosage varies depending on the source. Take with plenty of water.

FINAL THOUCHTS

To improve the management of heart disease, consider the following:

- Boost intake of soluble and insoluble fibre. Eat more fish, garlic, soy, yogurt, and nuts. Drink green tea.
- Minimize saturated fat, trans fats, sugar, and salt.
- Get regular exercise and reduce your stress.
- Don't smoke.
- Consider supplements of aged garlic extract, coenzyme Q10, fish oils, niacin, and stanols.

HEMORRHOIDS

Hemorrhoids, also known as piles, are a form of varicose veins—swollen, enlarged veins that develop in the anal and rectal area. They are very common; almost everyone will have them at some time in their life. They are particularly common during pregnancy and with aging. Approximately 50 percent of those over the age of 50 have them.

Hemorrhoids are usually caused by increased pressure on the veins in the pelvic and rectal area, which causes pooling of blood in the veins. The swelling veins stretch the surrounding tissue, leading to the development of hemorrhoids.

While they are uncomfortable and even painful at times, there are many natural remedies that can help shrink them and reduce symptoms. Lifestyle modifications can help reduce your risk of developing hemorrhoids.

SIGNS & SYMPTOMS

Hemorrhoids can develop either inside the rectum (internal) or outside (external). Symptoms vary and may include the following:

• Blue or purple skin in the rectal area

• Feeling of fullness in the rectum (with internal hemorrhoids)

• Itching, skin irritation, and discomfort

• Lumpy tissue protruding from the rectum

• Rectal bleeding (blood in stool or toilet paper)

• Swelling in rectal area.

Note: Rectal bleeding can also be a sign of serious conditions such as colorectal cancer. If you experience rectal bleeding, consult your doctor.

RISK FACTORS

Any factors that increase pressure in the veins in the rectal area can trigger hemorrhoids, including the following:

• Anal intercourse

• Chronic constipation or diarrhea (irritates rectal tissue)

• Dehydration: Not drinking enough fluids or drinking too many diuretic liquids, such as coffee or cola, can cause hard stools and irritate hemorrhoids.

• Diet (lack of dietary fibre; excess dairy consumption)

• Genetic factors (weak rectal vein walls or valves)

• Heavy lifting or straining

• Obesity

• Pregnancy and childbirth

• Sitting or standing for a prolonged time

DOCTOR'S ORDERS

There are several medical options for treating hemorrhoids. Hemorrhoid creams and suppositories contain ingredients such as hydrocortisone, zinc, mineral oil, shark liver oil, and witch hazel, which help shrink hemorrhoids and soothe the pain. Examples include Preparation H and Anusol.

Procedures to reduce or remove hemorrhoids include the following:

- **Banding** is a procedure in which a doctor places tiny rubber bands around the base of the hemorrhoid to cut off its circulation and it eventually falls off.
- **Sclerotherapy** involves injecting a solution into the vein to shrink the hemorrhoid.

For those with severe hemorrhoids, a surgeon will remove the hemorrhoid. This is usually done as an outpatient procedure and requires a few days for recovery.

HOMEOPATHIC RECOMMENDATIONS

Aesculus hippocastanum: Indicated when hemorrhoids cause sharp and shooting pains felt in the rectum and back.

Aloe: Indicated for hemorrhoids that are swollen and protrude like a bunch of grapes.

Graphites: Indicated for hemorrhoids caused by constipation or very large and dry stools. Individuals who respond to this treatment often experience a feeling of heaviness in the lower abdomen, along with anal itching and burning.

SHERRY'S NATURAL PRESCRIPTION

Dietary Recommendations

Foods to include:

- Pure aloe vera gel can be applied directly to hemorrhoids to help relieve itching and swelling.
- High-fibre foods help prevent constipation and ease bowel movements. Eat more fruits, vegetables, and whole grains. Blueberries and bilberries are particularly good because they are not only rich in fibre, but also contain antioxidant compounds that reduce inflammation and support the health of blood vessels. Add dried fruits (figs, prunes, raisins) to your yogurt or cereal along with ground flaxseed or chia seed. Aim for 21–38 g of fibre daily. Make sure to also increase your fluid intake so that the fibre can do its job.
- Yogurt, kefir, and tempeh contain beneficial bacteria that help improve digestion and elimination, and help your body absorb vitamin K, which helps prevent bleeding.

Foods to avoid:

- Caffeine (coffee and cola) is dehydrating.
- Fast/processed foods are low in fibre and high in saturated fats and chemicals that have a negative impact on bowel function.

Lifestyle Suggestions

- Develop good bowel habits. Go when you feel the urge; don't hold it in, as this can cause the stool to become dry and harder to pass. Don't strain to push a stool out.

- Exercise regularly to prevent constipation and improve bowel function.

- Don't lift heavy objects, as this can increase the pressure on the rectal veins.

- Avoid standing or sitting for a prolonged period of time. Move around. Use a doughnut cushion or pad on your chair.

- Bathe or shower daily to keep the area clean. Soak in a warm (not hot) sitz bath (a basin that fits over the toilet) with Epsom salts after a bowel movement and at night. Don't use soap, as it can irritate the skin.

- Use soft toilet paper or moist towelettes.

- Apply ice packs or cold compresses to external hemorrhoids to reduce swelling.

- Use creams with witch hazel to reduce swelling. Aloe vera, zinc, and calendula are soothing and promote skin healing.

Top Recommended Supplements

Diosmin: A flavonoid that improves vein health and reduces swelling, pain, itching, and bleeding. Numerous studies, including research on pregnant women, have found benefits for hemorrhoids. Dosage: 600–3,200 mg daily of a product standardized to 95 percent diosmin and 5 percent hesperidin.

Fibre: Supplements can be used to complement the diet. Look for a product that mixes well with water/juice, such as Benefibre, which contains inulin from chicory root, or Sunfiber, which contains hydrolyzed guar gum. These products are tasteless, dissolve completely in beverages, and don't thicken like other products. Sunfiber is a prebiotic fibre and thus less likely to cause gas and bloating. Increase fibre intake gradually and take regularly with plenty of water.

Complementary Supplements

Horse chestnut seed extract: Reduces swelling and pain and promotes vein health. It may take several weeks to notice benefits. Dosage: 300 mg orally three times per day, or use a cream or gel containing 2 percent aescin three or four times daily.

Probiotics: Supplements containing beneficial bacteria help to restore the normal gut flora and have been shown in studies to relieve constipation. Probiotics shown to be beneficial for constipation include BioGaia, VSL #3, and Kyo-Dophilus. Take as directed.

Witch hazel: Strengthens veins and reduces inflammation. It is available in teas, creams, and solutions (to make compresses). Safe for use during pregnancy and breastfeeding.

FINAL THOUGHTS

To prevent hemorrhoids or reduce symptoms, consider the following:

- Boost fibre intake from food or supplements; drink more fluids.
- Avoid prolonged sitting or standing; get regular exercise.
- Use cold compresses and creams or suppositories with witch hazel.
- Evidence is strongest for diosmin supplements.
- Probiotics and horse chestnut seed extract are also helpful.

HEPATITIS (VIRAL)

Hepatitis is an inflammation of the liver caused by one of the hepatitis viruses. Hepatitis can also be caused by drugs, alcohol, or autoimmune disease. The most common forms of viral hepatitis are A, B, and C. When you are first infected with hepatitis, it is called acute hepatitis. The virus attacks the liver, but there are often few or no initial symptoms. Hepatitis can also become a long-term disease known as chronic hepatitis. All forms of hepatitis cause jaundice, liver tenderness, and severe fatigue. In some cases hepatitis can cause severe symptoms and be fatal.

The hepatitis viruses differ in how they are transmitted (spread). Hepatitis A virus (HAV) is usually transmitted via the fecal–oral route. For example, someone with the virus could use the toilet, not wash his or her hands, and then handle the food you eat, thus passing the virus from their stool to your mouth. HAV can also be spread by drinking contaminated water, eating raw shellfish from water polluted with sewage, or being in close contact with a person who is infected. HAV only causes acute infection, which typically lasts a few months.

Hepatitis B virus (HBV) is transmitted through contact with the blood and body fluids of someone who is infected. Most commonly it is spread by sexual contact, sharing needles (IV drug abusers), and needle-stick injuries (nurses and hospital workers are susceptible). Women with HBV can pass the infection to their babies during childbirth. HBV can survive on personal items, such as toothbrushes and razors, for a few days and remain infectious. Most people infected as adults recover fully from HBV even if their signs and symptoms are severe. Infants and children are much more likely to develop a chronic infection.

Hepatitis C virus (HCV) is primarily spread by contact with blood. In the past it was transmitted by blood transfusions, but that is rare today because our blood supply is screened for the virus antibodies. Today it is spread by sharing needles, and less commonly from contaminated needles used in tattooing and body piercing. In rare cases, HCV may be transmitted sexually or through childbirth. HCV is one of the main causes of chronic liver disease. About 60 to 70 percent of people who have acute HCV go on to develop chronic hepatitis.

Other forms of hepatitis include the following:

- Hepatitis D virus (HDV): Caused by Delta agent, a type of virus, this form is only found in those who carry the hepatitis B virus, and it can make the hepatitis B liver disease worse.
- Hepatitis E virus (HEV): Has only been recognized since 1980. This virus is transmitted like hepatitis A (fecal–oral route) and is uncommon in North America.
- Hepatitis F and G viruses: Relatively new forms of the disease. HFV is thought to be transmitted by the oral–fecal route and HGV by blood. However, little is known about these forms.

Since there are no effective medical treatments for hepatitis, prevention is key—practising good hygiene and safe sex and taking necessary precautions when travelling to high-risk areas. For those who develop hepatitis, dietary approaches and supplements can help prevent liver damage and improve healing.

BE GOOD TO YOUR LIVER

The liver is the largest internal organ, and it performs more than 500 important functions in the body, including processing most of the nutrients absorbed from your intestines; removing drugs, alcohol, and other toxins from your bloodstream; manufacturing bile (the greenish fluid stored in your gallbladder that helps digest fats); and producing cholesterol, blood-clotting factors, and certain other proteins. The liver has an amazing ability to regenerate. It can heal itself by replacing or repairing injured cells. However, the liver is prone to a number of diseases, such as viral hepatitis, which can hamper its function. Take measures to protect yourself against contracting hepatitis by practising safe sex and good hygiene (hand washing) and not sharing needles.

SIGNS & SYMPTOMS

Some people with hepatitis have no signs or symptoms, especially in the acute (early) stages. When symptoms do occur, they may include the following:

- Clay-coloured stools

- Dark urine

- Fatigue

- Muscle and joint aches and pains

- Nausea and vomiting

- Poor appetite

- Tenderness in the area of your liver (right side beneath your lower ribs)

Note: Hepatitis B can damage your liver—and spread to other people—even if you don't have any signs and symptoms.

Most people infected with HCV develop chronic hepatitis. With chronic hepatitis, there may be no symptoms, or people may experience fatigue, yellowing of the skin and eyes (jaundice), and low-grade fever. Chronic hepatitis increases the risk of cirrhosis and liver cancer.

RISK FACTORS

Hepatitis A:

- Hemophilia or receive clotting-factor concentrates for another medical condition

- HIV positive

- Blood transfusions (although this is rare)

- Sexually active gay or bisexual man

- Sharing needles

- Travel or work in regions with high rates of hepatitis A

- Work in a research setting where you may be exposed to the virus

Hepatitis B:

- Being born to a mother who has hepatitis B

- Exposure to infected blood (health care workers)

- Having a sexually transmitted disease such as gonorrhea or chlamydia

- Having unprotected sex with someone who is infected with HBV

- Having received a blood transfusion or blood product before 1970, the year the blood supply began to be tested for HBV

- Receiving hemodialysis for end-stage kidney (renal) disease

- Sharing needles

- Travelling to regions with high infection rates of HBV, such as sub-Saharan Africa, Southeast Asia, the Amazon Basin, the Pacific Islands, and the Middle East

Hepatitis C:

- Being born to a mother who has hepatitis C

- Having an organ transplant before 1992

- HIV positive

- Health care worker who has been exposed to infected blood

- Having received clotting-factor concentrates before 1987 or have the clotting disease hemophilia and received blood before 1992

- Receiving hemodialysis for kidney failure

- Sharing needles or getting piercings or tattoo with unsterilized equipment

DOCTOR'S ORDERS

Conventional medicine has little in the way of treatment for acute hepatitis.

No specific treatment exists for hepatitis A. The goal is to ensure adequate nutrition and avoid permanent liver damage.

If you are exposed to HBV, call your doctor immediately. Receiving an injection of hepatitis B immune globulin within 24 hours of coming into contact with the virus may help protect you from developing hepatitis B. You should also receive the first in a series of three shots of the hepatitis B vaccine.

For those with chronic hepatitis B or C, the treatment depends on the severity of the signs and symptoms and liver damage. For those who have liver damage, doctors may recommend injections of a drug called interferon alpha combined with an oral antiviral drug to clear the virus from your bloodstream. Side effects from interferon include severe flu-like symptoms, irritability, depression, poor concentration, memory problems, and insomnia. Antiviral drugs can cause a low red blood cell count (anemia), gout, and birth defects. Both drugs can cause extreme fatigue.

For those with end-stage liver disease, a liver transplant may be necessary. This can be a risky procedure and difficult to have since there is a shortage of organs available to meet the demands. Newer procedures include the donation of liver segments from a relative. A liver transplant does not cure HCV; most people who have transplants will experience a recurrence of the virus. Transplant recipients are also at greater risk of developing cirrhosis within five years than are people with HCV who don't receive a transplant.

VACCINES FOR HEPATITIS

Vaccines are available for the prevention of hepatitis A and B. The hepatitis A vaccine (Havrix) may protect you for up to 20 years. It contains inactivated forms of HAV and is safe for children older than two years as well as for most adults, including those with compromised immune systems. The hepatitis B vaccine (Engerix-B) provides more than 90 percent protection for both adults and children. The vaccine generally protects against HBV for at least 15 years. Twinrix is a vaccine that protects people over the age of 18 against both HAV and HBV. Studies have shown Twinrix to be as effective as the separate HAV and HBV vaccines. The vaccines cause minor side effects (pain at injection site, headache, and fatigue), although allergic reactions can also occur.

SHERRY'S NATURAL PRESCRIPTION

A healthy diet is important to support liver function and protect against further damage.

Dietary Recommendations

Foods to include:

- Choose organics as much as possible to avoid ingesting pesticides and chemicals, which are hard on the liver.
- Drink vegetable juices—beets and carrots are particularly good.
- Eat small, frequent meals of brown rice, steamed vegetables, whole grains, fish, chicken, and legumes.
- Green tea contains catechins, which aid detoxification.

Foods to avoid:

- Alcohol is hard on the liver and speeds the progression to liver disease.
- Fast foods, processed foods, and snack foods contain chemicals that are taxing to the liver.
- Saturated and trans fats are hard on digestive function and stressful to the liver.

HEPATITIS PREVENTION

To avoid contracting any of the hepatitis viruses:

- Practise safe sex. Use condoms and ask your partner whether he or she has any of the viruses or has been tested.
- Don't share needles or other drug paraphernalia. Contaminated drug paraphernalia is responsible for more than half of all new hepatitis C cases.
- Avoid body piercing and tattooing, or if you do undergo piercing or tattooing, be absolutely certain the equipment is sterile.

- Talk to your doctor if you're travelling internationally to areas where hepatitis A or B is endemic, and discuss the benefits and risks of vaccination.

- If you're travelling in regions where hepatitis A outbreaks occur, you can help prevent infection by peeling and washing all your fresh fruits and vegetables yourself and by avoiding raw or undercooked meat and fish. Drink bottled water and avoid ice cubes in beverages. If bottled water isn't available, boil tap water for at least 10 minutes before drinking it. Don't forget to use bottled water for tooth brushing.

Lifestyle Suggestions

If you have hepatitis, consider the following to improve your health:

- Avoid medications that may cause liver damage, like Tylenol. Talk with your pharmacist before taking any over-the-counter (OTC) medications.

- Get regular exercise.

If you have hepatitis, take measures to prevent passing the virus to others:

- Tell your sexual partner if you have hepatitis and that he or she should be tested.

- Practise safe sex (use condoms). Avoid oral–anal contact.

- Wash your hands with soap and water after using the toilet.

- Those with hepatitis A should keep their utensils separate from those used by other members of their household. Wash utensils and dishes in a dishwasher or with plenty of hot, soapy water. Don't prepare food for others while you are actively infected.

- Help prevent others from coming into contact with your blood. Cover any wounds you may have and don't share razors or toothbrushes. Don't donate blood, body organs, or semen, and advise health care workers that you have the virus.

Top Recommended Supplements

Catechin: A type of flavonoid (an antioxidant plant compound) that has been shown to benefit those with acute viral hepatitis and chronic hepatitis. Dosage: 500–750 mg three times daily, under doctor supervision.

Milk thistle: Contains a compound called silymarin, which aids healing and regeneration of the liver. It stimulates the production of antioxidant enzymes that help the liver neutralize toxins. It also seems to increase the production of new liver cells and may even improve the severe scarring of cirrhosis. Dosage: 140 mg silymarin three times daily.

SAMe (S-adenosylmethionine): A nutrient that is naturally occurring and involved in numerous body processes, including detoxification. Studies show that it supports liver function and may help in the treatment of chronic hepatitis. Specifically it can help improve cholestasis, a problem that occurs when bile backs up into the liver. Dosage: 800–1,600 mg daily.

Complementary Supplements

Antioxidants: Play an important role in reducing oxidative stress, free radical damage, and inflammation, which is involved in the progress of the disease. Studies have shown that the livers of people with hepatitis have reduced levels of antioxidants, and there is some evidence that antioxidants, such as vitamins C and E and selenium, may help protect the liver from further damage.

H

Hepatitis (Viral)

Cordyceps: Helps reduce fibrosis and improve liver and immune function in those with chronic hepatitis B, including those with cirrhosis. Dosage: The usual amount taken is 34.5 g twice daily as capsules, or simmered for 10 to 15 minutes in water to make tea.

Thymus extracts: Made of proteins from the thymus gland; some research shows that these supplements can benefit those with chronic hepatitis B by improving liver function. Dosage: 200–300 mg three times daily, under doctor supervision.

Note: Various Chinese herbs and Ayurvedic products have been used to treat hepatitis. There is some science to support these products, but there are certain precautions and safety issues. Consult with a practitioner in these areas for advice prior to use.

FINAL THOUGHTS

To manage hepatitis, consider the following:

- Eat a healthy diet with lots of vegetables, brown rice, fish, chicken, and legumes. Choose organic foods.
- Drink vegetable juices and green tea.
- Avoid alcohol, processed foods, fast foods, and saturated and trans fats.
- Avoid medications that are hard on the liver, such as Tylenol.
- Consider supplements of catechins, milk thistle, or SAMe to promote healing.

HIGH BLOOD PRESSURE (HYPERTENSION)

Blood pressure is a measure of the force that blood exerts on the walls of arteries and veins as it is pumped through the body. It is determined by the amount of blood that the heart pumps and the amount of resistance to blood flow in the arteries. High blood pressure, or hypertension, occurs when the pressure on your blood vessels is elevated.

Our blood pressure is regulated by a complex system involving the heart, blood vessels, brain, kidneys, and adrenal glands. It fluctuates from moment to moment, typically increasing in response to physical activity or stress. When blood pressure stays elevated, even when you are at rest, it can damage the arteries and delicate organs like the brain, heart, and kidneys.

In about 90 to 95 percent of people with high blood pressure, there's no identifiable cause. This is referred to as essential hypertension or primary hypertension, which tends to develop gradually over many years. A combination of factors may be at play, such as diet, lifestyle, stress, and smoking.

The other 5 to 10 percent of high blood pressure cases are secondary hypertension as they are caused by an underlying condition, such as kidney or adrenal diseases or heart defects. Certain medications can also cause secondary hypertension, as noted on the next page.

High blood pressure is known as a silent killer because you can have it for years without knowing it, and then suddenly have a heart attack or stroke. Uncontrolled blood pressure can also cause organ damage, leading to increased risk of stroke, heart attack, and kidney failure. If you have high blood pressure, it is critical to be under a doctor's supervision. Do not stop taking any prescribed medications. The strategies outlined in this chapter are not meant as a substitute for medical care. Lifestyle approaches, such as proper nutrition, exercise, stress management, and supplements, can be used to complement your medical care.

SIGNS & SYMPTOMS

- Dizziness

- Dull headache

- Flushed cheeks

- Nosebleeds

- Sweating

- Visual disturbances

Many people have no symptoms of high blood pressure, even when levels are very high. Get your blood pressure checked regularly, beginning at age 18, and discuss the results with your doctor. The two numbers given when your blood pressure is taken are the systolic and diastolic pressure. Systolic is the top number, and it is the pressure when your heart contracts and pushes blood throughout your body.

Diastolic is the bottom number and it is the pressure when the heart relaxes between beats. Normal blood pressure is between 120/80 mm Hg and 129/84 mm Hg. A person's blood pressure reading along with their current and past medical history are used in determining treatment.

RISK FACTORS

- Age: It is more common with increased age; men often develop it between the ages of 35 and 55, and women are more likely to develop it after menopause.

- Chronic conditions such as high cholesterol, diabetes, kidney disease, and sleep apnea are associated with an increased risk of high blood pressure.

- Diet: High intake of sodium and alcohol; low intake of potassium and fibre. Research has also found a connection between low vitamin D intake and high blood pressure.

- Family history

- Illicit drugs such as cocaine and amphetamines

- Lack of physical activity

- Lack of sleep. Recent studies have found that chronic sleep deprivation (getting less than six hours' sleep at night) can increase blood pressure over time.

- Medications (birth control pills, cold remedies, and decongestants)

- Obesity: Those with a body mass index (BMI) of 30.0 or higher are more likely to develop high blood pressure.

- Race: It is more common in Black people.

- Smoking

- Stress

DOCTOR'S ORDERS

The first line of approach to the management of high blood pressure is lifestyle changes, including a healthy diet and regular exercise. If this is not successful, then your doctor will likely prescribe a medication. There are several types of medications that are used depending on the stage of your blood pressure and whether you have other medical conditions. A combination of medications may be necessary. All of these drugs can cause side effects and sometimes your doctor may change the drug or dose a few times to get your blood pressure properly regulated with the least amount of side effects.

The main classes of medications include the following:

- **Angiotensin-converting enzyme (ACE) inhibitors:** Relax the blood vessels, which reduces blood pressure. Examples include ramipril (Altace) and enalapril (Vasotec). A common side effect is chronic coughing.

- **Angiotensin II (A-II) receptor blockers (ARBs):** Work the same as the drugs above, but do not cause coughing. Examples include losartan (Cozaar) and valsartan (Diovan).
- **Beta-blockers:** Reduce the workload on the heart, slowing your heartbeat, which lowers the pressure. They are often given with a diuretic. Examples include propranolol and acebutolol.
- **Calcium channel blockers:** Relax the muscles of the blood vessels and some slow the heart rate. Examples include diltiazem (Cardizem) and nifedipine (Adalat).
- **Diuretics:** Act on the kidney to help your body eliminate sodium and water, thereby reducing blood volume. Examples include hydrochlorothiazide and furosemide.
- **Renin inhibitors:** Slow down the production of renin, an enzyme produced by the kidneys that is involved in raising blood pressure. Aliskiren (Rasilez) is the only drug in this category approved for treating hypertension. Due to serious health risks (stroke), this drug shouldn't be taken with ACE inhibitors or ARBs.

SHERRY'S NATURAL PRESCRIPTION

Dietary Recommendations

Foods to include:

- Cold-water fish contain beneficial fatty acids that can help reduce blood pressure and lower the risk of heart disease.

- Dark chocolate is rich in antioxidants, and several studies have found that regular consumption can help lower blood pressure and improve blood vessel health.

- Garlic and onions contain antioxidants that help lower blood pressure and cholesterol.

- Green tea contains antioxidants that offer benefits for the heart.

- Soy foods can help lower blood pressure. Incorporate soy milk, tofu, soy protein powder (make shakes), and soy nuts into your diet.

- Stevia is a natural, plant-based sweetener that can actually help lower blood pressure, according to some studies. Use stevia instead of sugar or artificial sweeteners. It is available in liquid or powder form for baking.

- Whole grains, vegetables, fruits, beans, and legumes contain lots of fibre, and there is research to show that a high-fibre diet can help lower blood pressure. High-fibre foods have a lower glycemic index (converted more slowly into sugar) and this can improve insulin response. Insulin plays a role in blood pressure regulation. Soluble fibre may also help increase the absorption of minerals like calcium, magnesium, and potassium, which also help lower blood pressure. Oranges, tomatoes, bananas, green beans, raisins, and dates are particularly good sources of potassium as well as fibre.

Foods to avoid:

- High caffeine intake can increase blood pressure in those who are caffeine sensitive. Limit yourself to one or two cups of coffee per day. Avoid soft drinks because they contain high amounts of caffeine and provide no nutritional value.

H

High Blood Pressure (Hypertension)

- Limit alcohol to one or two drinks per day; red wine can offer some health benefits because of the antioxidants it contains and is a better choice than beer or spirits.

- Reducing salt intake reduces blood pressure in most people. Salt causes water retention and increases the pressure inside your arteries. Avoid adding salt to foods and minimize eating processed and fast foods such as deli meats, snacks (chips, pretzels), french fries, and burgers. Limit salt intake to 2,300 mg per day, or less if advised by your doctor.

- Saturated fat (red meat and dairy) and trans fats (deep-fried and snack foods) can increase blood pressure and clog your arteries, increasing the risk of heart disease.

Lifestyle Suggestions

- Don't smoke, and avoid second-hand smoke. Smoking greatly increases the risk of high blood pressure.

- Get regular exercise—aim for one hour of moderate-intensity activity daily. Try brisk walking, biking, swimming, or dancing.

- Maintain a healthy body weight. Being overweight increases blood pressure and stress to the heart.

- Manage your stress levels by finding ways to promote calming and relaxation. Regular exercise, breathing techniques, or meditation are a few ways to reduce the effects of stress.

- Get adequate sleep at night. Aim for seven to eight hours.

- Acupuncture and yoga have been shown to lower blood pressure in many studies.

- See your doctor regularly. Get your blood pressure and cholesterol checked and discuss the results with your doctor. Consider purchasing a home blood pressure monitor; your pharmacist can help you choose a monitor suited to your needs.

Top Recommended Supplements

Coenzyme Q10: An antioxidant that has been widely studied and found to lower blood pressure and cholesterol and strengthen the function of the heart. Dosage: 60–100 mg twice daily.

Fish oils: Over 30 studies have shown that the omega-3 fatty acids in fish oil can help lower blood pressure, reduce atherosclerosis, and protect against heart attack. Dosage: 3 g of EPA plus DHA three times daily. Higher dosages are commonly used.

Garlic: Helps lower blood pressure and cholesterol, reduces clotting, and prevents plaque formation in the arteries. Most of the research showing benefits has been done on aged garlic extract (Kyolic). Dosage: 600 mg twice daily.

POTASSIUM LOWERS BLOOD PRESSURE

Numerous studies have shown that potassium can lower blood pressure, but the dose used in studies is quite high (2,400 mg daily). The highest dosage sold without a prescription in Canada is 100 mg. Potassium can cause stomach irritation in high doses and should not be combined with potassium-sparing diuretics or taken by those with kidney disease. Talk with your doctor about whether this is a good choice for you. Potassium is found naturally in apples, bananas, oranges, and tomatoes.

Complementary Supplements

Calcium and magnesium: Several studies have found that these minerals can promote modest reductions in blood pressure. Both are essential for proper muscle contractions and blood vessel health. Dosage: 800–1,200 mg calcium and 300–500 mg magnesium daily. Take in divided dosages with meals.

Polyphenols: Antioxidant compounds that relax (open up) blood vessels, reduce blood pressure, and improve blood vessel flexibility. Two clinically studied forms are MegaNatural BP, a patented form of grape seed extract (dosage: 150–300 mg daily) and Pycnogenol, a patented form of pine bark extract (dosage: 100–200 mg daily).

Green coffee bean extract: Contains antioxidants that have been shown in preliminary studies to lower blood pressure. Dosage: 185 mg daily.

Hawthorn: A few small studies have shown that this herb can modestly lower blood pressure. It may be particularly helpful in those with congestive heart failure and diabetes. Dosage: 1,200 mg daily.

Lycopene: A member of the carotenoid antioxidants. Preliminary research shows that it can lower blood pressure in those with mild hypertension and in those with moderate hypertension that are poorly controlled by medication. The most widely studied product is Lyc-O-Mato, a patented full spectrum lycopene complex. Dosage: 6–10 mg daily.

Vitamin C: Helps to lower blood pressure. Several studies have shown that it offers modest benefits. It also helps the body eliminate heavy metals, such as lead, which can contribute to high blood pressure. Dosage: 500 mg twice daily.

Vitamin D: A vitamin D deficiency is associated with high blood pressure. Supplements can help to ensure adequate intake and may play a role in preventing high blood pressure. Dosage: 800–1,000 IU daily. Higher dosages are often used for therapeutic purposes.

FINAL THOUGHTS

To improve the management of high blood pressure, consider the following:

- Boost your intake of fibre; eat more fish, potassium-rich foods, garlic, soy, and onions; and drink green tea.
- Get regular exercise. Aim for one hour of moderate-intensity activity daily.
- Don't smoke, and reduce your stress. Try acupuncture and yoga.
- Have your blood pressure checked regularly and know your results.
- Consider supplements of coenzyme Q10, fish oil, and garlic.

H

High Blood Pressure (Hypertension)

HIGH CHOLESTEROL

Cholesterol is a fatty substance that is found in every cell of our bodies. It is an important component of cell membranes and is used in the formation of various hormones such as estrogen, testosterone, progesterone, and cortisol as well as bile acids. The liver manufactures the cholesterol that the body needs. We get additional cholesterol from our diet when we eat foods containing saturated fat and cholesterol. About 80 percent of the body's cholesterol is made by the liver and the remaining 20 percent comes from diet.

Cholesterol is carried through the blood via proteins called lipoproteins. High-density lipoprotein (HDL) is known as "good" cholesterol because it picks up excess cholesterol in the blood and takes it back to the liver. Low-density lipoprotein (LDL) is called "bad" cholesterol because it can build up in the artery walls of the brain and heart, narrowing the passageways for blood flow, a process known as atherosclerosis, the precursor to heart disease and stroke.

High blood cholesterol, known as hypercholesterolemia, occurs when the liver produces too much cholesterol, the body cannot remove LDL cholesterol from the blood efficiently, or excess amounts of cholesterol or saturated fats are obtained from the diet.

Triglycerides are not a type of cholesterol, but they are a type of fat that is carried in the blood. High triglycerides also increase the risk of heart attack. Your triglyceride level is usually measured at the same time as your blood cholesterol.

Below are the current Canadian targets for cholesterol management:

- **Total cholesterol:** Less than 5.2 millimoles per litre (mmol/L) is ideal, and more than 6.2 mmol/L is considered high.
- **HDL cholesterol:** More than 1.3 mmol/L is desirable.
- **LDL cholesterol:** Less than 2.6 mmol/L is ideal and more than 4.0 mmol/L is high.
- **Triglycerides:** Below 1.7 mmol/L is desirable, 1.7–2.2 is borderline high, 2.3–5.6 is high, and above 5.6 is very high.

There are many natural ways to effectively lower cholesterol; following a healthy diet and getting regular exercise are essential. Lifestyle modifications and supplements, as discussed below, can help. In some cases, medication is necessary. Many of the strategies for lowering cholesterol are also effective for lowering triglycerides, and thus recommendations for lowering triglycerides are included here.

SIGNS & SYMPTOMS

There are no obvious signs or symptoms of high cholesterol. If left untreated, high cholesterol can form plaques inside the arteries (atherosclerosis). This reduces blood flow to the heart, which may cause chest pain and increases the risk of heart disease. The plaques can rupture and form a blood clot. If this blood clot blocks the flow of blood to the heart, a heart attack occurs; if it blocks blood flow to the brain, a stroke occurs.

- Diabetes: High blood sugar contributes to high LDL cholesterol and low HDL cholesterol, and also damages the lining of the arteries

- Family history: Genetic defects can cause the liver to produce too much cholesterol and impair the removal of cholesterol from the blood

- High blood pressure damages artery walls, which can increase the accumulation of fatty deposits

- Inactivity

- Obesity

- Poor diet: Eating too much saturated fat (meat, dairy) and cholesterol-rich foods

- Smoking damages the blood vessel walls, which makes them prone to cholesterol deposits; smoking also lowers HDL levels

- Risk factors for high triglycerides include poor diet (high intake of sugar and starches), obesity, excess alcohol consumption, and diabetes

DOCTOR'S ORDERS

The recommended first-line approach to the management of high cholesterol is lifestyle changes—a proper diet and regular exercise. Drugs are used when lifestyle changes are not enough or if the person is not willing to make the necessary changes. The most commonly used drugs include the following:

- **Bile acid-binding resins:** These drugs lower LDL cholesterol by working in the intestines to promote increased disposal of cholesterol via binding to bile acids, substances required for digestion. The liver uses cholesterol to make bile, so this process causes the liver to use excess cholesterol to make more bile acids, which reduces the level of cholesterol in the blood. Examples include cholestyramine (Questran) and colestipol (Colestid). Side effects include constipation, upset stomach, and increased risk of gallstones.

- **Cholesterol-absorption inhibitors:** This is a new class of drugs that reduces the absorption of dietary cholesterol and the storing of cholesterol in your liver and improves the way cholesterol is cleared from your blood. They are most effective at lowering the LDL cholesterol, but may also have modest effects on lowering triglycerides and raising HDL levels. The only drug in this class approved in Canada is ezetimibe (Zetia). Side effects include diarrhea, stomach pain, headache, and dizziness.

- **Fibrates:** These drugs are used primarily to lower triglycerides. They work by inhibiting the liver's production of VLDL (particles in the blood that carry triglycerides and lipoproteins) and by speeding up the removal of triglycerides from the blood. They have a modest effect on increasing HDL levels but are not effective in lowering LDL levels. For this reason they are sometimes combined with statins. Examples of

H

High Cholesterol

fibrates include gemfibrozil (Lopid), bezafibrate (Bezalip), and fenofibrate (Lipidil). Common side effects of fibrates include upset stomach, constipation or diarrhea, headache, and dizziness. Fibrates can also cause muscle and liver damage; these risks are higher when they are used with statins.

- **Statins:** These are the most commonly prescribed class of drugs for high cholesterol. They inhibit the action of an enzyme in the liver that is required for cholesterol production. They may also help the body reabsorb cholesterol from accumulated deposits on the artery walls. Statins effectively lower LDL cholesterol and they also modestly decrease triglycerides and raise HDL cholesterol. Examples include atorvastatin (Lipitor), fluvastatin (Lescol), lovastatin (Mevacor), pravastatin (Pravachol), rosuvastatin (Crestor), and simvastatin (Zocor). These drugs require close monitoring as they can cause liver toxicity and muscle inflammation and breakdown.

SHERRY'S NATURAL PRESCRIPTION

Dietary Recommendations

Foods to include:

- Fish contains beneficial omega-3 fatty acids, which help to reduce inflammation and LDL cholesterol levels and raise HDL cholesterol. Fatty fish like salmon, mackerel, and herring are particularly good sources. To reduce consumption of toxins, choose wild (not farmed) fish.

- Fruits and vegetables contain an array of antioxidants including flavonoids, which have been associated with a lower risk of heart disease. These compounds reduce inflammation, promote relaxation of blood vessels, lower cholesterol levels, and reduce blood clot formation. Some of the best choices are apples, berries, grapes, citrus, onions, tea, and cocoa.

- Garlic helps reduce cholesterol, thin the blood, and reduce plaque formation, and has antioxidant properties. Try to eat one fresh clove daily.

- Phytosterols (plant sterols) are plant compounds that are effective in lowering LDL cholesterol levels. They work by attaching to cholesterol in the digestive tract and carrying it out of the body. They are naturally present in small amounts in fruits, vegetables, nuts, seeds, and legumes. Manufacturers are now adding plant sterols to a variety of foods, such as orange juice (Minute Maid Heart Wise with CoroWise plant sterols), margarine (Becel pro. activ), and yogurt (Danacol).

- Moderate alcohol consumption (one drink daily for women and two for men) has been shown to have heart-protective effects. Alcohol increases protective HDL cholesterol and also helps to thin the blood. Higher amounts can be hard on the liver and increase blood pressure and the risk of heart disease.

- Nuts (almonds and walnuts) help lower cholesterol levels. Nuts contain fibre, plant sterols, and nutrients such as vitamin E, alpha-linolenic acid, magnesium, potassium, and arginine, which are important for heart health.

- Oat bran is rich in a soluble fibre called beta glucan, which has been shown to lower cholesterol levels. Beta glucan is also available in supplement form. The recommended intake is 10–15 g of beta glucan per day.

- Olive oil, which contains monounsaturated fatty acids, helps lower LDL cholesterol. Olive oil is best to add to foods after they are cooked or used in salad dressings.

- Palm fruit oil is rich in poly- and monounsaturated fatty acids and antioxidants like beta carotene and tocotrienols (a potent form of vitamin E). Research conducted on compounds found in Malaysian palm fruit oil has shown that it can help raise HDL cholesterol and lower LDL cholesterol. Palm fruit oil is heat stable, thus ideally suited for cooking. Many food companies have replaced the hydrogenated oils (trans fats) in their products with palm fruit oil. Pure (virgin) coconut oil has similar properties and benefits.

- Soluble fibre, which is found in oats, chia seed, flaxseed, beans, psyllium, and fruits, helps to lower cholesterol levels. Insoluble fibre, which is found in whole grains, vegetables, and fruits, does not lower cholesterol, but studies have shown that it helps protect against heart disease. Current Canadian guidelines recommend adults consume 21–38 g of fibre daily.

- Soy products (tofu, soybeans, miso, and soy protein powder) can help lower cholesterol and triglycerides. Substituting as little as 30 g (1 ounce) per day of soy protein for animal protein can significantly lower cholesterol.

- Tomatoes contain an antioxidant called lycopene, which has been shown to help reduce LDL cholesterol and slow the progression of atherosclerosis. Aim for 10 servings of tomato products weekly or consider a supplement.

- Yogurt and fermented milk products have been shown to lower cholesterol levels.

Foods to avoid:

- Foods high in cholesterol, such as organ meats, egg yolks, shrimp, squid, fatty meats, and whole milk products, may have a small effect on raising blood cholesterol levels in those with high blood cholesterol or type 2 diabetes. However, studies have shown that in healthy people with no history of heart disease, diabetes, or high blood cholesterol, eating an average of one egg per day does not increase the long-term risk of heart disease. If your cholesterol levels are normal you may eat up to seven eggs per week. If you have diabetes or high blood cholesterol, limit egg yolks to no more than four per week.

- Foods high in sugar and refined starches can raise triglyceride levels.

- Saturated fat, which is present in animal foods (beef, pork, and high-fat dairy), can raise cholesterol levels and is associated with increased heart disease risk. Vegetable and plant oils also contain some saturated fat, but much less than animal products. Limit consumption of saturated fat to 10 percent of total calories.

- Trans fatty acids are found in hydrogenated oils, which are present in some margarines, snack foods, microwave popcorn, and commercially prepared baked goods. These fats can raise cholesterol levels and increase the risk of heart disease. Avoid hard/stick margarines that contain hydrogenated oils. Look for non-hydrogenated margarines. Many snack food companies are now making products that are free of trans fatty acids.

Lifestyle Suggestions

- Lose excess weight. Losing even 5 to 10 percent of excess weight can lower cholesterol levels and reduce other risk factors for heart disease.

- Don't smoke. Smoking lowers the good HDL cholesterol and causes serious damage to blood vessels. It is never too late to quit. Within one year of quitting, your risk of heart

H

High Cholesterol

disease is half that of a smoker's. After 15 years, your risk is similar to that of someone who has never smoked.

• Exercise regularly. Moderate-intensity activities, such as brisk walking, biking, or swimming, can reduce cholesterol, support weight loss, and improve health.

• Reduce stress levels. Stress causes the liver to increase the production of cholesterol, which is used to make stress hormones. Try meditation, exercise, or yoga to promote calming and relaxation.

• Get your cholesterol levels checked regularly and discuss the results with your doctor.

Top Recommended Supplements

Fish oils: Contain the beneficial omega-3 fatty acids, eicosapentaenoic acid (EPA) and docosahexaenoic acid (DHA). Numerous studies show they can significantly lower triglycerides, modestly raise HDL cholesterol, and reduce inflammation and blood clotting. The typical dosage for lowering triglycerides is 3–6 g total of EPA and DHA daily, although higher amounts have been used in some studies.

Niacin (vitamin B3): Numerous studies have shown that niacin can lower LDL cholesterol, triglycerides, and lipoprotein-A levels and raise HDL cholesterol. Dosage: 1–4 g daily. Niacin can cause liver inflammation at higher dosages (more than 500 mg daily) and requires physician monitoring. Niacin at dosages of more than 100 mg daily frequently causes skin flushing, itching, upset stomach, and headache. These symptoms can usually be reduced by gradually increasing the dosage over several weeks or by using slow-release niacin. However, slow-release niacin may increase the risk of liver inflammation. Taking aspirin along with niacin can also reduce flushing.

Soluble fibre: Helps lower cholesterol levels. Those that have been studied and shown to offer benefits include glucomannan (PGX), partially hydrolyzed guar gum (Sunfiber), beta glucan, and psyllium (Metamucil). Dosage varies depending on the product and amount of fibre per serving. Add gradually to the diet to avoid gas and bloating. Take with plenty of water.

Phytosterols: Plant substances shown in many studies to lower total and LDL cholesterol, but have negligible effects on HDL and triglycerides. Studies have shown that plant sterols and plant sterol esters can lower total blood cholesterol by 6 to 10 percent and LDL cholesterol by 8 to 15 percent. They are safe to take with cholesterol-lowering medications. Look for a product that provides a daily dose of at least 1.3 g of phytosterol esters, such as ModuChol.

Complementary Supplements

Aged garlic extract: Helps to lower total and LDL cholesterol and triglycerides, reduces blood clotting, and prevents atherosclerosis. Dosage: 600–1,200 mg or more daily.

Flavonoids: Antioxidant compounds that can help lower cholesterol, and there is some evidence that they can help reduce atherosclerosis. Those that have been researched include Sytrinol (citrus and palm fruit extract) and Pycnogenol (pine bark extract). Follow label directions.

Policosanol: An extract from sugar cane that inhibits cholesterol production in the liver. Many studies have shown that it can significantly lower total and LDL cholesterol and raise HDL cholesterol. Dosage: 10–20 mg daily.

FINAL THOUGHTS
To lower cholesterol, consider the following:

- Eat more soluble fibre, soy, fish, nuts, and garlic.
- Minimize intake of saturated fat, trans fats, and processed and refined foods.
- Maintain a healthy body weight and don't smoke.
- Get regular exercise and reduce stress levels.
- Consider supplements of fish oils, niacin, stanols/sterols, and soluble fibre.

H

High Cholesterol

HYPOGLYCEMIA

Hypoglycemia occurs when your blood sugar (glucose) levels drop abnormally low. Blood sugar is the body's main source of energy, and when levels are too low it can cause fatigue and weakness.

During digestion, your body breaks down carbohydrates (which are present in vegetables, fruits, grains, and beans) into sugar molecules, such as glucose, which are absorbed directly into your bloodstream. As blood sugar levels rise, the pancreas secretes the hormone insulin, which ushers glucose into your cells to be used for energy. Blood sugar and insulin levels then return to normal.

Hypoglycemia most often occurs as a complication of diabetes. Diabetics take insulin or other medications to manage blood sugar levels, and if they take too much medication, eat too little, or exercise too much, blood sugar levels can drop off, causing hypoglycemia.

Hypoglycemia can also occur if the pancreas overproduces insulin. If too much insulin is released in response to a meal, then blood sugar levels can drop down very low. This is called reactive hypoglycemia and it may be caused by increased sensitivity to counter-regulating hormones like epinephrine, deficiency in glucagon release, polycystic ovarian syndrome, or a rare enzyme deficiency such as hereditary fructose intolerance or galactosemia. There are other factors that can lead to hypoglycemia and they are noted on the next page.

Hypoglycemia can be managed or prevented with lifestyle measures, primarily nutritional strategies that keep blood sugar levels within a normal range.

SIGNS & SYMPTOMS

- Anxiety
- Confusion and inability to think clearly
- Headache
- Heart palpitations
- Hunger
- Sweating
- Tremor and nervousness
- Visual disturbances, such as double vision and blurred vision

The symptoms may come on slowly or suddenly. As it becomes more severe, dizziness, weakness, confusion, seizures, and loss of consciousness can occur.

IS IT HYPOGLYCEMIA?

The signs and symptoms of hypoglycemia are vague and could be caused by other conditions. To determine whether you have hypoglycemia, your doctor can check your blood sugar levels and perform a glucose-tolerance test.

- Alcohol: Excessive consumption can trigger hypoglycemia.

- Chronic diseases: Liver disease, such as hepatitis, and kidney failure can reduce glucose production; disorders of the adrenal glands (Addison's disease) and the pituitary gland can result in a deficiency of hormones that regulate glucose production; tumours of the pancreas can cause excessive utilization of glucose and overproduction of insulin-like substances.

- Diabetes: Taking too much insulin or blood-sugar-lowering drugs like glyburide, not eating enough, or exercising too much

- Gender: Hypoglycemia is more common in women and older adults.

- Medications: Side effects of certain drugs such as quinine, isoniazid, phenylbutazone, propoxyphene, haloperidol, tricyclic antidepressants (amitriptyline), sulpha drugs, SSRIs (fluoxetine and sertraline), thiazide diuretics, ACE inhibitors, and others

- Overproduction of insulin (reactive hypoglycemia) may be caused by a disorder of the pancreas.

- Pregnancy

ALCOHOL AND HYPOGLYCEMIA

Avoid drinking alcohol on an empty stomach as this can trigger hypoglycemia. Heavy drinking can block glucose production and promote the release of insulin factors that will lower your blood sugar levels and induce hypoglycemia. When having an alcoholic beverage, do so with a meal as food delays the absorption of alcohol.

H

Hypoglycemia

DOCTOR'S ORDERS

The immediate treatment of hypoglycemia involves measures that raise blood sugar levels. Drinking a glass of juice or taking glucose tablets or candy will raise blood sugar levels within a few minutes. Those with diabetes or who are prone to hypoglycemia should carry some form of sugar with them at all times.

Those with severe symptoms who are unable to take anything by mouth will require immediate medical attention, which involves intravenous glucose or an injection of glucagon. If hypoglycemia is severe and untreated, it can result in serious consequences such as coma, heart problems, or death.

If hypoglycemia is not caused by diabetes or overproduction of insulin, it is important to work with your doctor to determine the underlying causes and develop a treatment. For example, if it is caused by a medication you are taking, your doctor may recommend changing the medication. If it is due to a tumour or glandular disorder, a surgical procedure may be necessary.

SHERRY'S NATURAL PRESCRIPTION

The recommendations in this section are geared toward diabetics and those with reactive hypoglycemia. Those with organ disease or other serious health problems need to work with their health care provider for specific recommendations.

Dietary Recommendations

Foods to include:

• Eat quality proteins (tofu, eggs, fish, and poultry) and healthy fats (fish, nuts, and seeds) with your carbohydrates as this will slow down the rate of digestion.

• Eat small, frequent meals (every two or three hours).

• High-fibre, low-glycemic carbohydrates such as fruits, vegetables, whole grains, and legumes are digested slowly and therefore promote better blood sugar balance. Refer to Appendix B for more information.

• Sweeteners such as xylitol and stevia have less of an impact on blood sugar.

MEASURING CARBOHYDRATES

The glycemic index (GI) is a measure of how quickly carbohydrates are broken down into sugar. Those that break down quickly have a high glycemic index and those that break down slowly have a low glycemic index. Eating low-GI foods helps to promote steady blood sugar levels and prevent hypoglycemia. Appendix B provides a list of the GI of common foods.

Foods to avoid:

• Alcohol can impair blood sugar control and trigger hypoglycemia by interfering with normal glucose utilization and increasing insulin secretion. Avoid drinking on an empty stomach, and limit alcohol to one drink per day.

• Caffeine can trigger hypoglycemia, so it should be minimized. Caffeine is found in coffee, tea, and soft drinks.

• Refined and processed flour products (white bread/bagels/pastries) and foods high in sugar break down quickly into sugar, and this can be followed by hypoglycemia.

Lifestyle Suggestions

• Regular exercise helps to improve blood sugar control and insulin sensitivity. Try brisk walking, swimming, or cycling for 30 minutes to an hour each day. Have a light snack 30 minutes before exercising to sustain your energy levels and prevent hypoglycemia.

• Reduce stress as this can trigger hypoglycemia. Try meditation, acupuncture, massage, and other relaxation techniques.

• Get adequate sleep to support overall health.

Top Recommended Supplements

B-vitamins: Play a role in metabolizing carbohydrates and converting blood glucose into energy. Look for a B-complex that provides 20–50 mg each of B1, B2, B3, B5, and B6, and 100 mcg of vitamin B12.

Chromium: A cofactor to insulin, chromium is essential for the body's utilization of glucose and helps prevent hypoglycemia. Look for chromium GTF or chromium picolinate. Dosage: 200 mcg daily.

Soluble fibre: Forms a gel in your stomach and slows the rate of digestion and absorption of food thus promoting better blood glucose control. Look for products that contain gluco-mannan (PGX), partially hydrolyzed guar gum (Sunfiber), or psyllium (Metamucil). Follow label directions. Mix with water and take two or three times daily.

Complementary Supplements

Fish oils: May help improve insulin sensitivity. Dosage: 1–3 g daily.

Magnesium: May help prevent blood sugar levels from falling low. Dosage: 300–400 mg daily.

Vitamin C: Plays an important role in blood sugar regulation; levels are depleted by chronic stress, which is a factor in hypoglycemia. Dosage: 500 mg three times daily.

FINAL THOUGHTS

To improve blood sugar control and prevent hypoglycemia, consider the following:

- Eat small, frequent meals of low-glycemic carbohydrates along with quality proteins and fats.
- Minimize or avoid alcohol and caffeine.
- Exercise regularly, but not on an empty stomach.
- Take B-vitamins, chromium, and soluble fibre supplements.
- Consider taking supplements of fish oils, magnesium, and vitamin C.

HYPOTHYROIDISM

The thyroid gland is located at the base of your neck, below your Adam's apple. It produces two hormones, triiodothyronine (T3) and thyroxine (T4), which circulate through your bloodstream. A significant amount of T4 is converted to T3, and T3 is the form that has the biological power to control metabolic activity in every cell in the body, from your heartbeat to body temperature to how fast you burn calories. Hypothyroidism, or an underactive thyroid, occurs when the thyroid gland cannot produce enough thyroid hormones to meet the body's demands. This causes all bodily functions to slow down and you feel tired, sluggish, and achy, and gain weight.

It is estimated that 30 percent of Canadians suffer from a thyroid condition. Of those, as many as 50 percent are undiagnosed. Many people do not realize that they have low thyroid because in the early stages the symptoms can be very mild and vague, such as fatigue.

Decades ago, the most common cause of hypothyroidism was iodine deficiency. Iodine is required for the production of thyroid hormone. When iodine was added to table salt, deficiency became a rare problem. However, today people are encouraged to reduce salt intake for health reasons (hypertension), and most of the salt that we get comes from processed foods that contain non-iodized sodium, so it is possible that low iodine levels are again partly contributing to thyroid disease.

The most common cause of hypothyroidism today is Hashimoto's disease, which is an autoimmune disorder in which the body makes antibodies that attack the thyroid gland, impairing the production of thyroid hormone. People with Hashimoto's develop a lump on their thyroid called a goiter.

Hypothyroidism can also result from treatment of Graves' disease (hyperthyroidism) with radioactive iodine, which destroys the thyroid gland, leaving it unable to produce hormones, and from surgical removal of the thyroid gland due to thyroid cancer.

A baby can be born without a thyroid gland or a defective thyroid (congenital hypothyroidism). In some cases, a genetic defect can lead to hypothyroidism in infants.

Diseases of the hypothalamus or pituitary gland can also cause hypothyroidism. These glands are involved in the regulation of the thyroid gland and the amount of thyroid hormone that is released. The hypothalamus releases thyrotropin-releasing hormone (TRH), which signals your pituitary gland to make thyroid-stimulating hormone (TSH). The amount of TSH released depends on how much T3 and T4 are in your blood. The thyroid gland regulates its production of hormones based on the amount of TSH it receives.

Hypothyroidism can also result as a side effect from taking the medication lithium. Lithium is a drug used to treat bipolar disorder. Use of lithium is also associated with goiter and chronic autoimmune thyroiditis.

Hypothyroidism is easily treated today with thyroid hormones, supplements, and various lifestyle approaches.

SIGNS & SYMPTOMS

- Anemia and easy bruising
- Cold intolerance (sensitivity to cold)
- Constipation
- Depression, irritability, and anxiety
- Dry, brittle nails
- Dry eyes and droopy eyelids
- Dry, itchy skin; dry hair and hair loss (including eyebrow hair loss)
- Fatigue and sluggishness
- Headaches
- High cholesterol
- Hoarse voice
- Infertility (hypothyroidism interferes with ovulation and diminishes egg quality)
- Insomnia
- Joint aching
- Low libido
- Memory loss
- Menstrual irregularities
- Muscle swelling or cramps
- Slow heart rate
- Slow reflexes
- Tingling or numbness in hands and feet
- Weight gain

Note: Hypothyroidism is rare in infants and young children. It may cause a large, protruding tongue, choking, yellowing of the skin and whites of the eyes (jaundice), constipation, poor muscle tone, and excessive sleepiness. If untreated it can lead to physical and mental retardation.

RISK FACTORS

- Age: It is most common after age 50.
- Family history
- Gender: It is five to ten times more common in women.
- History of autoimmune disease, hyperthyroidism, Graves' disease, or thyroid cancer

- Hormone imbalance (high estrogen and cortisol)

- Iodine deficiency

- Medication side effects (lithium, estrogen)

- Poor diet: Lack of iodine or selenium

- Pregnancy: The body produces antibodies that attack the thyroid gland, increasing the risk of miscarriage, premature delivery, pre-eclampsia, and damage to the fetus.

- Radiation to the neck and upper chest area

- Stress

DOCTOR'S ORDERS

Hypothyroidism is often a chronic problem that requires lifelong treatment. Doctors typically prescribe synthetic thyroid hormone (T4), such as Eltroxin or Synthroid. Blood tests are done to check your T3, T4, and TSH levels, and it often takes a few dosage adjustments to find your ideal level. Too much thyroid hormone can cause symptoms of racing heart, increased appetite, insomnia, and shakiness.

Some people do not convert T4 to T3 adequately and do better with a form of T3, which is called Cytomel. T3 does not circulate for long in the bloodstream, so it needs to be taken more frequently (three times daily). Some compounding pharmacies make a form of T3 that lasts longer and only needs to be taken once daily.

Thyroid hormones can be compounded by a pharmacist to provide T3 and T4 or just T3, depending on your needs. Compounded thyroid hormones are available through a compounding pharmacy with a doctor's prescription. The advantage of this form is that the dosage can be tailored to your needs and many people do better with the natural over the synthetic form.

Calcium and iron supplements and aluminum antacids may reduce the absorption of thyroid hormone, so take these products six hours away from your thyroid medication.

THYROID CHECK

Borderline hypothyroidism, also called compensated hypothyroidism, is very common and often undiagnosed. Blood tests may show thyroid hormone levels (T3 and T4) that are slightly low or even in the normal range, and normal or slightly elevated TSH levels. A person may have no symptoms or vague symptoms, such as fatigue, dry skin, or weight gain. Anyone at risk of hypothyroidism or who has any of the symptoms should consider testing beyond basic blood work. Measurement of T3 in a 24-hour urine sample correlate better with patient symptoms than serum TSH levels. These tests can be ordered through a doctor or pharmacy. See Appendix E for more information. You can also check your basal (resting) body temperature. The thyroid regulates metabolism, and low body temperature can indicate hypothyroidism. Here is what you do:

- Place a digital thermometer, paper, and pen beside your bed.

- When you wake up in the morning (before you get up or do anything), put the thermometer under your armpit and hold your elbow close to your side.

- Record the temperature and date.

- Repeat this for three mornings.

- A reading between 97.6°F and 98.2°F (36.4°C to 36.8°C) is normal. Readings below 97.6°F may indicate hypothyroidism.

SHERRY'S NATURAL PRESCRIPTION

Dietary Recommendations

Foods to include:

- Essential fatty acids are important for proper thyroid function and help reduce inflammation and support immune function. Eat more fish, chia seed, and flaxseed.

- Sea vegetables such as kelp, nori, dulse, and wakame contain iodine, which is used by the body to make thyroid hormone. Shellfish and salt-water fish also contain iodine. Iodine through food or supplements is helpful only if you are deficient in this nutrient.

Foods to avoid:

- Broccoli, Brussels sprouts, cabbage, cauliflower, collard greens, and kale contain goitrogens, which interfere with thyroid hormone synthesis. Cooking usually inactivates these goitrogens, so this is a rare case where cooked is preferred over raw.

- Gluten-containing foods may accelerate autoimmune thyroid disease, which is suspected when antibodies to thyroid hormones begin to rise. In some cases, removing gluten-containing grains from the diet may improve thyroid function.

- Soy contains isoflavones that have been shown in animal studies to suppress thyroid function. Soy may also have these effects in humans, although more research is needed. Other factors that may worsen the effects of soy on thyroid function are iodine deficiency, consumption of other goitrogens, and other problems synthesizing thyroid hormones. Soy can also reduce absorption of thyroid hormone. Until more is known, if you have hypothyroidism, limit intake of soy foods and avoid supplements containing soy.

- Most tap water contains fluorine and chlorine, which can inhibit the body's ability to absorb iodine.

Lifestyle Suggestions

- Don't smoke, as smoking can worsen hypothyroidism.

- Avoid fad dieting. Drastically reducing your calorie intake can lower metabolism, which can make weight management more difficult.

- Get regular exercise. Physical activity stimulates the thyroid to secrete more hormone and makes the body more sensitive to any thyroid hormone that is circulating.

- Manage your stress levels. Stress triggers the release of cortisol, which can suppress thyroid function.

Top Recommended Supplements

Guggul: Increases production of thyroid hormone (T3). Dosage: 25 mg of guggulsterones (the active component) three times daily.

Multivitamin/mineral complex: Many nutrients are required to produce thyroid hormone, such as vitamins C, E, and A and the B-vitamins. A deficiency of these vitamins and the minerals selenium and zinc has been associated with hypothyroidism, and there is evidence that supplements can help. Selenium is required for the conversion from T4 to the active form of thyroid, T3. Many people are deficient in selenium, which may hamper thyroid hormone levels, so a complete multivitamin can ensure that all essential nutrient requirements are met. A deficiency of vitamin D, which is quite common, may increase the risk of autoimmune thyroid disease.

Complementary Supplements

Ashwagandha: An herbal product that helps boost thyroid function and also reduces stress. Dosage: 500 mg three times daily.

Tyrosine: An amino acid involved in the synthesis of thyroid hormone. Dosage: 500 mg twice daily on an empty stomach. Do not combine with thyroid medication unless advised by your doctor.

H

Hypothyroidism

FINAL THOUGHTS

To manage hypothyroidism, consider the following:

- Eat more sea vegetables and salt-water fish if you are low in iodine. Fish, chia seed, and flaxseed provide essential fatty acids, which support immune health and reduce inflammation.
- Minimize eating raw goitrogens (broccoli, Brussels sprouts, etc.) and soy foods.
- Don't smoke, get regular exercise, and reduce your stress levels.
- Get your thyroid levels checked regularly and take medication as prescribed.
- Take a daily multivitamin/mineral complex and consider guggul extract.

INFERTILITY

Many couples take fertility for granted, assuming that it will happen once they start trying to conceive. However, the reality is that infertility is becoming a common concern. An estimated 10 to 15 percent of couples are infertile, which means they are unable to conceive after one year of frequent, unprotected intercourse. In healthy couples under the age of 30 who have sex regularly, the chance of getting pregnant is about 25 to 30 percent per month.

While once thought of as primarily a woman's problem, infertility can affect men, too. About one-third of infertility cases are due to male factors, one-third are due to female factors, and the remainder is caused by a combination of male and female factors.

Infertility may be due to a single cause in either you or your partner, or a combination of factors. To become pregnant, a woman's egg needs to connect with a man's sperm. When a woman's body is functioning as it should, each month the ovaries prepare an egg, which is released during ovulation. This occurs around day 14 of the menstrual cycle, and during this time a woman is fertile and can conceive. The egg travels through the fallopian tube and can be fertilized about 24 hours after its release. Conception is more likely to occur when intercourse takes place one to two days prior to ovulation. Sperm are capable of fertilizing the egg for up to 72 hours and must be present in the fallopian tube at the same time as the egg for conception to occur. If fertilized, the egg moves into the uterus where it attaches to the uterine lining and begins a nine-month process of growth.

If something in this whole process doesn't happen properly, it can affect the ability to conceive. Some of the most common causes of infertility in men are:

- Erectile dysfunction or retrograde ejaculation
- Genetic defects, such as blockage of epididymis or ejaculatory ducts
- Impaired production or function of sperm (low sperm count, impaired shape, or slow movement)
- Low testosterone levels
- Environmental pollution; drug or alcohol abuse; smoking
- Sexually transmitted disease (chlamydia and gonorrhea)
- Undescended testicle

In women, infertility can result from:

- Autoimmune disorders; diabetes; clotting disorders
- Benign uterine fibroids and pelvic adhesions
- Early menopause
- Eating disorders, poor nutrition; high alcohol intake
- Fallopian tube damage or blockage
- Hormonal problems: Elevated prolactin levels, low thyroid function, high estrogen-to-progesterone ratio

- No ovulation, or problems with ovulation
- Ovarian cysts and polycystic ovarian syndrome (PCOS)
- Scarring from endometriosis or sexually transmitted diseases

A woman's peak fertility occurs in her early twenties because there are a greater number of eggs in the ovaries and the quality of the eggs is better. After age 30 a woman's chance of getting pregnant is about 15 percent per month; after age 35 this drops to 10 percent, and after age 40 it is 5 percent. Since a woman is born with all of the eggs that she will have in her lifetime, the older she gets the fewer eggs that are left. In addition, as women age the percentage of genetically normal eggs remaining decreases. This is why women have a decreasing fertility rate, increased miscarriage rate, and increased chance of having babies with birth defects like Down syndrome as they age. Fertility in men also declines with age as the sperm quality, count, and motility is reduced.

In some cases the underlying cause of infertility is not known. However, there are a number of lifestyle, dietary, and supplemental approaches that can help improve fertility in both men and women.

SIGNS & SYMPTOMS

- Inability to get pregnant

RISK FACTORS

- Age: After about age 30, a woman's fertility gradually declines. There are hormonal changes and a reduced quantity and quality of eggs, older women are more likely to have health problems that may interfere with fertility, and the risk of miscarriage also increases with a woman's age. A gradual decline in fertility occurs in men older than 35.

- Alcohol: Heavy alcohol consumption (binge drinking) is toxic to sperm; alcohol also impairs female fertility.

- Caffeine: Some studies have linked caffeine to infertility, especially high amounts (greater than three cups of coffee per day); caffeine also increases the risk of miscarriage.

- Cancer or chemotherapy

- Drug abuse: Use of cocaine or marijuana

- Excessive exercise: Exercising more than seven hours a week can affect ovulation.

- Exposure to pesticides, xenoestrogens (environmental estrogens), heavy metals, and other chemicals that disrupt normal hormone levels

- Hypothyroidism in women

- Obesity causes hormonal changes that hamper fertility.

- Radiation and chemotherapy impair fertility in men and women.

- Smoking increases risk of infertility in both men and women.

- Stress interferes with hormones needed to produce sperm.

- Trauma to the reproductive organs

- Underweight: Women with eating disorders or very low body fat have hormonal problems and deficiencies of nutrients that can affect fertility.

AGING AND FERTILITY

According to several studies, by age 35 over one-third of women could not conceive within a year. Women are born with over one million eggs. Each month during the reproductive years, usually only a single egg matures. The quantity of eggs starts to diminish in childhood and continues into adulthood. Ovulation contributes to the decrease, but the majority of eggs are slowly absorbed by the body. By the fifth or sixth decade of life, most women will have depleted the egg supply they were born with.

DOCTOR'S ORDERS

The treatment of infertility depends on the underlying cause, your age, and personal preferences. For many couples, timing is the issue. To determine when you are ovulating, you can check your basal body temperature. Take your temperature when you wake up in the morning and record this every day. There is a slight rise in your body temperature when you ovulate. There are also ovulation kits available that measure hormones in urine to detect ovulation.

Fertility drugs can help women with ovulation disorders. The most commonly used drug is clomiphene (Clomid and Serophene), which stimulates the pituitary gland. There are also injectable drugs that can stimulate the ovaries to mature egg follicles. Fertility drugs can cause multiple births. Surgical procedures can correct blockages in the fallopian tubes.

For women with estrogen dominance (high estrogen-to-progesterone ratio), natural progesterone cream can be used to restore hormonal balance. This is available by prescription in compounding pharmacies. Saliva tests can be done to check hormone levels. Refer to Appendix E for more information.

Depending on the cause of male infertility, there are medications, hormones, and surgical options available.

For couples who are unable to conceive naturally, there are many other options available, such as in vitro fertilization. It is important to discuss all your options with your doctor.

HOMEOPATHIC RECOMMENDATIONS

Folliculinum: Women who have challenges getting pregnant could find success with this remedy if they have irregular menstrual cycles that are often weeks delayed, with a heavy, clotty flow. Often women in this state feel a loss of will and are full of self-denial. As the exception to the dosing recommendations for the rest of the homeopathics listed in this chapter, dissolve three pills of Folliculinum 30CH under your tongue once daily on days 0 to 10 unless otherwise directed.

Luteinum: Infertile women who need this remedy typically have either polycystic ovaries, fibroids, or endometriosis and often have estrogen dominance without even knowing it. Strong indications that this remedy is appropriate are early menstruation and short cycles, which represent a possible luteal phase defect. As the exception to the dosing recommendations for the rest of the homeopathics listed in this chapter, dissolve three pills of Luteinum 30CH under your tongue once daily on days 16 to menses unless otherwise directed.

SHERRY'S NATURAL PRESCRIPTION

Proper nutrition and a healthy lifestyle can make a difference in your ability to conceive.

Dietary Recommendations

Foods to include:

• Choose lean cuts of poultry (free range) and wild fish.

• Eat a healthy diet with whole grains, vegetables, fruits, nuts, and seeds. Choose organic as much as possible to avoid ingesting harmful pesticides.

• Men should eat pumpkin seeds as they contain zinc, which is important for male reproductive fluids.

Foods to avoid:

• Alcohol is toxic to sperm and can impair fertility in both men and women.

• Avoid farmed fish as it contains PCBs, dioxins, mercury, and other chemicals that can impair fertility.

• Caffeine may impair female fertility and also increase the risk of miscarriage. Minimize or avoid coffee, tea, and soft drinks.

• Fast foods and processed foods are full of chemicals that can cause hormonal imbalances.

Lifestyle Suggestions

• Reduce your stress, which can affect libido and cause hormonal changes that affect ovulation. Try yoga, tai chi, meditation, or massage.

• Acupuncture helps reduce stress and may improve fertility. It is particularly helpful for the treatment of female infertility due to problems with ovarian function.

• Get regular exercise to promote good circulation.

• Men should avoid hot tubs and wear boxers (not briefs).

- Maintain a healthy body weight. Being too thin or too heavy can impair fertility.

- Don't smoke. The more women smoke, the less likely they are to conceive.

- Avoid taking any unnecessary medications.

- Reduce your exposure to phthalates (chemicals used to make plastics soft), which can impair fertility by disrupting hormones. They are found in medical supplies (IV tubing), some flooring material, soft plastic food storage containers, and some cosmetics and perfumes. Contact the manufacturer to find out if their products contain phthalates.

Top Recommended Supplements

For men:

Antioxidants: Neutralize free radicals, which can be damaging to sperm. Some studies have found benefits with vitamins E and C and selenium for improving sperm count and activity. Dosage: 400 IU vitamin E, 1,000 mg vitamin C, and 100 mcg selenium. These are higher amounts than are typically found in multivitamin formulas. There is also evidence that the antioxidant coenzyme Q10 can help increase sperm count and motility.

L-carnitine: Numerous studies have shown that it can improve sperm function and enhance male fertility. Dosage: 3 g daily.

Zinc and folate: Essential nutrients for cell division, synthesis of genetic material, and numerous body processes. Zinc is critical for male fertility as it is involved in hormone metabolism, sperm formation, and sperm motility. Two studies of zinc combined with folate have found that the supplements can improve sperm count and the percentage of healthy sperm in men with impaired fertility. Dosage: 15 mg elemental zinc with 5 mg folate. Take along with a multivitamin/mineral complex containing copper to prevent copper deficiency.

For women:

Chasteberry (vitex): Helpful for infertility due to irregular ovulation. It works by increasing production of luteinizing hormone, which in turn boosts secretion of progesterone during the last 14 days of the menstrual cycle. It also suppresses production of the lactation hormone prolactin, creating a hormonal environment more conducive to ovulation. One study combined chasteberry with arginine, green tea, and multivitamins with positive results. Dosage: 160–246 mg daily. Discontinue if conception occurs.

Multivitamin/mineral complex: Ensures that your body gets all essential nutrients. The B-vitamins play a key role in reproductive health and also in early fetal development. Folic acid, especially, can prevent certain birth defects. Even a subtle deficiency of nutrients such as iron can impair fertility. Look for a formula designed for women of childbearing age and take daily.

Vitamin C: Supplements may be helpful for women with infertility due to luteal phase defect. With this hormonal abnormality the uterine lining does not develop and mature properly, likely because of a deficiency of progesterone. One study of women with luteal phase defect found significant benefits with vitamin C supplements over six months. Dosage: 750 mg daily.

Complementary Supplements

For men:

L-arginine: Needed for sperm production. Research shows that several months of L-arginine supplementation increases sperm count, quality, and fertility. Dosage: 4 g daily.

Infertility

Panax ginseng: Preliminary research found that it improved sperm function. Dosage: 100–200 mg daily.

Tongkat ali: Also known as *Eurycoma longifolia*. Several clinical studies on a patented form of this plant called Physta show that it can increase testosterone and DHEA levels, improve sexual performance, and boost energy levels in men. It also has antioxidant properties. Recent research has also found that it can improve sperm count, quality, and motility. Dosage: 200–600 mg daily.

Vitamin B12: A vitamin B12 deficiency can lead to reduced sperm counts and lowered sperm mobility. Studies have found vitamin B12 supplementation helpful for improving fertility in men with abnormal sperm production. Dosage: 400 mcg sublingually daily.

For women:

Bee propolis: Recommended for women with endometriosis. Preliminary research found that supplementing with 500 mg twice a day for six months significantly increased pregnancy rate in a group of women with infertility and mild endometriosis. The mechanism is not known; more research is needed.

Chirositol: A nutrient derived from carob juice that may help women with infertility caused by polycystic ovarian syndrome. Preliminary studies show it can help improve blood glucose metabolism and insulin sensitivity, aid weight loss, and improve ovulation. Dosage: 600–1,200 mg daily.

Coenzyme Q10: Preliminary research suggests it can improve egg quality and the number of healthy follicles Dosage: 1,200 mg is the dosage being studied.

Essential fatty acids: Fish oils and primrose or borage oil should be taken daily by women to promote the healthy functioning of the uterus and help regulate hormone production. Dosage: 1 g three times daily.

FINAL THOUGHTS

To improve your chances of conceiving, consider the following:

- Eat a healthy diet with organic whole grains, vegetables, fruits, nuts, seeds, wild fish, and free-range poultry.
- Minimize caffeine; avoid alcohol and fast foods, processed foods, and junk foods.
- Get regular exercise, reduce stress, and don't smoke.
- Men should take antioxidants, L-carnitine, and a multivitamin/mineral complex containing adequate zinc and folate.
- Women should take a multivitamin/mineral complex and consider extra vitamin C, coenzyme Q10, and chasteberry.

INSOMNIA

Insomnia is characterized by persistent difficulty falling asleep, waking up too early, awakening frequently during the night, or waking feeling tired and not refreshed. According to recent reports, approximately 40 percent of adults suffer occasionally from insomnia and 10 percent experience chronic insomnia.

Sleep is vital for physical and mental health, yet it often gets sacrificed when we are busy. While it is thought that sleep is relaxing and passive, actually quite a lot happens in the body during sleep. During the deepest stages of sleep our bodies' major organs and regulatory systems are busy working on repair and regeneration and secreting certain hormones.

Short-term or transient insomnia is common and usually lasts only a few days. This may result from temporary situations, such as jet lag, stress at work, a brief illness, or a change in environment. When the precipitating factor disappears, the condition goes away, usually without medical treatment.

Insomnia is classified as long term or chronic when it lasts more than three weeks. Possible causes include stress; depression; chronic pain; use of alcohol, caffeine, or nicotine; snoring or sleep apnea; and other medical conditions as noted below.

The exact amount of sleep needed varies among individuals, but is between seven and nine hours. Getting less than six hours is associated with health problems, such as memory loss, poor concentration, depression, headache, irritability, increased response to stress, high blood pressure, depressed immune function, low libido, and weight gain.

SIGNS & SYMPTOMS

- Daytime fatigue, irritability, difficulty concentrating and focusing
- Difficulty falling asleep or staying asleep
- Waking too early
- Waking feeling tired and fatigued

RISK FACTORS

- Age (the incidence increases with age; those over 60 are most often affected)
- Diet (high intake of refined and processed foods; overeating)
- Exposure to noise and light
- Gender: Women are more likely to suffer insomnia; this may be due to hormonal changes that occur during the menstrual cycle, pregnancy, and menopause.
- High caffeine consumption (coffee, soft drinks, energy drinks)
- Lack of exercise

- Medical conditions (depression, anxiety, cancer, alcoholism, restless legs, hypothyroidism, sleep apnea, bladder problems)

- Medications (heart and blood pressure drugs, antidepressants, decongestants, stimulants like Ritalin, long-term use of sleeping pills)

- Pain (back pain, headaches, arthritis, fibromyalgia)

- Poor sleep habits (going to bed at different times)

- Smoking (nicotine is a stimulant)

- Snoring (disrupts deep sleep)

- Stress and muscle tension

- Travelling to a different time zone or working shifts can upset one's internal clock and lead to sleep disturbances.

- Vitamin deficiencies (vitamin B12 and iron)

DOCTOR'S ORDERS

There are several types of medications that are used to promote sleep, called sedatives and tranquilizers. The most commonly used class is the benzodiazepines, including lorazepam (Ativan), temazepam (Restoril), and diazepam (Valium). These drugs are recommended only for short-term use (a few weeks), as they cause a number of side effects, including next day drowsiness and difficulty thinking and concentrating, sleep walking, and loss of short-term memory. When used over the long term, they become less effective, can result in dependency, and can actually worsen sleep quality. Abruptly stopping use of these drugs can cause withdrawal symptoms, therefore they should be weaned off slowly (reduce dosage and take every other night) under doctor supervision.

There are also over-the-counter products for insomnia like Nytol and Unisom. These drugs actually contain an antihistamine that is marketed for its side effect—drowsiness. While these drugs may make you fall asleep easier, they also cause a range of side effects including next day drowsiness, dry mouth, and blurred vision.

HOMEOPATHIC RECOMMENDATIONS

Coffea cruda: This remedy relieves sleeplessness due to worries, overactive thoughts, and hypersensitivity to pain.

Nux vomica: This remedy relieves sleeplessness from irritability that wakes the person. Typical presentation also includes digestive troubles associated with overindulgence in food and alcohol.

Staphysagria: This remedy helps relieve physical symptoms, sleeplessness, and irritability caused by grief, repressed anger, or vexation.

SHERRY'S NATURAL PRESCRIPTION

There are a number of lifestyle tips and natural remedies that can greatly improve sleep quality. In most cases insomnia is temporary and can be improved with good sleep hygiene habits.

Dietary Recommendations

Foods to include:

• A small snack before bed that contains tryptophan (an amino acid) stimulates the release of serotonin, a brain chemical that facilitates sleep. Good food sources of tryptophan include turkey, soybeans, nuts, seeds, and dairy products (milk, cheese, yogurt). Dairy products also contain calcium, which helps the brain use tryptophan and promotes relaxation.

• Chamomile tea has been used traditionally to promote calming and relaxation.

Foods to avoid:

• Caffeine (coffee, tea, soft drinks, and chocolate) can affect sleep quality, and should be avoided eight hours before bed.

• Alcohol may help you fall asleep, but it causes nighttime wakening and reduces sleep quality, so minimize or avoid completely.

• Go easy on sugary foods, especially in the evening, as they can cause a sugar rush and affect your ability to fall asleep.

• Avoid big meals close to bedtime because this can interfere with sleep.

Lifestyle Suggestions

• Set aside at least seven to eight hours for sleep. Leaving only five or six hours may make you feel stressed and affect your ability to fall asleep.

• Establish a regular bedtime and wake time.

• Do relaxing activities before bed—read a book, have a warm bath, or meditate.

• Reserve your bedroom for intimacy and sleep only; don't work in your bedroom.

• Limit naps to a half hour and avoid napping after 3 p.m. as this can interfere with your ability to fall asleep at night.

• Make your bedroom dark, quiet, and comfortable.

• Exercise regularly early in the day. Vigorous exercise too close to bedtime is stimulating and can affect your ability to fall asleep.

• Don't smoke, as nicotine is a stimulant and impairs your ability to fall asleep and have a restful sleep.

• Consider acupuncture, massage, yoga, or meditation for relaxation.

• Try cognitive therapy, which involves changing your thoughts about sleep, replacing worry with positive thoughts.

Top Recommended Supplements

Melatonin: A hormone that is naturally secreted by the brain in response to darkness and regulates sleep/wake cycles. Supplements reduce the time needed to fall asleep, reduce nighttime wakening, and improve sleep quality. It is particularly helpful for those who work shifts or travel to different time zones (jet lag). Dosage: 1–6 mg one hour before bed. Dosages up to 10 mg have been used in studies.

L-theanine: An amino acid naturally present in green tea in small amounts. A patented form of L-theanine called Suntheanine has been found in research to help improve sleep quality and reduce stress. This product can be taken by children and adults. Dosage: 50–200 mg 30 minutes before bed.

Valerlan: An herb that is widely used for insomnia; it improves many aspects of sleep and is non-addictive. Some formulas combine valerian with hops, passion flower, and other herbs that promote relaxation. Dosage: 600 mg half an hour to one hour before bed, or 2 mL of a tincture.

Complementary Supplements

5-hydroxytryptophan (5-HTP): Increases serotonin and melatonin levels, which promote relaxation and improved sleep. Dosage: 100–200 mg one hour before bed.

Magnesium: An important mineral for muscle and nervous system relaxation. It may be particularly helpful in those with muscle tension or inadequate dietary intake and in the elderly. Dosage: 250 mg after evening meal.

Seditol: A patented blend of magnolia bark and jujube seed, two herbal extracts that have a calming effect. Preliminary research found that Seditol promotes better sleep and does not cause next day drowsiness. Dosage: 1 capsule 30 minutes before bedtime.

Note: Supplements that promote sleep should be used only occasionally, as it is important to address the underlying factors causing insomnia.

FINAL THOUGHTS

For a good night sleep, consider the following:

- Set aside at least seven hours for sleep and try to go to bed at the same time.
- Get regular exercise early in the day.
- Avoid alcohol, caffeine, and smoking.
- Relax before bed with meditation or stretching.
- Consider supplements of melatonin, valerian, and Suntheanine.

IRRITABLE BOWEL SYNDROME (IBS)

Irritable bowel syndrome (IBS) is a common disorder, affecting about one in five Canadians. It is also one of the most common reasons for a doctor's appointment, especially among women. It is characterized by abdominal pain or cramping and changes in bowel function, such as bloating, gas, diarrhea, and constipation, which makes it a sensitive topic to discuss. In the past IBS has been called mucous colitis, spastic colon, and irritable colon, but these terms are misleading because the problem is not limited to the colon.

The walls of the intestines are lined with layers of muscle that contract and relax as they move food from your stomach through your intestinal tract to your rectum. Normally, these muscles contract and relax in a coordinated rhythm. With irritable bowel syndrome, the contractions are stronger and last longer, causing food to be forced through your intestines more quickly. This causes gas, bloating, and diarrhea. In some cases, the opposite occurs and food passage slows, causing dry, hard stools and constipation.

Several factors have been implicated in causing IBS, such as infection, food intolerances, abnormal bowel motility, imbalance of good bacteria in the intestine, abnormal serotonin levels, and nervous system dysfunction. Since women are two or three times as likely as men to have IBS, hormonal changes may also play a role. In many cases of IBS, the disorder is increased and intensified by stress.

For most people, IBS is a chronic condition, although there are times when the symptoms will disappear for weeks or months. Although there is no known cure, there are a number of dietary strategies, supplements, and lifestyle measures that can greatly help to manage this condition.

SIGNS & SYMPTOMS

- Abdominal pain or cramping
- Depression and anxiety
- Diarrhea or constipation that may alternate
- Gas and bloating
- Headache and fatigue
- Mucus in the stool
- Nausea

The severity and type of symptoms can vary from one episode to another.

RISK FACTORS

- Age: IBS typically begins around age 20 and rarely appears after age 50.
- Gender: Two to three times as many women as men have the condition.
- Genetics: Many with IBS have a family member with the disorder, suggesting a possible genetic cause.

> There are also a variety of factors that can trigger an episode, like emotional stress. Many people find that their symptoms worsen when they eat certain foods, such as milk, caffeine, wheat, alcohol, carbonated beverages, artificial sweeteners, or food preservatives. Other illnesses, such as an infection, can trigger IBS.

DOCTOR'S ORDERS

The medical treatment of IBS focuses on dietary strategies and drug therapy to reduce symptoms. Drugs that regulate gut motility, namely pinaverium bromide (Dicetel) and trimebutine maleate (Modulon), are often prescribed. They are well tolerated and help to restore normal contractions of the bowel.

Antidiarrheal medications like loperamide (Imodium) and laxatives should be used cautiously and only occasionally when recommended by your doctor.

Fibre supplements, when taken along with adequate fluids, can help control constipation and improve bowel function.

Antispasmodic drugs, such as dicyclomine (Bentylol) and hyoscine (Buscopan), block the transmission of nerve impulses and reduce muscle activity, thus slowing the movement of food through the intestinal tract.

HOMEOPATHIC RECOMMENDATIONS

Podophyllum: This remedy is useful when abdominal pain and cramping with a gurgling, sinking, empty feeling are followed by watery, offensive-smelling diarrhea. The individual that benefits from this remedy often also has alternating constipation or pasty yellow bowel movements containing mucus.

SHERRY'S NATURAL PRESCRIPTION

Dietary Recommendations

Foods to include:

- Cultured products, such as live yogurt, kefir, and sauerkraut, can help restore normal gut flora, aid digestion, and reduce symptoms of IBS. Activia yogurt has been studied and found to be beneficial for improving IBS symptoms.

- Drink lots of fluids, such as water, herbal tea, and vegetable and fruit juices, throughout the day. Chamomile tea contains essential oils that can help ease intestinal cramps. Fennel, ginger, and peppermint tea are also helpful.

- Eat small, frequent meals (four or five meals daily), chew food thoroughly, and eat slowly. This will help regulate bowel function and improve digestion.

- Fibre can help regulate bowel function and reduce constipation, but it can also cause gas and cramping. Add high-fibre foods to the diet gradually to minimize gas and bloating, and drink plenty of water. Recommended fibre-rich foods include oats, brown rice, milled flaxseed, psyllium, and vegetables. Ground flaxseed also contains fatty acids that help reduce inflammation. One study found that flaxseed reduced constipation, abdominal pain, and bloating in those with IBS. Try adding 1–2 tbsp to your diet. Mix with water or sprinkle on yogurt or cereal.

Foods to avoid:

- Alcohol, caffeinated beverages, and spicy foods stimulate the intestines and can make diarrhea and pain worse.

- Artificial sweeteners, such as sorbitol or mannitol, cause reactions (gas and diarrhea) in some people. Sorbitol and mannitol are found mainly in diabetic and low-carbohydrate foods and snacks.

- Carbonated drinks (soft drinks and soda water) can produce gas and should be avoided.

- Chewing gum causes ingestion of swallowed air, which contributes to intestinal gas.

- Concentrated amounts of fructose (fruit sugar) in dried fruit and fruit juice can ferment in the colon, causing gas and bloating.

- Gas-producing foods, such as beans, lentils, onions, broccoli, cabbage, cauliflower, pickles, and peppers, should be minimized.

- High-fat foods, such as whole milk, cream, cheese, ice cream, butter, and fatty meats (prime rib, sausage, deli meats), can trigger IBS in some people.

- Wheat and lactose-containing foods (dairy) are common food allergens that can trigger reactions in those with IBS.

Several studies have drawn a correlation between food sensitivities and IBS. The most commonly implicated foods include wheat, dairy, sugar, and artificial sweeteners. Standard blood tests to evaluate allergies are usually not helpful because IBS food sensitivities may not be true allergies but rather an intestinal reaction. Following an elimination diet (see Appendix D) and using a food and symptom diary can help determine which foods should be avoided.

Lifestyle Suggestions

- Stress can trigger and worsen IBS symptoms so it is critical to find ways to reduce stress, such as deep breathing, meditation, or counselling.

- Acupuncture can provide relief from chronic pain, promote relaxation, and improve bowel function.

- Regular exercise will help reduce stress and also stimulate normal contraction of the intestines. Try walking, biking, yoga, or stretching.

- Don't smoke, as nicotine can irritate the stomach lining.

- Get adequate sleep. Lack of sleep can worsen symptoms.

Top Recommended Supplements

Peppermint oil: Contains oils that directly affect the smooth muscle of the digestive tract and reduce spasms. Several studies have found it helpful for reducing pain, bloating, stool frequency, and gas. Take one to three capsules of peppermint oil three times daily, about 15 minutes before meals. Choose a product that is enteric-coated to reduce the risk of heartburn, such as Peppermint Plus by Enzymatic Therapy. Take one capsule three times daily between meals.

Probiotics: Beneficial bacteria are part of normal gut flora and may be depleted in those with IBS. Probiotics aid digestion and offer a range of benefits for gut health. Research on a particular probiotic called TuZen (*Lactobacillus plantarum 299V*) found that it reduced symptoms of IBS, such as gas, bloating, constipation, diarrhea, and abdominal pain. Initial dosage is one capsule twice daily. Benefits are often found within four to six weeks.

Soluble fibre: Helps regulate bowel activity and improve symptoms of both constipation and diarrhea. Sunfiber is a prebiotic fibre made from hydrolyzed guar gum. This is a truly regulating fibre that has been shown to help with both constipation and diarrhea and relieve abdominal pain. Sunfiber also mixes well with fluids. There is some evidence that psyllium (Metamucil) can help improve some IBS symptoms, although it can also cause bloating and does not mix as well with liquids as other types of soluble fibre.

Complementary Supplements

Digestive enzymes: Help improve food digestion and reduce bloating and gas. Look for a full-spectrum enzyme that contains proteolytic enzymes, lipase, amylase, and lactase. Gluten Defense is a broad spectrum enzyme that may be particularly helpful for those with gluten sensitivity. Dosage: One or two capsules with each meal.

Evening primrose oil: Contains gamma linolenic acid, a fatty acid that helps reduce inflammation. Preliminary research has shown that it can help reduce pain. Dosage: 1,000 mg three times daily.

Melatonin: Plays a role in the regulation of gastrointestinal function and sensation. A few small studies have shown that it can reduce pain and improve sleep in those with IBS. Dosage: 3 mg at bedtime.

FINAL THOUGHTS

To reduce the symptoms of IBS, consider the following:

- Eat small, frequent meals and eat slowly.
- Gradually increase fibre intake. Try milled flaxseed.
- Avoid caffeine, alcohol, carbonated beverages, fatty or spicy foods, and other known food triggers.
- Reduce stress levels and get regular exercise.
- Try peppermint oil capsules, probiotics (TuZen), and soluble fibre.

KIDNEY STONES

The kidneys are two bean-shaped organs, about the size of your fist, that are located behind your abdomen on each side of your spine. The main function of the kidneys is to remove excess fluid and wastes from your blood in the form of urine. Kidney stones, known medically as renal lithiasis, occur when minerals and other substances in the urine form crystals inside your kidneys. Over time, these crystals may combine to form a small, hard mass or stone.

Kidney stones have become increasingly common today. It is estimated that 10 percent of North Americans are affected by kidney stones. Poor diet and lack of fluids are the major underlying causes. Crystals can form in the urine when there is a high concentration of substances such as calcium, oxalate, uric acid, and, rarely, cystine or phosphate, or a low level of substances that help prevent crystal formation, such as citrate and magnesium. Crystals also may form if your urine becomes too concentrated or is too acidic or too alkaline.

Roughly 70 to 80 percent of all kidney stones contain a combination of calcium and oxalate. Oxalates are compounds naturally occurring in some fruits and vegetables, such as rhubarb, spinach, and tomatoes. Eating lots of these foods may increase your risk for stone formation.

Some people have higher levels of calcium in their urine than others, increasing the risk of stone formation. Genetics may play a role. Calcium levels may also be higher in those with cancer or kidney disease, or those taking certain diuretics and thyroid hormones. It was once thought that a diet high in calcium, or that taking calcium supplements, increased your risk for developing kidney stones, but this has been disproven. Recent studies have shown that high-calcium diets actually help prevent stones because dietary calcium binds with oxalates in the gastrointestinal tract so that oxalates can't be absorbed from the intestine and excreted by the kidney to form stones.

Kidney stones can range in size from a grain of sand to a pearl or a golf ball. Most stones are small and pass into your bladder without causing any pain or symptoms. However, larger stones cause excruciating pain and bleeding in the urine, and can even cause permanent damage. Fortunately, there are a number of medical interventions and natural products that can help eliminate kidney stones, as well as lifestyle measures that can be undertaken to prevent them from occurring.

SIGNS & SYMPTOMS

- Bloody, cloudy, or foul-smelling urine

- Fever and chills (if there is infection)

- Frequent need to urinate

- Intense pain that may be intermittent and can occur in your lower back or your side (under your ribs); it may radiate to your lower abdomen, groin, and genitals.

- Nausea and vomiting

Note: If a large kidney stone is left untreated, it could block the flow of urine, causing pain, bleeding, infection, and the risk of kidney damage. Small kidney stones can partially block the ureters (thin tubes that connect each kidney to the bladder) or the urethra (the tube that carries urine out of the body). If left untreated, these stones may also cause recurrent urinary tract infection or kidney damage.

RISK FACTORS

- Climate: Living in hot, dry areas or working in a hot environment increases risk due to increased likelihood of dehydration; kidney stones are also more common during the summer months.

- Dehydration: Not drinking enough fluids, especially water, makes the urine more concentrated.

- Diet: Consuming foods high in oxalate (naturally occurring in some fruits and vegetables, such as rhubarb, spinach, and tomatoes). High intake of animal protein and salt and a low intake of calcium and magnesium increases the risk of some types of stones.

- Gender: Men are at greater risk.

- History of kidney stones: If you have had a stone in the past, you're at greater risk; having a family history also increases your risk.

- Imbalance in urinary pH (acid and base balance).

- Lack of activity: A lack of activity causes your bones to release more calcium, which can increase the risk of calcium stones.

- Medical conditions: Having kidney disease, gout, chronic urinary tract infections, and hyperparathyroidism.

- Medications: Certain diuretics can increase your risk.

- Race: Caucasians are at greater risk.

DOCTOR'S ORDERS

The treatment of kidney stones depends on the type of stone, the underlying cause, and the severity of symptoms. In some cases, a small stone can easily be passed by drinking lots of water (2 L to 3 L) and being physically active.

Stones that are too large to pass or that cause bleeding, infection, or kidney damage may require treatment by a urologist, a doctor who specializes in the treatment of urinary tract problems. There are various procedures that can break up and remove a kidney stone. Extracorporeal shock wave lithotripsy uses shock waves to break up the stone. Percutaneous nephrolithotomy involves removal of the stone through a small incision in your back using a nephroscope. A stone that is lodged in a ureter can be broken down with ultrasound or laser energy and removed with a small instrument called a ureteroscope.

Depending on the type of stone, there are medications that can be used to change the pH of your urine to prevent and treat the problem.

SHERRY'S NATURAL PRESCRIPTION

Dietary Recommendations

Foods to include:

- Apples, green leafy vegetables, kelp, seeds, legumes, and figs are good sources of magnesium. Ensuring adequate magnesium intake is important because a magnesium deficiency can increase the risk of stones.

- Drink lots of water to help flush out your kidneys and prevent dehydration. Add some lemon slices or juice to your water. Lemon contains citric acid, which acidifies the urine and can help assist the passage of calcium oxalate stones.

- Eat lots of vegetables, fruits, and whole grains. Fish, beans, seeds, and poultry provide good sources of protein.

- Oranges, bananas, raisins, avocados, and artichokes contain potassium, which reduces the amount of calcium lost in the urine. Boosting intake of potassium has been shown to reduce the risk of stones.

- Pumpkin seeds have been shown in preliminary research to reduce the risk of stone formation.

Foods to avoid:

- Foods high in oxalic acid increase the risk of stone formation, so minimize intake of spinach, rhubarb, beet greens, nuts, chocolate, tea, bran, almonds, peanuts, and strawberries. Other foods contain some oxalic acid, but only these have been found to be a problem.

- Grapefruit juice has been linked to increased risk of kidney stones.

- Limit caffeine (coffee, tea, soft drinks) because it promotes fluid loss.

- Studies have shown that a diet high in animal protein increases the risk of stone formation. Animal protein increases the excretion of calcium, causing a buildup of calcium in the urine. On the other hand, a vegetarian diet is protective against stone formation.

- Reduce sodium intake as a high sodium intake can promote calcium excretion and also lead to dehydration. Limit sodium to 2,000 mg daily. Foods high in sodium include snack foods, deli meats, condiments, and processed foods. Avoid using the salt shaker.

- Sugar has been linked to increased risk of oxalate stones. Limit intake of sweets, candy, and soft drinks. Soft drinks also contain phosphoric acid, which also increases the risk of stones.

Lifestyle Suggestions

- Get regular exercise. Physical activity and having good circulation may help in prevention. Vigorous exercise can also help dislodge a stone.

- Acupuncture may help reduce pain and ease the passage of a stone.

- Have a warm bath with mineral salts and add a few drops of lavender or chamomile oil to promote relaxation and ease pain.

- If you suspect that you are passing a kidney stone, urinate through a strainer so that the stone can be analyzed.

Top Recommended Supplements

IP6: Inositol hexaphosphate (Inocell) is a naturally occurring component of plant fibre. Studies have shown that it reduces urinary calcium levels and may reduce the risk of forming a kidney stone. Dosage: 120 mg daily.

Potassium citrate: Helps prevent stone formation by various mechanisms. Citrate binds with calcium in the urine, thereby reducing the amount available to form calcium oxalate stones. It also prevents calcium oxalate crystals from forming into larger stones. Finally, it makes the urine less acidic, which inhibits the development of both calcium oxalate and uric acid stones. Several studies have demonstrated significant benefits in those at risk of stone formation. Consult your health care provider for individualized dosage recommendations as too much potassium can cause side effects (upset stomach) and interact with medications.

CALCIUM SUPPLEMENTS AND KIDNEY STONES

For years, those with or at risk of calcium oxalate stones were told to avoid calcium-rich foods and supplements. However, recent studies have shown that high-calcium diets actually help prevent stones because dietary calcium binds with oxalates in the gastrointestinal tract so that oxalates can't be absorbed from the intestine and excreted by the kidney to form stones. Calcium supplements seem to have the same protective effect as dietary calcium, but only if taken with meals. When taken on an empty stomach, the calcium can't bind with the oxalates in food, thus increasing the risk of stone formation.

Complementary Supplements

Calcium: Helps bind to oxalate and reduce the risk of calcium oxalate stones. Dosage: 500 mg with meals three times daily. Choose calcium citrate as the citrate also has a protective effect.

Magnesium: May help prevent calcium oxalate stone development. Dosage: 100–200 mg twice daily with meals. Choose magnesium citrate.

Vitamin B6: May help prevent calcium oxalate stones. A deficiency of vitamin B6 increases the amount of oxalate in the urine, and some research has shown that those with a high intake of B6 are at a lower risk of stone formation. Dosage: 50 mg daily as part of a B-complex.

FINAL THOUGHTS

To manage kidney stones and prevent them from occurring, consider the following:

- Drink plenty of water (2 L to 3 L) with lemon. This is important for treatment and prevention.
- Boost intake of potassium- and magnesium-rich foods (oranges, bananas, raisins, apples, and leafy green vegetables).
- Reduce intake of foods high in oxalic acid, such as rhubarb, spinach, and beet greens.
- Get regular exercise.
- For prevention, consider IP6 and potassium citrate supplements.

LICE

For parents of school-aged children, head lice are an inconvenient fact of life. One in ten Canadian schoolchildren get head lice each year. Head lice are not a sign of poor hygiene, but rather a common societal problem.

Head lice are small insects approximately 2 mm to 4 mm in length. Head lice bite and consume the blood of their host, causing itching and irritation. An adult louse looks like a small, brown-black, flat-backed beetle. Younger lice, called nymphs, are miniscule and have a spider-like appearance. The eggs or nits are extremely tiny, often shiny or translucent globules found cemented to the hair shaft, usually close to the scalp for food (blood), moisture, warmth, and shelter. While adult lice and some nymphs may be removed using a fine-toothed or special lice comb, the eggs must be manually removed by pinching them and drawing them off the entire length of the hair strand.

The life cycle of a louse is approximately one month. Only female lice can reproduce. Eggs take 9 to 10 days to hatch, and the nymphs take a week to become adults, at which point they can reproduce for the remaining two weeks of their lifespan. Adult females may lay five or more eggs per day. To stop the spread of head lice, the adults, nymphs, and nits must all be killed and removed from the hair.

Head lice live only on the scalps of their human hosts (no other area). Off the head, they will die within 48 to 72 hours unless they find a new host. Head lice have strong legs and claws, which help them cling to the hair during exposure to showers, combs, brushes, and hair dryers. Head lice cannot fly or jump and can pass to others only through direct human contact—direct head-to-head or hair-to-hair contact. They do not infect family pets.

There are many things that can be done to prevent the spread of head lice and to get rid of this problem.

SIGNS & SYMPTOMS

- Itching: Persistent scratching of the scalp (especially behind the ears and base of the neck) in young children may indicate lice.
- Red bumps on scalp or neck
- Seeing adult lice or nits (eggs) in the hair, on a brush, or in the tub after a bath or shower
- In severe cases, a secondary bacterial infection can occur.

RISK FACTORS

- Head lice are more common in girls likely because girls are more likely to have close contact during play (not because they have longer hair).
- Head-to-head contact (cuddling, hugging, wrestling, etc.)
- Sharing brushes, combs, hats, shirts, head scarves, and personal items.

DOCTOR'S ORDERS

Most health professionals recommend using an over-the-counter pharmaceutical lice treatment shampoo at the first sign of lice infestation.

Products such as Nix, Resultz, and R & C are commonly used. Nix and R & C are made with strong chemicals (pesticides) that are designed to kill the lice. Lindane is another option, but it is not used often because of risk of neurotoxicity and seizures. None of these pesticides are 100 percent effective in killing the eggs, so a second treatment is often required after 7 to 10 days. Another problem is that lice can be resistant to these pesticides. Use them only if you or your child have a confirmed case of head lice. Follow the product instructions carefully. After application use a fine tooth comb to remove the nits. Possible side effects of Nix and R & C include dry scalp, itching, and irritation. They can also trigger asthma and allergies in certain individuals.

Resultz doesn't contain pesticides, but it does contain chemicals that work to dissolve the wax that covers the head lice, dehydrating them and causing them to die. It is highly effective and better tolerated than the pesticides. The product is applied to dry hair and left on for 10 minutes, then rinsed away with warm water. The application is repeated seven days later.

Those who prefer to avoid using chemicals or products can simply use a fine tooth comb to remove the nits and live lice. This is the method that is advocated by the National Pediculosis Association. It is time-consuming and you may have to repeat the procedure for several days to remove them all, but this approach is also the safest.

SHERRY'S NATURAL PRESCRIPTION

Lifestyle Suggestions

- All school-aged children should be educated about the spread of lice and taught to avoid sharing articles of clothing, combs, and brushes.

- Get into the habit of inspecting school-aged children once a week for lice. Breaking the cycle of lice is significantly easier if it is caught in the early stages when fewer eggs have been laid on the hair follicles.

- Use a natural shampoo and conditioner containing tea tree (if tolerated) or the essential oils of citronella, eucalyptus, marjoram, and rosemary to help prevent an outbreak.

- Spray a combination of water and lavender essential oil, which is a natural insect repellant, on the base of the neck and hair each day.

BEATING LICE

Whether you are using a pesticide or natural product to control a lice outbreak, take the following steps:

1. Treat the infected person immediately, according to the product instructions.

2. After treatment, use a lice comb to remove any remaining lice and nymphs. Be patient as this may take up to two hours depending on the length of hair. For children with very

fine hair, a lice comb may not be adequate to remove all the eggs. In this case, you can loop a piece of thread through the comb to help pull out the eggs.

3. Examine the scalp of all other members in the household. Treat only those with confirmed cases.

4. Strip all bedding in the home and wash in hot water. Dry in a hot dryer for at least 45 minutes.

5. Items that come in close contact with the head, including hats worn in the last week, combs, and brushes, should be washed in hot water and dried thoroughly.

6. For any items that cannot be washed—such as blankets or pillows or large sleeping bags, quilts, or bulky coats—seal tightly in garbage bags and place in a cold environment such as the garage or basement for at least one week.

7. Inspect the hair daily for at least two weeks to ensure that all nits and lice have been removed; a magnifying glass and bright light may be helpful. Whether you use the pharmaceutical or the natural treatment, the key to success is diligence in removal of all lice and eggs.

Natural Treatments

Citronella: A volatile oil extracted from *Cymbopogon nardus* or *Cymbopogon winterianus*. Preliminary research has shown that it can help eliminate lice and prevent recurrence. In this study, a lotion containing 3.7 percent citronella or placebo was sprayed on the hair of children with head lice every morning for six days each week. After two and four months, those using citronella lotion had significantly fewer cases of head lice compared to the placebo group.

One small study found that a natural product containing coconut oil, anise oil, and ylang ylang oil, applied to hair three times a day at five-day intervals, was as successful as the control pediculicide in eliminating lice. But this research is considered preliminary.

Tea tree: Heavily promoted for head lice, but the scientific evidence is preliminary. Tea tree may work by degrading the bond of the lice to the hair shaft and helping dislodge them from the scalp. Regular use may help prevent an outbreak, but there are some concerns with using this on the scalp as it can cause adverse effects (skin rash and irritation). Do not use at full strength; add a few drops to regular shampoo. Test a small patch of skin prior to use.

LICE HOME REMEDIES

Various home remedies have been tried over the years to get rid of lice, such as applying mayonnaise, petroleum jelly, olive oil, or thick hair gel. Applying these thick products to the hair and scalp and leaving on overnight will theoretically suffocate and reduce the attachment of lice. There are numerous case reports suggesting benefits, but there are no clinical studies supporting the efficacy of these products.

FINAL THOUGHTS

The best way to prevent and cope with an outbreak of lice is to stay vigilant.

- Check school-aged children once a week for lice. Use a fine-toothed lice comb.
- Keep a natural lice treatment product in your medicine cabinet.
- Use shampoos and conditioners containing tea tree oil (if tolerated) or citronella regularly for prevention.
- Spray the base of the neck, as well as jackets and knapsacks, with a combination of water and essential oil of lavender.
- To eliminate head lice without the use of pesticides, try citronella or Resultz.

LOW LIBIDO

Low libido is an absence or deficiency of sexual fantasy and desire for sexual activity. This is also referred to as inhibited sexual desire. It is difficult to define "normal" sexual desire, as it varies among individuals, gender, and age. However, surveys have found that approximately 30 to 40 percent of all adults complain of a low sex drive.

This may be a primary condition (a person never felt much sexual desire) or secondary (a person used to possess sexual desire, but no longer has an interest).

There are many factors that affect one's libido—psychological, physical, medical, and even lifestyle. While this is a sensitive topic for some to discuss, it is an important one because lack of desire for a partner can have troubling consequences for the relationship. As well, studies have found a correlation between sexual desire and overall happiness.

SIGNS & SYMPTOMS

• Loss of interest in or desire for sex

RISK FACTORS

There are many potential causes and risk factors for low libido, including the following:

• Health conditions: Cushing's syndrome, fatigue, menopause, postpartum depression, diabetes, hysterectomy, and obesity

• Hormonal imbalance: Low thyroid, estrogen, testosterone, or DHEA

• Nutritional deficiency in zinc

• Physical problems: Vaginal dryness, vulvodynia, impotence (erectile dysfunction), and inability to reach climax

• Prescription drugs: Beta-blockers (for blood pressure), birth control pills, antidepressants, tranquilizers, Proscar (for prostate enlargement), Tamoxifen (for breast cancer)

• Psychological issues: Stress, depression, relationship conflict (feelings of anger or resentment), negative or traumatic sexual experiences

• Use of alcohol or marijuana

Note: Low libido affects more women than men. This could be due to hormonal changes (PMS, child birth, and menopause) and the fact that female libido is more complex and influenced by a variety of physical and emotional factors.

DOCTOR'S ORDERS

Consult with your doctor if you are taking medications or have a condition that could be affecting your libido, as this could be easily remedied by a change in therapy.

There are no specific drugs to treat low libido. However, there are medications that can treat the underlying cause. For example, hormones such as thyroid, estrogen, testosterone, or DHEA can be given to those deficient. For women with low estrogen, testosterone, or progesterone, a compounding pharmacy can prepare a topical cream in an appropriate dosage that is better tolerated than oral pills.

SHERRY'S NATURAL PRESCRIPTION

Dietary Recommendations

Foods to include:

• Eat a healthy, whole foods diet as outlined in Chapter 4.

• Many foods are claimed to enhance libido, but science is lacking in this area. For example, oysters are high in zinc, which raises sperm and testosterone production, yet studies showing that oysters raise libido have not been done.

Foods to avoid:

• Refined carbohydrates, sugar, processed and fast foods, and caffeine can trigger mood swings, irritability, and anxiety.

• Saturated and trans fats (red meat, high-fat dairy, deep-fried and processed foods) can impair blood vessel health.

• Alcohol may reduce inhibitions; however, it can also act as a depressant and negatively affect sexual function.

APHRODISIACS

An aphrodisiac is a food, drink, drug, scent, or device that can arouse or increase sexual desire. Named after Aphrodite, the Greek goddess of sexual love and beauty, there is a long list of purported aphrodisiacs, including anchovies, oysters, adrenaline, licorice, chocolate, and Spanish fly. However, there is no scientific proof that any foods can treat sexual dysfunction.

Lifestyle Suggestions

• Exercise: Aerobic activities such as walking and cycling can reduce stress, improve mood, increase energy, and improve circulation (improved blood supply to the pelvic area may help to improve sexual sensation and satisfaction).

• Maintain a healthy body weight.

• Women with vaginal dryness can try a lubricant such as Replens or Astroglide.

• Don't smoke, as smoking causes damage to nerves and blood vessels, which can affect sensation.

• Relax—try massage, meditation, yoga, breathing exercises, or a warm bath. Aromatherapy oils known to inspire romance include rose, clary sage, sandalwood, and jasmine.

• Set aside time to be intimate with your partner and work on improving communication.

Top Recommended Supplements

Arginine: An amino acid that is involved in many body processes including hormone secretion and the production of nitrous oxide (a substance that relaxes blood vessels). Several studies have found it helpful for improving sexual desire and function in both men and women. It is often combined with other products such as yohimbe, ginkgo biloba, ginseng, and damiana. Dosage: 2–8 g per day.

Ginkgo biloba: Increases blood flow to the brain and sexual organs (improves sexual sensation); has been shown to alleviate sexual problems caused by antidepressant drugs, such as low libido, arousal, and orgasm. Dosage: 120 mg daily.

Muira puama: Also known as potency wood, clinical studies have found it beneficial for enhancing libido and other aspects of sexual function in both men and women. One particular study, which evaluated the effects of muira puama and ginkgo biloba in women with low sex drive, found significant improvement in the frequency of sexual desires, sexual intercourse, sexual fantasies, satisfaction with sex life, intensity of sexual desires, excitement of fantasies, ability to reach orgasm, and intensity of orgasm. Tincture dosage: 2–4 mL of a 4:1 extract twice daily.

Tongkat ali: Also known as *Eurycoma longifolia*. Several clinical studies on a patented form of this plant called Physta show that it can raise testosterone and DHEA to normal levels, lower cortisol (stress hormone), improve sexual performance and satisfaction, and boost energy levels in men. Preliminary research in women suggests it will offer similar benefits. Dosage: 50–100 mg daily.

Complementary Supplements

Zinc: Required for the production of testosterone; levels are depleted by many drugs, including ACE inhibitors, oral contraceptives, and methotrexate. Dosage: 25–50 mg daily.

Note: Several products, including maca and horny goat weed, are promoted as libido enhancers, yet evidence to support these claims is lacking.

Supplements for erectile dysfunction are listed under that condition in this book.

FINAL THOUGHTS

There are many factors that affect one's libido, so it is important to seek help and identify the underlying cause. Here are some general tips to consider:

- Eat a healthy diet and reduce intake of processed and refined foods and alcohol.
- Exercise regularly to improve mood and blood flow.
- Don't smoke.
- Promote relaxation with massage, meditation, and essential oils.
- Supplements of arginine, ginkgo biloba, muira puama, and tongkat ali may help improve several aspects of sexual interest and function.

LUPUS

Lupus is an autoimmune disease, meaning that the immune system produces antibodies that attack the body's own tissues, causing pain and inflammation. It most commonly affects your skin, joints, kidneys, blood cells, heart, and lungs.

The word "lupus" comes from the Latin word for "wolf," because doctors once thought the classic lupus rash resembled a wolf's face. It appears across the cheeks and bridge of the nose and is actually more of a butterfly-shaped rash. About 50 percent of people with systemic lupus erythematosus will have this rash.

There are three main types of lupus:

Discoid lupus erythematosus (DLE): A less serious form that causes only skin rash, triggered most often by sun sensitivity.

Drug-induced lupus: Results from the long-term use of certain prescription drugs, such as the antipsychotic chlorpromazine, high blood pressure medications (hydralazine), the tuberculosis drug isoniazid, and the heart medication procainamide. Beta-blockers and arthritis and ulcer drugs have also been associated with lupus. Symptoms (joint pain, swelling, fever, and fatigue) usually disappear after the drug is stopped.

Systemic lupus erythematosus (SLE): The most common and most serious form of the disease. This form causes inflammation and pain throughout the body, affecting the joints, muscles, and skin. Infection with a bacteria or virus is a common trigger.

The underlying cause of DLE and SLE is not known, but researchers believe that it results from a combination of factors, including genetics, environment (sunlight), and hormones.

Mounting research suggests that vitamin D deficiency may be involved in triggering lupus. Vitamin D modulates the activity of immune cells, and several studies have identified widespread vitamin D deficiency in those with lupus.

Lupus is a treatable condition. In recent decades, early diagnosis and treatment have greatly improved the life expectancy and quality of life for those with lupus. Proper medical care and lifestyle strategies can help to manage the symptoms and put the disease into remission.

SIGNS & SYMPTOMS

The signs and symptoms vary greatly among individuals. They may appear suddenly or develop slowly, and may be mild or severe. Most people experience intermittent periods of flare-ups and remission. Typical symptoms include the following:

• Arthritis: Joint pain, particularly in the fingers, hands, wrists, and knees

• Blood vessel inflammation

• Digestive problems: Abdominal pain, weight loss, nausea, and vomiting

• Fatigue and fever

• Hair loss

- Headaches, dizziness, visual problems, and depression

- Heart problems: Inflammation of the sac around the heart (pericarditis), which causes shortness of breath and chest pain

- Kidney damage: Symptoms may include swelling in the legs

- Lung problems: Pleuritis (inflammation of the lining of the lungs)

- Muscle pain and weakness

- Raynaud's phenomenon: Fingers, toes, nose, and ears turn pale and numb when exposed to cold temperatures

- Skin lesions: Small pimples or flat lesions that can become scaly, crusty, or itchy

- Skin rash (affects one in three people with lupus)

- Sun sensitivity (photosensitivity)

- Swollen glands or swelling around the eyes

- Ulcers in the mouth or nose

Without treatment, complications from lupus can be life-threatening. The disease can cause significant damage to the kidneys, heart, central nervous system, and lungs. Lupus also increases the risk of infection because many of the drugs used to treat the disease suppress the immune system.

RISK FACTORS

- Age: Lupus affects people of all ages, but it is most often diagnosed between the ages of 15 and 45.

- Family history

- Gender: Women are approximately nine times as likely to develop the disease as men, with the exception of drug-induced lupus, which affects more men than women; this is likely because men are more likely to develop chronic conditions that require long-term treatment.

- Hormones: In women, lupus often comes on during or right after pregnancy, which leads researchers to believe that estrogen and progesterone may have a role in the disease. Many people with lupus also have low levels of the hormone DHEA.

- Race: Blacks are at increased risk of developing lupus; they also tend to develop lupus at a younger age and have more serious complications; Hispanics, Asians, and Aboriginals also are at higher risk of developing lupus.

- Recurrent infection with Epstein-Barr virus

- Sunlight: Exposure can trigger the disease and flare-ups.

- Researchers are continuing to learn about the factors that are thought to play a role in this disease, which include stress, certain foods, the artificial sweetener aspartame, silicone breast implants, mercury dental fillings, hair dye, and pesticides and other toxic chemicals. To date, no clear link has been found between these factors and lupus.

DOCTOR'S ORDERS

The treatment of lupus depends on the severity of your symptoms. Drugs can help manage symptoms and prevent complications, but they all carry the risk of side effects, and some drugs can actually worsen lupus symptoms, so it is important to discuss the benefits and risks with your doctor. Here are some of the most commonly used drugs for managing lupus:

- Anti-malarials, such as hydroxychloroquine (Plaquenil) and chloroquine (Aralen), are commonly used. There is no relationship between lupus and malaria; however, these drugs have minor immune suppression and anti-inflammatory effects, which can help with the management of the skin and joint problems and ulcers and may also help reduce flare-ups. Side effects include upset stomach, diarrhea, and visual problems.
- Corticosteroids, such as prednisone, help reduce inflammation and suppress the activity of the immune system. They can cause serious side effects, including weight gain, high blood pressure, and increased risk of glaucoma and infection. Corticosteroids interfere with the absorption of calcium, which can lead to osteoporosis. These drugs can also reduce the absorption of nutrients such as vitamins B6, C, and D, zinc, and potassium, and interfere with cells' ability to use them. In addition, corticosteroids can cause loss of muscle protein, change the body's ability to handle blood sugar (increasing diabetes risk), and increase fat deposits and sodium retention.
- Immunosuppressants, such as azathioprine (Imuran), methotrexate (Rheumatrex), and cyclophosphamide (Cytoxan), suppress the immune system and help to bring lupus into remission. These drugs are used only for severe cases as they cause anemia and increase the risk of infection and cancer.
- Non-steroidal anti-inflammatory drugs help to reduce joint and muscle pain and inflammation. Examples include ibuprofen (Motrin), naproxen (Naprosyn), and celecoxib (Celebrex). These drugs can be hard on the stomach and may cause stomach ulcers. Celebrex has also been linked to heart problems.
- Monoclonal antibodies are the newest class of drugs for treating lupus and they are considered groundbreaking because they provide targeted therapy. These antibodies are targeted toward receptors on the surface of B-cells, which destroy self-reactive B-cells involved in causing lupus. The only monoclonal antibody drug approved in Canada so far is belimumab (Benlysta), which is given intravenously.

SHERRY'S NATURAL PRESCRIPTION

Dietary Recommendations

Below are dietary recommendations that can help offset nutrient deficiencies caused by lupus drugs and support overall health.

Foods to include:

- Cranberries and cranberry juice can help prevent urinary tract infections in those at risk.

- Fish contain beneficial fatty acids that help reduce inflammation. Choose wild (not farmed) fish such as salmon, mackerel, herring, and sardines. Flaxseed, chia seed, wheat germ, olive oil, nuts, and seeds also contain good fatty acids.

- Include rich sources of calcium, especially if you take corticosteroids, which interfere with the absorption of calcium and can lead to osteoporosis. Foods high in calcium include dairy products and, to a lesser extent, broccoli, greens (chard, okra, kale, and spinach), sauerkraut, cabbage, rutabaga, and salmon (with bones).

- Tomato products, especially tomato paste, have high levels of lycopene, which may decrease the risk of heart disease and certain kinds of cancer.

- Vegetables, fruits, and whole grains contain essential vitamins and minerals.

- Vitamin C supports immune function and is essential for the health of our skin, heart, and lungs. Foods high in vitamin C include fresh tomatoes, broccoli, citrus fruits, strawberries, cauliflower, cantaloupe, cabbage, and green peppers.

- Vitamin D aids in the absorption of calcium and reduces the risk of osteoporosis. It also supports immune function and may protect against certain cancers. Good food sources include eggs, fish oils, and whole-grain cereals.

Foods to avoid:

- Alcohol hampers immune function; has negative effects on your liver, kidneys, heart, and muscles; and may interact with your medications.

- Caffeine can affect your sleep, so minimize or avoid coffee, soft drinks, and caffeinated teas.

- Saturated fat (meat and high-fat dairy) and trans fats (snack and processed foods) can worsen inflammation and also increase the risk of heart disease.

- Soy, alfalfa sprouts, mushrooms, and beans contain compounds that can aggravate lupus symptoms.

- Sugar can hamper immune function and increase the risk of infections. Avoid candy, sweets, soft drinks, and other high-sugar foods.

Lifestyle Suggestions

- Get adequate sleep. Lack of sleep can worsen immune function and stress.

- Wear sunscreen with at least SPF 30 on any sun-exposed areas. Make sure the product provides both UVA and UVB protection. Wear sunglasses and a wide-brimmed hat when outdoors. Limit time outdoors between 11 a.m. and 4 p.m., when the sun's rays are most intense.

- Get regular moderate-intensity exercise, such as walking. Aim for one hour daily. Regular exercise improves heart and lung function and joint mobility, helps reduce stress, and gives you more energy. Weight-bearing activities such as walking also help to improve bone strength and ward off osteoporosis. Start slowly and gradually increase your time and intensity.

- Find ways to manage your stress. Stress can trigger flare-ups and worsen the disease. Exercise helps, as does meditation, yoga, and deep breathing. Acupuncture can reduce pain and stress.

- Hot paraffin baths, therapeutic mud treatments, baths with Epsom/mineral salts, and sauna can ease pain and inflammation.

- Light massage with botanical oils (camphor, eucalyptus, pine needle, or rosemary) can help reduce pain and promote relaxation.

- Don't smoke. Smoking causes lung and heart damage, and those with lupus are already at risk of these problems.

Top Recommended Supplements

DHEA (dehydroepiandrosterone): A naturally occurring hormone that is used to make all sex hormones (estrogen, progesterone, and testosterone). Levels are often depleted in those with SLE. Several studies have shown that supplementing with DHEA can reduce symptoms and the frequency of flare-ups. In Canada, DHEA is available only by prescription from a doctor and has to be prepared in a compounding pharmacy. Dosage: The typical dosage for SLE is 50–200 mg daily.

Gamma linoleic acid (GLA): A beneficial fatty acid found in evening primrose, borage, and black currant oils that may help to reduce skin inflammation. Dosage: 1 g three times daily.

Fish oils: Contain omega-3 fatty acids, which have anti-inflammatory and immune balancing properties. Fish oils have been found useful for rheumatoid arthritis, and two studies also found it effective for reducing the symptoms of SLE. In particular it may help reduce joint pain and swelling. Fish oil can also protect against heart disease. Dosage: 6–10 g of EPA plus DHA daily.

Vitamin D: Required for proper immune function and bone health (prevention of osteoporosis). Those with lupus are often deficient in vitamin D, which can be compounded by use of sunscreens. Dosage: 1,000–10,000 IU as advised by your health care provider.

Complementary Supplements

Antioxidants: Help to quench free radicals, which are generated by inflammation. Many people with lupus have low levels of antioxidants, such as beta carotene and vitamin C. These antioxidants are essential for good health, immune function, and disease protection. Antioxidants may play a protective role against lupus complication such as joint, muscle, and organ damage. Vitamin E has been shown in some research to decrease lupus activity. Look for a product that contains vitamins C and E, beta carotene, and selenium. Preliminary research suggests that the antioxidant Pycnogenol (pine bark extract) can help improve lupus symptoms.

Calcium: Essential for bone health. Those with lupus who are taking corticosteroids are at significant risk of osteoporosis. Supplementing with calcium can help protect against bone loss. Dosage: 1,000–1,500 mg. Look for a product that also contains vitamin D, magnesium, and zinc, which are also essential for bone health.

Celadrin: A patented blend of fatty acids that reduces inflammation and pain, lubricates joints, and promotes healing. Several clinical studies have shown benefits for joint health. Celadrin is available in capsules and cream; there are no known side effects. Dosage: 1,500 mg daily; cream is applied twice daily.

Flaxseed oil: Some preliminary research suggests that flaxseed might help prevent or treat lupus nephritis. Dosage: 1 g three times daily.

Moducare: A combination of beta-sitosterol and beta-sitosterolin, which help to balance immune function. It does not stimulate the immune system. Studies show that Moducare is helpful for reducing pain and inflammation associated with rheumatoid arthritis. While it has not been specifically studied for SLE, it may offer similar benefits. Dosage: One capsule three times daily on a regular basis.

NATURAL PRODUCTS THAT WORSEN SLE

The herb alfalfa contains a substance called L-canavanine, which can worsen SLE or bring it out of remission. People with SLE should avoid alfalfa completely. Echinacea and soy can also aggravate lupus. If you are taking medications to manage your lupus, consult with your doctor and pharmacist before you start taking any new herbal or other supplements to avoid any potential interactions.

FINAL THOUGHTS

To improve the management of lupus, consider the following:

- Eat a healthy diet of vegetables, fruits, whole grains, fish, nuts, and seeds.
- Avoid soy, alfalfa, mushrooms, beans, alcohol, saturated and trans fats, sugar, and caffeine.
- Get adequate sleep and find ways to reduce stress.
- Wear sunscreen; don't smoke.
- Consider supplements of fish oils, vitamin D, and GLA, and talk to your doctor about whether you can benefit from DHEA.

MACULAR DEGENERATION

Macular degeneration is a chronic disease that occurs when the macula of the eye breaks down or is damaged. The macula is part of the retina, which is located on the inside back wall of the eyeball and is responsible for central vision. Deterioration of the macula results in blurring and loss of central vision, which worsens over time, leading to blindness.

This condition most commonly affects older adults, so it is referred to as age-related macular degeneration (ARMD). Macular degeneration is the leading cause of visual loss in people over 60 years of age and the second leading cause of blindness (after cataracts) in those over age 65.

There are two forms of macular degeneration:

- **Dry:** This is the most common form and is responsible for 90 percent of cases. It occurs when the macula breaks down and thins over time due to aging, free radical damage, inflammation, poor vascular health, and lack of blood and oxygen to the macula. Cellular debris accumulates under the retina and central vision slowly deteriorates over time.
- **Wet:** Also known as hemorrhagic macular degeneration, this is less common but more serious as it develops suddenly and progresses fast. It occurs when blood vessels grow under the macula, pushing against it and leaking fluid, which causes scarring of the macula and permanent damage to central vision.

Early detection and intervention can help reduce visual loss from macular degeneration. It is possible to slow down the progression and prevent macular degeneration with lifestyle measures and supplements.

SIGNS & SYMPTOMS

The symptoms of dry macular degeneration develop slowly over time, while symptoms of the wet form develop suddenly and worsen rapidly. They include the following:

- Increasing need for light to do close work
- Difficulty reading fine print
- Words, straight lines, and signs appear crooked and wavy
- Colours appear less bright
- Blurring and loss of central vision; grey or blank spots in the centre of the visual field

RISK FACTORS

- Age (most common in those over 60)
- Diet (high consumption of saturated and trans fats and sugar; nutritional deficiencies of vitamins A, C, E, zinc, lutein, and zeaxanthin)
- Environmental toxin exposure

- Family history (having a close relative with AMD increases your risk by about 50 percent)

- Gender (women are at greater risk)

- Heart disease (high blood pressure, high cholesterol, coronary artery disease, and stroke)

- Light-coloured eyes (green or blue)

- Obesity

- Race (more common among Caucasians)

- Smoking (the most preventable cause of macular degeneration; smoking a pack of cigarettes a day more than doubles a person's risk of developing macular degeneration)

- UV light exposure

DOCTOR'S ORDERS

There are a few surgical procedures, such as laser and photodynamic therapy, that can be done for wet macular degeneration, with limited success. These procedures prevent further damage to the macula and further visual loss, but they do not restore vision that is lost. Recently, a new class of medications called antivascular endothelial growth factor drugs has become available for treating wet AMD. These drugs help promote regression of the abnormal blood vessels and improve vision. They are injected directly into the vitreous humour of the eye.

Currently, there are no medical treatments for dry macular degeneration. A number of treatments are being investigated, including photocoagulation. Research has shown that antioxidant supplements can prevent worsening of this condition and further vision loss; this is discussed below.

SHERRY'S NATURAL PRESCRIPTION

Dietary Recommendations

Foods to include:

- Numerous studies have found that those with high intakes of carotenoids have a lower risk of macular degeneration. Carotenoids are antioxidants found in yellow, orange, and dark green fruits and vegetables. They include beta carotene, lutein, and zeaxanthin. It is thought that these plant pigments protect the macula against UV light damage by dying the macula yellow (acting as natural sunglasses) and by neutralizing free radicals. These nutrients are not only important for prevention but they can also help slow progression and protect against further visual loss. Carrots are an excellent source of beta carotene. Kale, collard greens, spinach, and broccoli are the best sources of lutein and zeaxanthin.

- Vitamins C and E and selenium can protect against macular degeneration. In one study, those with the highest levels of these antioxidants had a 70 percent lower risk of developing macular degeneration. The best food sources of vitamin C are berries (acai, blueberry, and cranberry), grapes, tomatoes, peppers, and citrus fruits. Vitamin E is found in nuts, seeds, whole grains, and vegetable oils. Selenium is found in meat, seafood, grains, and vegetables.

- Fish is rich in omega-3 fatty acids, which help reduce inflammation and are protective against AMD and other blood vessel diseases like heart disease. Some research has found that eating fish at least twice a week can significantly reduce the risk of macular degeneration.

- There is some evidence that a low-glycemic diet (eating slow-release carbohydrates) can help improve macular degeneration; eat more high-fibre foods that are low in the glycemic index. Refer to Appendix B.

Foods to avoid:

- Fast foods and processed foods contain hydrogenated fats (trans fats), saturated fats, and chemicals that can generate free radicals, which are associated with an increased risk of macular degeneration.

- High-glycemic carbohydrates (refined starches like white flour) raise blood sugar levels, which can worsen macular degeneration.

Lifestyle Suggestions

- Wear sunglasses with UV protection to shield your eyes from the sun's harmful rays. Wide-brimmed hats are also recommended.

- Don't smoke, and avoid exposure to second-hand smoke, as this is a major risk factor for macular degeneration.

- Use magnifying glasses to read, and have proper light in your home.

- Avoid driving at night and during bad weather conditions.

Top Recommended Supplements

Antioxidants: Research on a specific combination and dosage of antioxidant vitamins and minerals found that they significantly reduced the progression of macular degeneration and the risk of further visual loss, and they may help improve visual acuity. These nutrients are 500 mg of vitamin C, 400 IU of vitamin E, 15 mg of beta carotene, 80 mg of zinc (as zinc oxide), and 2 mg of copper (as cupric oxide). Look for a product that contains these ingredients and dosages. *Note:* 80 mg of zinc is a high dose, and can impair copper absorption, which is why it is important to also supplement with copper.

Fish oils: Mounting evidence supports the benefits of fish oil for reducing the risk of macular degeneration and preventing progression to advanced AMD in those with the disease. Dosage: 1–3 g daily.

Lutein: Studies have found that supplements can prevent disease progression and improve vision in those with both early and advanced macular degeneration. Dosage: 6–10 mg daily.

Complementary Supplements

Bilberry: Preliminary research suggests that bilberry can help prevent macular degeneration. Bilberry contains anthocyanidins, which are powerful antioxidants that support blood vessel health.

B-vitamins: Help lower homocysteine levels, a biomarker of inflammation. Low levels of certain B-vitamins (B6, B12, and folic acid) are associated with increased risk of AMD, and recent research has found that supplementing with these vitamins can reduce the risk of

AMD in adults with cardiovascular risk factors. Dosage: 50 mg B6, 1 mg B12, and 2.5 mg folic acid.

Ginkgo biloba: Some research has shown that it can improve vision in those with macular degeneration. Ginkgo has antioxidant properties and improves circulation and blood vessel health. Dosage: 60 mg three or four times daily.

FINAL THOUGHTS

To help prevent macular degeneration, consider the following:

- Don't smoke, and avoid second-hand smoke and chemical exposure.
- Wear sunglasses with UV protection and wide-brimmed hats while outdoors.
- Eat more eye-healthy foods: carrots, spinach, broccoli, kale, collard greens, berries, peppers, citrus fruits, nuts, seeds, whole grains, and fish.
- Maintain a healthy body weight.
- Take antioxidant supplements and lutein.

MEMORY LOSS

Occasionally forgetting a person's name or an appointment is normal, especially when we are busy multitasking in our daily lives. These temporary lapses in memory are usually not a cause for concern. However, when you or your loved ones notice increasing episodes of memory loss and forgetfulness, this needs to be addressed.

While many people fear Alzheimer's disease, only a small percentage of people over the age of 65 develop this disease. More commonly, people experience non-Alzheimer's decline in memory as they get older. And while memory loss is more common with age, it is not a consequence of aging, but rather a result of changes that occur in the brain that are more common as we age. For our memory to function well, the brain requires healthy nerve cells and adequate supplies of blood, nutrients, and neurotransmitters (chemicals that relay messages between nerve cells). As we age, nerve cells shrink, and damage to blood vessels can hamper circulation, which hampers the supply of blood and nutrients to the brain. This reduces the production of neurotransmitters. Stress, pollution, smoking, poor diet, and lack of exercise also take a toll on the health of our brain and our memory. Memory loss can also result from a stroke, heart disease, and damaged blood vessels from uncontrolled diabetes. In some cases, this type of loss is reversible with therapy.

There are many things that can be done to prevent age-related memory loss, such as physical and mental exercise, supplements, and dietary changes. Even those who are elderly and have experienced memory loss can take steps to improve their memory.

SIGNS & SYMPTOMS

- Difficulty remembering names, places, and events
- Forgetfulness
- Lack of concentration
- Poor mental focus

RISK FACTORS

- Alcohol and illicit drug use can alter chemicals in the brain and impair memory
- Allergies
- Atherosclerosis, the buildup of plaque in the blood vessels, is a major cause of memory loss
- Head injury or trauma
- Fatigue: Not getting enough sleep at night can affect your memory the next day
- High fever
- Hormonal problems, such as thyroid deficiency or menopause

- Low blood sugar

- Medications (sleeping pills, antihistamines, antidepressants, pain relievers)

- Poor nutrition: A diet high in fat and refined carbohydrates and low in nutrients; deficiencies of vitamins B1 and B12 can affect memory

- Stress increases cortisol levels, which impairs memory

DOCTOR'S ORDERS

It is important to discuss memory loss with your doctor so that tests can be done to rule out Alzheimer's or stroke. Even a small stroke can impair memory, and a proper diagnosis and treatment are necessary to prevent further strokes.

There are a few prescription medications that are used to help improve memory:

Ergoloid mesylates (Hydergine) is thought to improve oxygen flow to the brain and improve memory and cognitive impairment.

Selegiline (Eldepryl) is a drug commonly used for treating Parkinson's disease, but it also offers benefits for memory and brain function. Eldepryl enhances neurotransmitter levels and helps protect neurons.

SMART PILL

A "smart pill" is known medically as a nootropic drug, a substance that enhances cognitive ability and memory, and facilitates learning. The word "nootropic" comes from the Greek words *noos,* which means "mind," and *tropos,* which means "changed" or "turn." One drug that is used for this purpose is Hydergine.

SHERRY'S NATURAL PRESCRIPTION

Diet and lifestyle have a major impact on the function of our brain and our memory.

Dietary Recommendations

Foods to include:

- Brewer's yeast, wheat germs, spirulina, and eggs contain B-complex vitamins, which are essential for memory and cognitive function. Wheat germ and whole grains also contain the antioxidant vitamin E, which helps protect against free radical damage.

- Colourful fruits and vegetables, such as berries, peppers, citrus fruits, spinach, and leafy greens, contain a range of antioxidants, which help protect against free radical damage and support brain health.

- Cold-water fish (salmon, mackerel, and sardines) contain beneficial omega-3 fatty acids (DHA). Eat wild or organic fish; avoid farmed fish because of toxins.

- Palm fruit oil contains tocotrienols (a potent form of vitamin E) along with other antioxidants that are neuro-protective. Palm fruit oil is stable for cooking, and it is also found in commercially prepared foods such as peanut butter, hazelnut spread, and some non-hydrogenated margarines.

- Add turmeric to recipes. This spice contains curcumin, which is a powerful antioxidant and helps reduce inflammation. There is also some evidence that curcumin may help protect the brain against cognitive decline.

Foods to avoid:

- Alcohol destroys brain cells and alters brain chemistry, causing memory loss; minimize or avoid completely.

- Diets high in saturated fat can increase the risk of atherosclerosis, which damages blood vessels and reduces blood flow to the brain and heart.

- Refined carbohydrates (white bread/rice/baked goods) and sugary foods can cause blood sugar imbalances that can worsen memory and cognitive function.

- To determine whether food allergies are affecting your memory, refer to Appendix D for information on how to do an elimination diet.

Lifestyle Suggestions

- Don't smoke, as smoking damages blood vessels and hampers memory.

- Get regular physical exercise to maintain blood flow to the brain. Research has found that regular aerobic exercise, such as brisk walking, can improve attention, reasoning, and memory.

- Reduce stress with meditation, breathing exercises, or relaxation techniques. Staying calm and relaxed helps improve concentration and memory. Yoga has been found to improve memory and prevent memory loss.

- Keep your brain active. Challenging the brain with activities such as reading, writing, doing puzzles and crosswords, and playing games stimulates brain cells and the connections between the cells, and may help improve memory and prevent cognitive decline.

- Maintain social interactions, which help to reduce stress and improve mental well-being. Studies have found that loneliness increases the risk of late-life dementia.

- Try acupuncture. Some studies have found that stimulating acupuncture points can improve memory.

- Maintain an ideal body weight. Being overweight increases the risk of high blood pressure and cholesterol, factors associated with memory loss.

Top Recommended Supplements

Acetyl-L-carnitine: An amino acid derivative that crosses into the brain and increases the levels of acetylcholine, a brain neurotransmitter essential for memory and learning. Studies have found it helpful for improving memory and cognitive function in the elderly. Dosage: 1 g two or three times daily.

Fish oils: Contain omega-3 essential fatty acids, such as DHA (docosahexaenoic acid), which reduce inflammation and promote efficient transmittal of electrical signals between nerve cells. DHA also stabilizes and protects against the natural breakdown of cell membranes, a process that can compromise brain cells and nerves. In addition, DHA seems to improve concentration and may help reverse memory loss. Dosage: 3–9 g daily. Look for a product that provides at least 400 mg EPA and 200 mg DHA per dosage.

Ginkgo biloba: Improves memory and cognitive function by increasing blood flow to the brain. It may also help to prevent or delay cognitive decline with aging. It has been shown to be beneficial in those with Alzheimer's and non-Alzheimer's dementia and memory loss. Dosage: 120–240 mg daily, standardized to 6 percent terpene lactones and 24 percent flavone glycosides. It may take six weeks to notice benefits.

Phosphatidylserine: An amino acid–like substance that helps support the structure and health of cell membranes. Several studies involving more than 1,000 people have found it effective in improving memory in both college-age individuals and the elderly. Dosage: 300 mg daily.

Vinpocetine: A compound derived from periwinkle leaves; several studies have shown that it can improve memory and mental function in those with mild to moderate dementia and Alzheimer's disease. Dosage: 10 mg three times daily.

Complementary Supplements

Bacopa monnieri: An herb that has been shown to enhance several aspects of mental function. It increases availability of acetylcholine in the brain, which improves memory and cognition. Antioxidant properties help protect brain cells. Dosage: 200–450 mg daily standardized to contain bacosides.

B-vitamins: Play an important role in brain and nerve function. A deficiency of B1, B6, and B12 is more common among the elderly and can hamper memory and cognitive function. Take a B-complex vitamin daily. Those with poor intestinal health may require monthly injections of vitamin B12.

Melatonin: A hormone that regulates sleep/wake cycles; having adequate sleep is important for cognitive function. Supplements of melatonin have been found to improve sleep quality, mood, and memory. Dosage: 3–6 mg one hour before bed.

Tocotrienols: A potent form of the antioxidant vitamin E that protects the brain from damage caused by oxidative stress and inflammation. Studies in older adults have found that those with higher blood levels of vitamin E have better brain function. Preliminary research on tocotrienols derived from Malaysian palm fruit oil suggest it can protect the brain from damage that occurs with stroke. Supplements at higher dosages have been found to slow cognitive decline. Dosage: 1,000–2,000 IU daily.

FINAL THOUGHTS

To prevent memory loss and improve cognitive function, consider the following:

- Eat more fish, vegetables, nuts, seeds, and olive/palm fruit oil.
- Avoid saturated and trans fats.
- Get regular exercise such as brisk walking. Don't smoke.
- Keep your brain active with games, puzzles, and exercises.
- Consider supplements of acetyl-L-carnitine, fish oils, ginkgo biloba, and phosphatidylserine.

MENOPAUSE

Menopause is a natural phase in a woman's life that can be thought of as a time of ovarian retirement. At birth women have over 1 million eggs in their ovaries. At puberty ovulation starts and eggs are released by the ovaries each month for the purpose of conception. As the years go by, the amount of eggs gradually declines until menopause, when the ovaries shut down and stop producing estrogen and progesterone, the two main female sex hormones. Menopause occurs when ovulation ceases and a woman can no longer conceive naturally.

A woman is considered to be in menopause when she goes one year without a menstrual period. The average age for menopause is about 51 years, but it can occur naturally between ages 40 and 55. The decade or so before menopause is called perimenopause. During this time hormone levels fluctuate and the menstrual cycle becomes erratic, yet conception can still occur.

After menopause the adrenal glands, which supply some sex hormones throughout life, become the primary source. Women who have poor adrenal function, which can be caused by chronic stress, poor diet, lack of sleep, or excessive caffeine, are not able to provide adequate hormone amounts, and may have more severe menopausal symptoms. Estrogen can also be produced in the fat cells from androgens. This is why obese women often experience fewer menopausal symptoms.

There are many lifestyle measures and supplements that can promote hormone balance and ease menopausal concerns.

SIGNS & SYMPTOMS

Menopausal symptoms are caused primarily by an imbalance of the hormones estrogen, progesterone, and/or testosterone. High cortisol levels caused by stress can negatively impact these hormones as well. The severity and duration of symptoms experienced vary because of genetics, ethnicity, cultural factors, and even attitude. They include the following:

- Fatigue, foggy head, headache, memory loss

- Fluid retention and weight gain

- Hot flashes and night sweats

- Incontinence, bladder infections

- Low libido

- Mood swings, irritability, anxiety, depression

- Vaginal dryness

- Weight gain: linked to hormonal imbalance, stress, and lowered metabolic rate

RISK FACTORS

Menopause usually happens naturally as women age; however, certain medical treatments can bring it on sooner than expected:

- Exposure to radiation or chemotherapy

- Premature ovarian failure: Approximately 1 percent of women experience menopause before the age of 40; this may be due to genetic factors or autoimmune disease.

- Removal of both ovaries

DOCTOR'S ORDERS

Hormone replacement therapy (HRT) is no longer routinely recommended for women in menopause because several large studies have found that HRT can increase the risk of heart attack, stroke, blood clots, and breast cancer. One study also found that estrogen caused cognitive decline and dementia in older women.

HRT is now used only for women experiencing severe symptoms that cannot be helped by other measures. When it is necessary, it should be used at the lowest dose for the shortest periods of time (less than five years).

Bioidentical hormones are becoming more widely used. They are thought to be a safer alternative to synthetic hormones because they are associated with fewer side effects while still providing symptom relief. Bioidentical means that the hormones are exactly the same as the ones your body produces. Compounding pharmacists can make customized hormones in various dosages and forms (creams, suppositories, and capsules) to suit your individual needs. Bioidentical hormones are available in compounding pharmacies, by a doctor's prescription.

Women who experience serious emotional symptoms are sometimes prescribed antidepressants and tranquilizers. However, there are many side effects and risks with these drugs, and it is best to try natural methods first.

Bone-building drugs such as bisphosphonates (Didrocal, Fosamax, and Actonel) or selective estrogen receptor modulators (Evista) are often given to women with osteoporosis or those at great risk. It is still important that women taking these drugs get adequate calcium intake and do weight-bearing exercises for optimal bone health.

HORMONE CHECK

Many hormones can be unbalanced during menopause (estrogen, progesterone, testosterone, dehydroepiandrosterone, and cortisol) leading to troublesome symptoms. Blood or saliva tests can be done to find out which hormones are causing your symptoms. See Appendix E for more information.

HOMEOPATHIC RECOMMENDATIONS

Lachesis: Intense hot flashes with purple-red flushing, palpitations, and feelings of pressure, congestion, and constriction may indicate a need for this remedy. Tight clothing around the neck and waist may be impossible to tolerate. The person may be very talkative and tend to feel suspicious.

Sepia: This remedy can be helpful if a woman's periods are sometimes late and scanty. It is best used from the middle to the end of menopause (12 to 24 months after the last period). During the wind-down, menses can be heavy. The uterus feels weak and saggy, and there may be cravings for vinegar and sour foods. Women who need this remedy usually feel dragged-out and weary, emotionally distraught, and fatigued.

Combination recommendation: PascoeFemin by Pascoe

SHERRY'S NATURAL PRESCRIPTION

Dietary Recommendations

Foods to include:

• Vegetables, fruit, whole grains, and legumes provide essential vitamins, minerals, anti-oxidants, fibre, and compounds that can reduce the risk of cancer and heart disease and improve overall health. In particular, load up on broccoli, Brussels sprouts, cauliflower, and cabbage, as these vegetables contain compounds that help the liver process hormones while reducing the risk of breast cancer.

• Soy foods (tofu, soy milk, soybeans, tempeh, and soy nuts) contain isoflavones (plant-based estrogens), which help minimize menopausal symptoms, offer protection against breast cancer and heart disease (lower cholesterol, protect against atherosclerosis, and decrease blood pressure), and improve bone health (modestly increase bone density). Aim for two servings of these foods daily. It may take several weeks to notice benefits for menopausal symptoms such as hot flashes.

• Flaxseed is a rich source of fibre, which promotes bowel regularity, reduces the risk of colon and breast cancer, and lowers cholesterol. It also contains lignans (phytoestrogens), which may help balance estrogens and reduce menopausal symptoms.

• Fish, nuts, and seeds (chia) contain essential fatty acids that are important for heart and skin health.

Foods to avoid:

• Alcohol, caffeine, and spicy foods can worsen hot flashes.

• Saturated fats (red meat) and trans fats (processed, deep-fried, and fast foods) increase the risk of heart disease.

Lifestyle Suggestions

• Address your stress. Stress can make menopausal symptoms more pronounced and affect your adrenal gland function, reducing hormone production. Meditation, yoga, and breathing techniques can help reduce stress. Massage and acupuncture promote relaxation, and studies have shown that acupuncture can reduce hot flashes.

- Get regular exercise. Studies have shown that regular exercise reduces the frequency and severity of hot flashes. It also improves mood and sleep and protects against heart disease, and weight-bearing activities strengthen the bones.
- Don't smoke. Smoking can worsen hot flashes and symptoms of anxiety, irritability, and depression.
- Dress in layers so that you can peel off clothing during a hot flash.
- Consider a support group; it may help to share your experience with others.
- Laughter is good medicine. Watch funny movies, go to comedy shows, and spend time with people who make you happy and laugh.

Top Recommended Supplements

Black cohosh: An herb that has been found in many studies to reduce hot flashes, night sweats, insomnia, nervousness, and irritability. Some research has found it beneficial when combined with St. John's wort to relieve symptoms of depression and anxiety. Dosage: 20–40 mg twice daily. Consult with your doctor if you have liver disease. St. John's wort interacts with many medications.

Calcium and magnesium: Important minerals for bone health; women over 50 years should have 1,200 mg of calcium and 320 mg of magnesium daily, or more if they have osteoporosis. It is difficult to get this amount from diet alone, so supplements are often necessary. Look for a formula that also contains vitamin D and zinc.

Fish oils: Help protect against heart disease by lowering cholesterol and triglycerides, reducing inflammation, and protecting against heart attack and stroke. Dosage: 1,000–3,000 mg daily.

Complementary Supplements

Chasteberry: An herb that helps balance hormones and is particularly helpful during peri-menopause. Dosage: 160–240 mg daily.

Ginkgo biloba: An herb that helps improve memory and cognitive function by increasing blood flow to the brain. It is also an antioxidant. Dosage: 40 mg three times daily.

Melatonin: A hormone that regulates our sleep/wake cycles. Supplements help improve sleep quality by reducing the time needed to fall asleep and nighttime wakening. Dosage: 3–6 mg one hour before bed. Dosages up to 10 mg have been used in studies.

Red clover: A phytoestrogen that has been shown to reduce hot flashes. It also offers benefits for bone and heart health. Dosage: 80 mg daily.

FINAL THOUGHTS

To reduce the symptoms of menopause and improve health during menopausal years, consider the following:

- Reduce stress: Try meditation, yoga, or massage.
- Get regular exercise, and don't smoke.
- Eat a diet rich in soy foods, fish, whole grains, fruits, and vegetables.
- Ensure adequate calcium intake or take a mineral supplement for bone health; consider fish oils for heart health.
- Consider black cohosh as a first-line approach for relief of menopausal symptoms.

METABOLIC SYNDROME

Metabolic syndrome, formerly known as Syndrome X, is a cluster of conditions (abdominal obesity, elevated blood pressure, triglycerides, high cholesterol and/or fasting glucose, and insulin resistance) that occur together, increasing your risk for heart disease, stroke, and diabetes. Having just one of these conditions increases your risk of disease, but having them in combination multiplies the risk significantly. According to research, those who have three features of metabolic syndrome are nearly twice as likely to have a heart attack or stroke and more than three times as likely to develop heart disease as are those with no features.

There is a great deal of research focused on this problem, as it is affecting a growing number of our population. According to reports, over half of people over the age of 60 meet the criteria for metabolic syndrome, and overall about 25 percent of the entire Canadian population are classified as having metabolic syndrome.

Researchers believe that insulin resistance is the key underlying cause of this syndrome and responsible for the metabolic changes that occur. Insulin is the hormone secreted by the pancreas that takes glucose from your blood and moves it into the cells to be used for energy. In people with insulin resistance, cells don't respond to insulin and glucose can't enter the cells. The pancreas reacts by releasing more and more insulin to help glucose get into your cells. This results in higher than normal levels of insulin and glucose in the blood. High insulin levels cause triglycerides and cholesterol levels to rise. It also interferes with kidney function, leading to increased blood pressure. High insulin levels also promote fat storage around the belly, leading to abdominal obesity. These combined factors greatly increase one's risk of heart disease, stroke, diabetes, and other conditions.

The key to the management of metabolic syndrome and the prevention of its consequences is to address insulin resistance. This can be done effectively with lifestyle strategies (diet, exercise, and supplements).

SIGNS & SYMPTOMS

- Abdominal obesity (a pot belly): Waist circumference of 40 inches (102 cm) or more for men and 35 inches (89 cm) or more for women

- Elevated blood pressure: Systolic greater than 130 mmHg; diastolic greater than 85 mmHg

- Elevated fasting glucose: Greater than 5.6 mmol/L

- Elevated triglycerides and low HDL (good) cholesterol: Triglycerides greater than 1.7 mmol/L and HDL less than 1.04 mmol/L for men or 1.3 mmol/L for women

- Insulin resistance

- Those with metabolic syndrome often have elevated levels of C-reactive protein, a marker of inflammation.

RISK FACTORS

- Age: Metabolic syndrome is more common in those over the age of 60; it is not caused by aging, but factors that lead to insulin resistance (lack of activity and obesity) are more common among older adults.

- Having high blood pressure, heart disease, or polycystic ovarian syndrome

- History of diabetes: Those with a family history of diabetes or women who experienced gestational diabetes are at greater risk.

- Lack of exercise reduces insulin sensitivity.

- Obesity: Having a body mass index (BMI) greater than 25 or having an apple-shaped body (pot belly) increases risk.

- Poor diet: Eating a high-glycemic diet (refined starches and sugars)

- Race: Hispanics and Asians are at greater risk.

CHILDREN AND METABOLIC SYNDROME

Metabolic syndrome is a rising problem among youth, due in large part to the obesity epidemic. Over half of children who are obese have the features of metabolic syndrome, putting them at significant risk of heart disease, diabetes, and premature death. Studies have shown, however, that in as little as 12 weeks, regular exercise and healthy eating can facilitate weight loss and improve blood pressure, cholesterol, and blood sugar. (*Pediatrics,* 2006, 118(5): 1390–1398)

DOCTOR'S ORDERS

The treatment of metabolic syndrome varies depending on which features a person has. Medications can be used to lower blood pressure, cholesterol, triglycerides, and blood sugar and to improve insulin sensitivity. These medications are discussed in the respective chapters. However, lifestyle changes are absolutely critical. As discussed below, a low-glycemic diet and regular activity can greatly improve insulin sensitivity and the other features of this syndrome.

SHERRY'S NATURAL PRESCRIPTION

Dietary Recommendations

Foods to include:

- Add cinnamon to your cereal, oatmeal, or breakfast shakes. Cinnamon contains compounds that work with insulin to reduce blood sugar levels. One study found benefits with just ½ tsp daily.

- Chromium is essential for blood glucose regulation. It is found in brewer's yeast, whole grains (especially wheat germ), onions, and garlic.

- Eat lean animal protein (poultry, fish) and healthy fats (olive oil, nuts, and seeds) with each meal to further slow the rate of digestion.

- For a natural and healthy sugar substitute, try stevia or xylitol.

- Low-glycemic (slow-release), high-fibre carbohydrates such as whole grains (sprouted and multigrain bread, oats, quinoa), vegetables, fruits, and beans help promote better blood sugar control. Refer to Appendix B.

Foods to avoid:

- Alcohol can cause either high or low blood sugar depending on how much you drink and if you are eating while drinking. Limit alcohol intake to no more than two drinks daily.

- Avoid high-fructose corn syrup, which is found in many processed, convenience foods and in drinks, including soda and juice cocktails.

- Avoid processed and junk foods as they are high in calories (especially from fat and refined starches) and low in nutritional value.

- High-glycemic (quick-release) carbohydrates such as white bread and baked goods, refined cereals, potatoes, white rice, and sugar (candy, cookies, soda) cause rapid and profound increases in blood sugar and insulin levels.

- Minimize table salt as it can worsen high blood pressure. Try herbal seasonings instead.

- Saturated fat (animal products such as meat and dairy), trans fats (hydrogenated margarine), and deep-fried foods can worsen blood glucose control.

Lifestyle Suggestions

- Exercise regularly as this can help improve insulin sensitivity and help with weight loss. Aim for 30 minutes to one hour of moderate-intensity activity daily such as brisk walking, cycling, or swimming.

- Incorporate resistance training. Muscle burns more calories than fat and helps your body use blood sugar and insulin more efficiently. Try different strength-training exercises that focus on the core muscle groups: chest, back, shoulders, abdominals, and quadriceps.

- Lose excess weight. Losing even 5 to 10 percent of excess weight can help improve insulin sensitivity and reduce blood pressure and cholesterol.

- Don't smoke as smoking worsens insulin resistance and also increases the risk of heart disease and stroke.

- Manage your stress. Stress triggers the release of hormones that impair insulin sensitivity. Try yoga, meditation, or other relaxation techniques.

Top Recommended Supplements

Since metabolic syndrome is a collection of medical disorders, recommendations vary depending on which factors are present. Below are some general recommendations for supplements that address a few of the features of metabolic syndrome. For specific recommendations on supplements for obesity, diabetes (insulin resistance), high blood pressure, and cholesterol, refer to those sections of this book.

Fish oils: Help improve glucose tolerance, reduce triglycerides and cholesterol levels, and reduce inflammation. Studies have shown that fish oils play an important role in protection against heart disease and stroke. Dosage: 1–3 g daily.

Soluble fibre: Helps improve blood glucose control, cholesterol levels, and weight management. Research on psyllium (Metamucil), oat bran, partially hydrolyzed guar gum (Sunfiber), and glucomannan (PGX) have shown benefits for blood sugar, lowering cholesterol, and weight management. Dosage: Varies with product and formulation. Most fibre products (with the exception of Sunfiber) cause some bloating and gas, especially during initial consumption. To minimize this effect, gradually increase the amount you consume and take with plenty of water.

Complementary Supplements

Alpha lipoic acid: A potent antioxidant that reduces free radical damage. Studies have shown that it can improve blood glucose control and reduce diabetic complications. Dosage: 100–200 mg three times daily.

Chirositol: A nutrient derived from carob that helps improve insulin sensitivity and glucose levels. It has also been shown to reduce appetite and support weight management. Studies have found it particularly helpful in women with insulin resistance and polycystic ovarian syndrome. Dosage: 600 mg daily.

Chromium: Improves blood sugar regulation and insulin sensitivity. It may also help lower cholesterol levels. There are several different forms of chromium. Most research has been done with chromium picolinate. Dosage: 400–1,000 mcg daily.

Phase 2: A white kidney bean extract that reduces starch digestion. Studies have shown that it can lower after-meal blood sugar levels, reduce triglycerides, and help promote weight loss. Dosage: 500–1,000 mg before starchy meals.

Vitamin E: Helps improve glucose tolerance and insulin sensitivity and reduce glycosylation (binding of sugar to proteins in blood vessels). It also helps reduce blood clotting, and as an antioxidant it fights free radical damage. Dosage: 400–1,200 IU daily.

FINAL THOUGHTS

To reduce the risks of metabolic syndrome, consider the following:

- Eat small, frequent meals with low-glycemic, high-fibre carbohydrates, protein, and healthy fats. Add cinnamon to your diet.
- Avoid eating fast/processed/refined/deep-fried foods, alcohol, and saturated fat.
- Reduce your stress with yoga or relaxation techniques.
- Boost your activity level. Aim for at least 30 minutes of exercise daily.
- Consider supplements of fish oil and soluble fibre.

MIGRAINE HEADACHES

Migraines are intense, severe, pounding headaches that affect over 3 million adults and one-quarter of a million children in Canada. They can be overwhelming and debilitating, affecting one's quality of life. They also cost the Canadian economy over $500 million annually.

The name "migraine" comes from the Greek word *hemikrania,* meaning "half the skull," because migraines usually begin on one side of the head. Migraines can also affect the entire head, including the sinus area. For some people, migraines are preceded or accompanied by a sensory warning sign, called an aura, such as flashes of light, wavy lines, blind spots, or tingling in your arm or leg. A migraine attack may last for just a few minutes or continue for up to several days. Episodes can vary in frequency from several times in one week to once every few years. Typically, the intensity and frequency of migraines diminishes with age.

It is thought that a variety of factors contribute to causing migraines, including constriction and dilation of the blood vessels in the brain, changes in the nervous system (affecting the trigeminal nerve pathway), and imbalances in hormones and neurotransmitters (brain chemicals) such as serotonin, which plays a regulatory role for pain messages going through this pathway. During a migraine, serotonin levels drop. Researchers believe this causes the trigeminal nerve to release substances called neuropeptides, which travel to your brain's outer covering (meninges) and cause blood vessels to become dilated and inflamed. The result is headache pain.

There is also evidence that imbalances in the hormones estrogen and progesterone can cause migraines. Many women experience migraine attacks around their menses, when estrogen is dominant. Researchers have found that women with higher levels of progesterone had less severe menstrual headaches compared to those with lower progesterone levels. Hormone replacement therapy (use of synthetic estrogens) can also cause and worsen migraines for many women.

Melatonin is another hormone implicated in causing migraines. Melatonin is secreted from the pineal gland in the brain, and research has shown that the pineal gland in migraine sufferers is depressed, which leads to low levels of both serotonin and melatonin during migraine headaches.

There have been many advances in the treatment of migraines. There are drugs that can abort and help prevent headaches, and various natural products that can reduce the severity and frequency of headaches. Dietary and lifestyle changes, as discussed below, can also be very helpful.

SIGNS & SYMPTOMS

- Nausea or vomiting

- Sensitivity to light and sound

- Moderate to severe pain that can be throbbing or pulsating, usually on one side of the head

- Visual disturbances that precede or accompany the headache

A migraine typically lasts from 4 to 72 hours, but can go away faster with treatment. Some people experience an aura 15 to 30 minutes before the headache begins. An aura may cause you to see sparkling flashes of light, changes in vision (wavy lines and blind spots), tingling, a pins and needles sensation in one arm or leg, and, less commonly, weakness or difficulty in speaking. Several hours or a day before the headache, some people experience a prodrome—feelings of elation or intense energy, cravings for sweets, thirst, drowsiness, irritability, or depression.

RISK FACTORS

- Age: Most common between ages 20 and 55, although young children and adolescents can also be affected

- Family history: More than 50 percent of sufferers have a close relative who suffers from migraines.

- Gender: Women are three times more likely to be affected.

- Migraines occur more frequently in those with anxiety, depression, neurotic personality, or epilepsy. Recent research suggests a connection between cardiovascular disease (heart disease and stroke) and migraine headaches.

Migraines can be triggered by the following:

- Alcohol, particularly red wine and beer

- Bright lights or sun glare

- Change in weather (humidity) and changes in altitude

- Foods: Aged cheese; eggs; yeast; chocolate; aspartame; caffeine; fermented, pickled, or marinated foods; food additives and preservatives, such as monosodium glutamate, sulphites, benzoic acid, and tartrazine; and colouring agents

- Hormonal changes: In women, migraines often begin around the onset of menstruation; they may get better or worse with pregnancy or menopause; use of birth control pills can worsen migraine headaches.

- Lack of sleep

- Medications: Estrogen, progestins, blood pressure drugs, antihistamines, and decongestants

- Smells: Perfumes, flowers, smoke, and strong chemical odours such as gasoline or paint thinner

- Stress: Emotional (worrying) or physical (intense exercise)

DOCTOR'S ORDERS

There are a variety of drugs that can be used to treat and prevent migraines. The choice of treatment depends on the frequency and severity of your headaches and other existing medical problems.

For a mild migraine, a pain reliever such as Tylenol or Motrin may be helpful. For more severe pain, drugs containing codeine may be prescribed. Codeine and other narcotic pain relievers can be addictive and cause constipation and other problems, so they should be used only when absolutely necessary.

To manage nausea and vomiting associated with a migraine, dimenhydrinate (Gravol) is helpful. This is available in tablets and suppositories; the latter are a better delivery route when someone is vomiting.

The triptans are a class of drugs that has revolutionized migraine treatment. These drugs are rapid acting and effective in relieving pain, nausea, and sensitivity to light. Examples include sumatriptan (Imitrex), rizatriptan (Maxalt), naratriptan (Amerge), and zolmitriptan (Zomig). Usually a single dose of these drugs will provide relief.

There are drugs that can be taken regularly to prevent migraines (reduce the frequency). They don't work to relieve a migraine that does occur. Examples include beta-blockers (propranolol), calcium channel blockers (verapamil), and antidepressants (amitriptyline and nortriptyline). These drugs are only effective in about half of migraine sufferers and they can cause serious side effects, so speak to your doctor and pharmacist.

One of the latest drug approaches for migraine prevention and treatment is the use of botulinum toxin type A (Botox) injections. It is thought that Botox works by inhibiting release of transmitters from the pain-sensitive nerve endings. Several studies found that Botox is effective in reducing migraine severity and frequency.

HOMEOPATHIC RECOMMENDATIONS

Belladonna: Major throbbing or pounding head pain that starts at the back of the skull or upper neck and spreads to the forehead and temple (especially on the right) may indicate a need for this remedy. Pain is worse from jarring, light, and noise. For some reason, headaches that require Belladonna are worse around 3 p.m. Pupils may be dilated, with sensitivity to light, and the person may either feel delirious or drowsy.

Spigelia: Excruciating headaches usually present on the left side of the head, with violent throbbing, or stabbing pains above or through the eyeball. Pain extends through the face and is worse from any movement or touch. The person may feel better from lying on the right side with the head supported, and keeping very still.

Combination recommendation: Antimigren by Pascoe

SHERRY'S NATURAL PRESCRIPTION

Dietary Recommendations

Foods to include:

• Drink plenty of water (dehydration can cause a headache).

• Eat small, frequent meals; skipping meals can cause blood sugar levels to drop, which can trigger a migraine.

• Fish (salmon, mackerel, and herring) contain omega-3 fatty acids, which can help prevent migraines.

- Ginger tea may help reduce nausea that accompanies a migraine.

- Whole grains, nuts, seeds, and green leafy vegetables contain good sources of magnesium, which can help prevent migraines.

Foods to avoid:

- Food additives, preservatives (benzoic acid), and dyes (tartrazine) can trigger migraines.

- Phenylalanine, which is found in MSG, aspartame, and nitrates (hot dogs and deli meats), is a common trigger.

- Sodium can also be a trigger. Limit foods high in salt (snack foods, deli meats) and avoid using the salt shaker.

- Sugary foods (candy, sweets, and soft drinks) and high-glycemic carbohydrates (white bread/rice and refined grains) can cause rapid blood sugar changes, which may trigger a headache.

- Tyramine—which is found in cheese, chocolate, deli meats, smoked fish, wine, sausage, sour cream, fermented foods, and vinegar—is a common trigger.

Try an elimination diet to determine if food sensitivities are triggering your migraines (see Appendix D).

Lifestyle Suggestions

- Get adequate sleep (seven to nine hours per night).

- Reduce stress with yoga, breathing exercises, meditation, or massage. Biofeedback is also helpful for alleviating migraines. This relaxation technique uses special equipment to teach you how to monitor and control certain physical responses, such as muscle tension.

- Exercise regularly to help prevent migraines. Do moderate-intensity activities (walking, swimming, and cycling) and warm up slowly because sudden, intense activity can trigger a headache.

- Acupuncture can help relieve headache pain.

- During a migraine, go into a dark, quiet room and apply an ice pack wrapped in a towel to the back of your neck and head for 10 to 15 minutes.

• •

KEEP A DIARY

Keeping a diary of your migraines can help you identify your triggers. Make a note when your headaches start and how long they last. Record what you ate that day and any factors that you feel could have triggered the event, such as stress, reaction to a smell, or light. Also note what you took to relieve your headache. This information will also be helpful to your doctor in determining a treatment strategy.

• •

Top Recommended Supplements

Butterbur: Reduces inflammation and spasms in cerebral blood vessels. Studies have found that it significantly reduces the frequency of migraine attacks. Dosage: 50–75 mg twice daily with meals as a preventive. Look for a product standardized to contain at least 15 percent petasins, the main active ingredient.

Feverfew: Several studies have shown that it can reduce the pain, severity, and frequency of migraines, and it may also reduce the nausea, vomiting, and light/sound sensitivity. It is believed to work by modulating serotonin release and reducing production of inflammatory substances in the brain. Dosage: Take a product that provides 0.25–0.5 mg parthenolide twice daily for prevention. Recent research on a combination of feverfew and ginger (LipiGesic M) found that it was effective in halting a migraine and preventing it from becoming severe when taken at the first onset of symptoms. This product is available as a gel and is taken under the tongue (sublingually).

Magnesium: Those with migraines often have low magnesium levels during an acute attack, which can lead to brain hyperexcitability and cerebral artery spasm and increase the release of substances that cause pain. Three studies have found that magnesium supplements can significantly reduce the frequency of migraine attacks. It may be particularly helpful in preventing menstrual migraines. Dosage: 100–200 mg three times daily with meals.

Complementary Supplements

Coenzyme Q10: Several small studies have found that it can reduce the frequency and number of days with migraine headache. Dosage: 100–300 mg daily.

Fish oils: Reduce inflammation and blood vessel spasms and support healthy brain function. Preliminary research shows that supplements can reduce frequency and severity of migraines. Dosage: 1 g three times daily of EPA and DHA.

5-HTP: Increases serotonin levels and has been shown to reduce the frequency and severity of migraines. Dosage: 200–300 mg twice daily.

Melatonin: Several studies have demonstrated that melatonin effectively relieves migraine pain, decreases frequency of migraines, reduces intensity of migraines, and shortens migraine duration. Dosage: 3–5 mg one hour before bed.

Vitamin B2 (riboflavin): Shown to reduce the frequency, duration, and severity of migraine headaches. Dosage: 400 mg daily; take along with a B-complex vitamin.

FINAL THOUGHTS

To manage migraines and help prevent them, consider the following:

- Eat small, frequent meals and include more whole grains, nuts, seeds, and fish in your diet. Drink lots of fluids. Try ginger tea to relieve nausea.
- Get adequate sleep, exercise regularly, and reduce your stress.
- Keep a diary of your migraines to identify and avoid your triggers.
- When suffering with a migraine, use cold packs on the head and neck, rest in a dark room, and use medications only if necessary.
- Try butterbur, feverfew, and magnesium for prevention or LipiGesic M to halt an attack.

MULTIPLE SCLEROSIS (MS)

Multiple sclerosis (MS) is a chronic, often disabling disease that affects your central nervous system (the brain and spinal cord). It is generally believed that MS is an autoimmune disease; the body mistakenly directs antibodies and white blood cells against proteins in the myelin sheath, a fatty substance that insulates nerve fibres in your brain and spinal cord. This results in inflammation and injury to the sheath and ultimately to the nerves that it surrounds, resulting in multiple areas of scarring (sclerosis). Over time this damage can slow or block the nerve signals that control muscle coordination, strength, sensation, and vision, causing fatigue, numbness, loss of balance, impaired vision, and disability.

The actual cause for this autoimmune reaction is not known. It is thought that several factors may be involved, such as genetic predisposition, environment, and exposure to a viral infection. Many researchers believe that MS is related to a protein that mimics the myelin protein, which may be introduced into the body by a virus. Other researchers believe that the immune system overreacts toward myelin proteins in people with MS, which leads to an abnormal tendency to develop autoimmune disease. It is known that lifestyle factors, such as stress, poor nutrition, and hormonal changes, can exacerbate symptoms. Exposure to environmental toxins (pesticides, heavy metals, and chemicals) can bring on symptoms and cause damage to myelin and DNA. Food allergies can worsen symptoms in some people.

MS occurs in four main patterns:

Primary progressive: People with this form experience a gradual decline in function without periods of remission. This form is not as common, and it often strikes after the age of 40.

Progressive relapsing: This is primary progressive MS with the addition of sudden episodes of new symptoms or worsened existing ones. This form is rare.

Relapsing remitting: About 70 percent of people with MS have this form, which is characterized by periods of sudden flare-ups followed by periods of near-normal health (remission) that can last for months or years.

Secondary progressive: More than half the people with relapsing remitting MS eventually enter a stage of continuous deterioration referred to as secondary progressive MS.

Canada has one of the highest rates of MS in the world, and MS is the most common neurological disease affecting young adults in Canada. Every day, three more people in Canada are diagnosed with MS. An estimated 55,000 to 75,000 Canadians have the disease. MS can affect anyone, at any age, although it is most commonly diagnosed between the ages of 15 and 40.

Great progress has been made over the years in our understanding of MS. Today, people with MS can live healthy, productive lives. There are medications, dietary approaches, and supplements that can help reduce symptoms and promote remission.

SIGNS & SYMPTOMS

Signs and symptoms of MS vary widely, depending on the location of affected nerve fibres, and may include the following:

• Bladder or bowel incontinence

• Blurred vision, visual loss, and eye pain

• Constipation

• Dizziness

• Electric-shock sensations that occur with certain head movements

• Extreme fatigue

• Forgetfulness, lack of concentration

• Loss of balance and coordination

• Muscle stiffness or spasticity

• Numbness or weakness in one or more limbs

• Paralysis

• Slurred speech

• Tingling or pain

• Tremors

RISK FACTORS

• Dietary factors: Deficiency of vitamin D, a diet high in saturated (animal) fat, food allergies, and digestive problems

• Environmental toxins: Exposure to organic solvents, heavy metals (mercury), pesticides, and X-rays

• Ethnicity: MS is more common in Caucasian people of northern European origin, especially those of Scottish descent; it is extremely rare among Asians, Africans, and Native Americans.

• Exposure to a virus, in particular human herpesvirus type 6, *varicella zoster*, and retroviruses

• Gender: Women are three times as likely as men to get MS.

• Genetics: Represent a small risk; if one of your parents has MS, the risk of you developing it over a lifetime is less than 5 percent; researchers suspect that the tendency to develop MS is inherited, but the disease manifests only when environmental triggers are present.

• Geographical location: Rates of MS are about 10 times greater in higher latitudes and lowest among those who live close to the equator; it is most common in Europe, Canada, the northern United States, and southeastern Australia; researchers suspect a connection between low levels of sunshine and vitamin D deficiency, which is common in MS.

- Having other autoimmune diseases, such as thyroid disease, type 1 diabetes, or inflammatory bowel disease, is associated with an increased risk of developing MS.

- Smoking: Smokers are nearly twice as likely to develop multiple sclerosis as people who have never smoked.

••

COW'S MILK AND MULTIPLE SCLEROSIS

There is evidence that infants fed only cow's milk during infancy may have a higher risk of MS later in life. Studies have also shown that populations that drink cow's milk have a greater prevalence of MS. Whole milk contains a high amount of saturated fat, which has been shown to worsen or trigger MS symptoms. However, researchers believe that the problem with milk extends beyond the fat. Certain proteins in milk mimic a particular protein affiliated with human myelin. These milk proteins can elicit an autoimmune response to myelin, triggering an MS episode. This has been demonstrated in animal studies. Overall the evidence is not conclusive, but it does appear there is a link that requires further study.

••

DOCTOR'S ORDERS

The main classes of drugs used to treat MS are drugs that treat an attack and symptoms, and drugs that can slow the progression.

Steroids, such as prednisone, are used to reduce inflammation and decrease the severity and duration of MS relapses. Side effects include increased blood pressure and weight gain, and long-term use can lead to cataracts, high blood sugar, and increased risk of infections.

If you have a relapsing form of the disease, depending on the severity and frequency of your attacks, your doctor may recommend a disease-modifying medication. These drugs are also called immunomodulatory therapies and they work by targeting some aspect of the inflammatory process of MS, with an aim of preventing inflammation, which causes relapses. These drugs also help slow progression of the disease. They cannot be taken if you are pregnant or may become pregnant. Examples include the following:

- **Beta interferons:** Interferon beta-lb (Betaseron) and interferon beta-1a (Avonex, Rebif) are genetically engineered copies of proteins that occur naturally in your body. They are taken by injection and help fight viral infection and regulate your immune system. These drugs reduce but don't eliminate flare-ups, they don't reverse damage, and they haven't been proven to significantly alter long-term development of permanent disability. Some people develop antibodies to beta interferons, which may make them less effective. Other people can't tolerate the side effects (flu-like symptoms).

- **Glatiramer (Copaxone):** This drug is an alternative to beta interferons for those with relapsing remitting MS. Glatiramer is thought to work by blocking your immune system's attack on myelin. It is injected once daily. Side effects may include flushing, shortness of breath after injection, bacterial infection, lymphadenopathy, edema, weight gain, and nausea.

Muscle relaxants, pain medications, antidepressants, and drugs to help with bladder and bowel control may be also be prescribed.

SHERRY'S NATURAL PRESCRIPTION

As with many chronic diseases, diet and lifestyle changes, dietary supplementation, and moderate physical exercise all contribute to better quality of life with MS.

Dietary Recommendations

Foods to include:

- Drink plenty of water.

- Drinking pure (unsweetened) cranberry juice can help protect against urinary tract infections.

- Eat fresh, whole, unprocessed foods; choose organic as much as possible to avoid ingestion of pesticides and harmful chemicals.

- Eat lots of fruits, vegetables, and whole grains. These foods are rich in nutrients that can help offset deficiencies and are also high in fibre, which helps to prevent constipation.

- Ensure adequate protein intake. Weight loss is a common concern for many people with MS. Protein is essential to support healthy muscles. Choose beans, legumes, nuts, seeds, fish, and lean poultry.

- Eat more foods that contain beneficial polyunsaturated fatty acids, namely omega-3 and omega-6 fatty acids, which support proper nerve function and also reduce inflammation. Choose wild (not farmed) cold-water fish such as salmon, cod, herring, and mackerel. Chia seed and flaxseed also provide some omega-3 fatty acids. Sunflower and safflower oil contain linoleic acid, an omega-6 fatty acid. There is some evidence that these beneficial fats can lessen the severity of MS attacks (see box below).

- Yogurt contains beneficial bacteria that aid digestion and improve intestinal flora.

. . . .

SATURATED FAT AND MS: THE SWANK DIET

There is some evidence that changing the type and amount of fat in the diet might alter the course of MS. A survey of people in 36 countries found that people with MS who ate foods high in polyunsaturated and monounsaturated fatty acids were likely to live longer than those who ate more saturated fats. (*American Journal of Epidemiology*, 1995, 142: 733–737)

In another survey, researchers gathered information from nearly 400 people over three years. They found that people who ate more fish were less likely to develop MS, while those who ate pork, hot dogs, and other foods high in saturated (animal) fats were at greater risk. Saturated fats trigger inflammation and alter immune function while polyunsaturated fats (essential fatty acids) reduce inflammation. (*International Journal of Epidemiology*, 1998, 5: 845–852)

Based on observations from population studies linking diets lower in saturated fat to lower rates of MS, Dr. R.L. Swank, a professor of neurology at University of Oregon Medical School, developed a special low-fat diet and tested it in 150 MS patients. This program, now called the Swank diet, involved significantly reducing hydrogenated oils, peanut butter, and animal fat (meat and dairy). Cod liver oil (5 g per day) and linoleic acid (an essential fatty acid) from vegetable oil was allowed. After 34 years, the mortality rate among people consuming an average of 17 g of saturated fat per day was only 31 percent, compared with 79 percent among those who consumed a higher average of 25 g of saturated fat per day. People who began to follow the low-fat diet early in the disease did better than those who changed their eating habits after the disease had progressed. (*Nutrition*, 1991, 7: 368–376)

Foods to avoid:

• Consider an elimination diet to detect and avoid potential allergens. See Appendix D.

• Gluten may trigger or worsen MS symptoms in those with sensitivity. Antibodies to gluten are more common in those with MS, and MS is more prevalent in geographical areas where consumption of gluten is high. Foods containing gluten include wheat, rye, barley, and products made with these grains such as most breads, pastas, and baked goods. Refer to the section on celiac disease for more information on a gluten-free diet.

• Saturated fats trigger inflammation and can worsen the disease progression. Trans fats are also detrimental to health. Minimize meat, full-fat dairy, and deep-fried and processed foods.

• Sugar can hamper immune function, increasing the susceptibility to infection. Limit sweets, candy, and soft drinks.

Lifestyle Suggestions

• Manage your stress levels. Stress can trigger a flare-up. Try yoga, tai chi, meditation, or breathing exercises. Massage and acupuncture can help promote relaxation and may help reduce pain and muscle stiffness and improve sleep quality.

• Get adequate rest to allow your body to recuperate and to improve your ability to handle stress.

• Don't smoke, as smoking contributes to the progression of the disease. It is thought that nitrous oxide, a chemical present in cigarette smoke, may hasten degeneration of nerve fibres. Chemicals in cigarette smoke could also damage the cells that create myelin, a protective coating for neurons, or may predispose smokers to autoimmune responses.

• Get regular exercise, which can help improve strength, flexibility, balance, and coordination. It also helps to relieve stress. Swimming is a good activity for those with MS who are sensitive to heat. Regular exercise can reduce the risk of certain complications, such as bladder and bowel dysfunction, osteoporosis, permanent muscle contractions, ulcerations of the skin, or abnormal blood clotting.

- Physical and occupational therapy can help with mobility, self-care, and improving overall activity and quality of life.

- Avoid extreme heat, which can cause muscle weakness and worsen symptoms in some people with MS.

- Avoid exposure to pesticides, heavy metals (mercury, lead), and other chemicals.

- There is some evidence that treatments involving transcutaneous nerve stimulation (TENS) can decrease pain and muscle spasticity and lessen depression.

- Magnet therapy has shown promise for treating MS. Preliminary research has found that treatments with pulsed electromagnetic field therapy improved hand function, muscle spasticity, and bladder function.

- Consider having mercury dental amalgams removed and replaced with mercury-free material. Several reports have linked mercury-containing amalgams to an increased risk of MS and worsening of symptoms in those with the disease.

- Consider hyperbaric oxygen therapy, which involves exposure to oxygen at higher pressures in multiple sessions. Some reports have shown that treatments weekly or every other week over a period of several years can reduce disease progression.

Top Recommended Supplements

Fish oils: Research has found that those with MS have lower levels of omega-3 fatty acids. These beneficial fats can help reduce inflammation and support healthy nerve function. Research suggests benefits for reducing urinary incontinence, improving eyesight, and reducing risk of relapse. Studies have found benefits from using a dosage of 6–20 g daily. Consult with your health care provider for guidance.

GLA: An essential fatty acid available in primrose, borage, and black currant oil. It helps reduce inflammation, and preliminary studies have shown that it can reduce symptoms and improve peripheral blood flow and hand-grip strength. Dosage: 500 mg three times daily.

Vitamin B12: Essential for supporting myelin formation; deficiency is common in people with MS, and a lack of B12 can cause neurological problems. B12 has been used for decades for MS to alleviate symptoms and boost energy levels. Dosage: 1 mL by injection (from your health care provider) monthly. Sublingual B12 tablets are an alternative. Dosage: 5–40 mg of B12 daily in the form of sublingual methylcobalamin.

Vitamin D: Has immune-modulating activity. Most people with MS are deficient in vitamin D, and studies have shown that low levels of vitamin D increase the risk of MS. As well, research suggests that vitamin D may help those who already have MS by reducing inflammation and relapses. Dosage: Typical dosages used for MS are 5,000–10,000 IU daily, as advised by your health care provider. Studies have used dosages of 28,000 IU and more.

··

AVOID IMMUNE BOOSTERS WITH MS

Immune-boosting herbs can worsen MS as they enhance auto-antibody production responsible for demyelinating nerve fibres. Avoid taking echinacea, Asian ginseng, licorice, and other immune-boosting herbs.

··

Complementary Supplements

Antioxidants: People with MS tend to have lower levels of key antioxidants that are necessary to reduce oxidative stress. Free radicals may contribute to the tissue damage and progression of MS. Supplemental antioxidants support cellular antioxidant defences by scavenging free radicals. Look for a formula that contains vitamins C and E, coenzyme Q10, lipoic acid, beta carotene, and selenium. Dosage: Take daily.

Digestive enzymes: Many people with MS have poor digestion and inadequate digestive enzyme secretion. Supplements can help improve digestion and gut function. Dosage: Take a broad spectrum enzyme before each meal.

L-carnitine: An amino acid that is important for heart health and energy production. Some drugs that are used to treat MS appear to deplete carnitine. In one trial, supplementing with L-carnitine significantly improved fatigue in 63 percent of drug-treated MS patients. Dosage: 3–6 g daily.

Phosphatidylcholine: Necessary for optimal brain and nerve function. It helps protect the myelin sheath and also increases acetylcholine, which is important for muscle function. Dosage: 500 mg twice daily.

Probiotics: Beneficial bacteria that promote healthy GI flora. Some people with MS have reduced levels of beneficial bacteria and *Candida* overgrowth. Dosage: Take one to three capsules daily with meals.

Threonine: A naturally occurring amino acid that might help reduce the muscle spasticity that often occurs with MS. Two studies have demonstrated positive effects. Dosage: 6 g daily.

FINAL THOUGHTS

To improve the management of MS, consider the following:

- Eat a healthy diet with fruits, vegetables, whole grains, fish, and yogurt.
- Avoid or minimize saturated fat, trans fats, and sugar.
- Reduce stress, get adequate sleep, and exercise regularly.
- Don't smoke, and avoid extreme heat exposure.
- Consider supplements of fish oils, GLA, vitamin B12, and vitamin D.

OBESITY

Obesity has become one of the greatest health threats facing Canadians, as it is linked to many serious diseases that result in premature death. Over two-thirds of adults are overweight and nearly one-quarter are obese. This health crisis is having a significant impact on youth, with just over one-quarter of all children and adolescents being overweight or obese, resulting in dangerous diseases and a predicted shortened life expectancy.

Many factors contribute to obesity, most notably poor diet (excess calorie intake and consuming unhealthy foods) and lack of physical activity. However, other factors can contribute to weight gain and obesity including excess carbohydrate consumption, stress, hormonal disorders, and side effects of medications.

Carrying extra weight can impact a person's physical and emotional well-being. Obesity is associated with numerous consequences and health risks, including type 2 diabetes, heart disease, certain cancers, gallbladder disease, sleep apnea, osteoarthritis, depression, and more.

Numerous studies have found that those who maintain a lean body live longer, suffer less disease, and enjoy a better quality of life. If you are overweight or obese, it is important to know that even small losses can improve your health. Studies have shown that losing 10 to 15 percent of excess weight can reduce blood pressure, blood sugar, cholesterol, and triglycerides. The key to successful weight loss is a lifestyle program that includes proper eating and regular exercise. Nutritional supplements can help complement your lifestyle approaches.

SIGNS & SYMPTOMS

- Fatigue and lethargy

- Shortness of breath

- Increased body fat

There are several methods used to determine whether a person is overweight or obese, including the body mass index (BMI) and body fat percentage. BMI is the most commonly used method; it compares your height and weight to a standard. To calculate your BMI, take your weight in kilograms and divide that by your height in metres squared (kg/m^2).

A BMI between 18.9 and 24.9 is considered normal, a BMI between 25 and 29.9 is classified as overweight, and a BMI greater than 30 indicates obesity. Studies have shown that the greater the BMI, the greater the risk of developing health problems, such as heart disease and diabetes. A drawback of this method is that it does not look at body composition (amount of fat), which is an important determinant of disease risk.

Body fat percentage can also be checked by various methods (as described in Appendix A). Men with greater than 25 percent and women with more than 30 percent body fat are considered obese and at significant risk of developing health problems. Recommended ranges of body fat are 15 to 25 percent for women and 10 to 20 percent for

Note: Those carrying excess weight are at increased risk of inflammatory disorders and developing heart disease, cancer, diabetes, and the complications that come with these diseases. Excess weight also increases one's risk of breathing disorders, gall bladder disease, sexual dysfunction, osteoarthritis, and stroke. The emotional consequences— low self-esteem, depression, and anxiety—can be just as serious.

APPLES VS. PEARS: WHERE'S YOUR FAT?

An "apple"-shaped body (pot belly) is associated with more health risks compared to a "pear"-shaped body (larger hips and thighs). These risks include: type 2 diabetes, high cortisol, high cholesterol and blood pressure, coronary heart disease, stroke, and early death. Men with a waist circumference greater than 40 inches (102 cm) and women with greater than 35 inches (89 cm) have a substantially increased risk of developing these diseases. Abdominal obesity is influenced by a number of factors, including low sex hormone levels (especially testosterone in men), genetics, and lifestyle choices. Stress and eating a high-glycemic diet (refined carbohydrates) promote belly fat storage. Increased physical activity, not smoking, following a low-glycemic diet, and using unsaturated fat over saturated fat have been shown to reduce abdominal obesity.

RISK FACTORS

- Excess calorie intake; poor dietary choices

- Genetics

- Hormonal imbalances (high insulin; low thyroid, testosterone, DHEA, or growth hormone)

- Lack of physical activity

- Lack of sleep (increases appetite and promotes food cravings)

- Low metabolic rate (rate at which calories are burned at rest; this is often secondary to a hormonal imbalance)

- Medications (antidepressants, antiseizure medications, steroids [prednisone], hormones, diabetic medications)

- Stress (causes hormonal alterations that increase appetite, reduce metabolism, and stimulate abdominal fat accumulation)

DOCTOR'S ORDERS

Lifestyle changes should be the first approach to a weight-loss program. In cases where this isn't enough, your doctor may prescribe a drug to help promote weight loss. The only drug approved in Canada to support weight loss is orlistat (Xenical). This drug works as a fat blocker, reducing absorption of fat from meals. This product may cause loose stools, fecal incontinence, abdominal cramps, and nausea.

If a hormonal disorder (such as low thyroid) is suspected, you may be referred to an endocrinologist.

For individuals who are extremely obese and at risk of serious health consequences, and where lifestyle changes or drugs have not helped, a surgical procedure may be done to reduce the size of the stomach. Surgery is associated with various health risks, thus it is reserved for severe cases that have not responded to lifestyle changes.

SHERRY'S NATURAL PRESCRIPTION

Dietary Recommendations

Avoid fad diets. There is no good evidence supporting safety and efficacy, and some can be dangerous. For example, the once popular low-carb diets lead to nutrient deficiencies, constipation, depression, and bad breath.

A detoxification program, such as a juice cleanse, can eliminate stored toxins and help the body recover from addictions, such as sugar. This should be done only for a few days and under the supervision of a health professional because drastically reducing calorie intake can lead to nutrient deficiencies, muscle wasting, fatigue, and a reduced metabolism. Refer to Appendix C for more information.

Foods to include:

- Quality proteins, such as lean meat, poultry, fish, beans, soy products, nuts, and seeds, are essential for building and maintaining muscle mass, which drives our metabolism. Adequate protein is also important for helping to control appetite. The recommended amount of protein is based on body weight and activity level. For the average person, a daily intake of 0.8 g to 1 g per kilogram, or 0.5 g per pound of body weight is adequate. Bodybuilders and those involved in intense exercise require more protein. Consider a protein supplement to complement your diet.

- Nutrient-dense, low-glycemic carbohydrates such as fresh fruits, vegetables, legumes (beans, peas, and lentils) and whole grains (multigrain breads, brown rice/pasta, quinoa, oats, chia seed, and flaxseed) are high in fibre, which fills us up and aids digestion and elimination. Fibre also balances blood sugar and insulin levels, which is important in regulating appetite and energy levels. Aim for 8 to 10 servings of fruits, vegetables, and legumes. Refer to Appendix B for more information on the glycemic index.

- Healthy fats such as those found in cold-water fish, olive oil, nuts, and seeds provide us with essential fatty acids (healthy fats), which are essential for health and disease prevention. Other fats found in tropical oils like palm fruit and coconut have been shown to help support a healthy metabolism.

- Chili peppers contain compounds called capsinoids and capsaicinoids that can increase energy expenditures (amount of calorie burned). Several studies have found that regular consumption can reduce appetite and body fat levels.

- Green tea contains antioxidants that help boost metabolism, reduce inflammation, and reduce blood pressure and cholesterol levels.

Foods to avoid:

- Processed and fast foods, candy, cookies, and sweets are high in sugar and fat calories and low in nutritional value.

- Limit refined grains (white bread/pasta/rice) as these foods are broken down quickly into sugar, causing fluctuations in blood sugar and insulin levels, which can increase appetite and promote fat storage.

- Minimize saturated (from meat and full-fat dairy) and hydrogenated fats, which are high in calories, promote weight gain, and are linked to heart disease and cancer.

- Reduce alcohol intake as these drinks are high in empty calories.

- Cut down on salt as using the salt shaker and eating salty snack foods and processed foods can cause fluid retention.

Lifestyle Suggestions

- Eat five times daily: three small meals and two snacks between meals. This will help keep metabolism and energy levels high. Do not skip meals as this can increase appetite, reduce metabolism, and lead to binge eating.

- To facilitate weight loss of one pound per week (a safe and manageable goal), reduce caloric intake by 500 calories per day.

- Boost your activity level: Regular physical activity is essential to achieving a healthy body weight. Aim for one hour of moderate-intensity activity daily. Do a combination of the following:

  - Cardiovascular activities such as walking, cycling, and swimming, which promote fat loss by burning calories and stored fat.

  - Resistance activities (working out with weights, exercise bands/tubes, or machines) help to build lean muscle mass, which will elevate your metabolic rate so that you burn more calories.

  - Stretching promotes flexibility and relaxation, and reduces injuries. Spend at least five minutes stretching your muscles after a workout.

- Reduce stress, which can trigger appetite and food cravings and increases the production of cortisol, a hormone that promotes fat storage around the abdomen.

- Get adequate sleep as lack of sleep increases production of the hormone ghrelin, which stimulates appetite and can also reduce production of growth hormone, an important regulator of our metabolism.

- Consider counselling or support groups: If you find that your eating habits are tied to your emotions, you may benefit from counselling or a support group.

Top Recommended Supplements

Conjugated linoleic acid (CLA): A fatty acid that stimulates the breakdown of stored fat, reduces the number of existing fat cells, and prevents fat storage. Dosage: 3–4 g daily; may cause oily skin and loose stool, but no serious side effects.

Fibre supplements: Soluble fibre helps reduce appetite and cravings, improve blood sugar balance, and promote weight loss. Those that have been studied and found beneficial include glucomannan (PGX), guar, psyllium, and pectin. Recent research conducted on an alginate supplement derived from brown seaweed extract, which contains a significant amount of fibre, has found that it can enhance satiety (increase fullness), slow stomach emptying, and reduce overall calorie intake. Follow label directions and take with lots of water.

Green coffee bean extract: Inhibits an enzyme (glucose-6-phosphatase), which is responsible for the release of glucose stored in the liver. This causes glucose to be taken from deposits in fat tissue instead and helps stimulate weight loss. Several small trials have shown benefits. Dosage: 700–1,050 mg of a product standardized to 30 to 50 percent chlorogenic acid.

Phase 2: A white kidney bean extract that promotes weight loss by neutralizing starch from the diet. Foods high in starch include bread, pasta, potatoes, and rice. Phase 2 inhibits the enzyme alpha-amylase, which breaks down starches into sugar. Studies show that it reduces the amount of sugar absorbed from starchy meals, lowers after-meal blood sugar levels, and promotes fat loss. Dosage: 1,000–1,500 mg before starchy meals; no known side effects.

Complementary Supplements

Xanthigen: a proprietary blend of fucoxanthin (a carotenoid found naturally in edible brown seaweed) and pomegranate oil that has been shown to increase fat-burning and promote weight loss. One particular product called fücoTHIN has been shown in preliminary research to increase metabolism and reduce body fat and waist circumference. Dosage: 200 mg three times daily.

Green tea: Promotes weight loss by increasing thermogenesis (the rate of calorie burning) due to an interaction between antioxidants (EGCG) and caffeine. There are no serious side effects; however, high amounts of caffeine may cause restlessness, insomnia, and increased heart rate in some individuals. Supplements vary in potency, so check labels for dosage.

Hydroxycitric acid (HCA): A compound derived from the fruit *Garcinia cambogia*, which supports weight loss by reducing appetite, enhancing the breakdown of fat, and inhibiting fat storage. Dosage: 2,800 mg per day; no known side effects.

Raspberry ketones: Compounds present in raspberries that are responsible for the berry's characteristic aroma. Preliminary research suggests that raspberry ketones can promote fat weight loss. It is thought to do this by increasing levels of adiponectin, a protein used by the body to regulate metabolism, and by increasing lipolysis (fat breakdown). Dosage: 100 mg once or twice daily with meals.

FINAL THOUGHTS

If you have decided to lose weight, set reasonable goals, make small, gradual changes to your lifestyle, and be patient as it takes time to lose weight, but the rewards are worthwhile. Here are the key points to keep in mind:

- Know your risk—check your BMI and body fat percentage.
- Develop a regular exercise program, including cardiovascular, resistance activities, and stretching.
- Eat small, frequent meals with quality proteins, high-fibre carbohydrates, and good fats.
- Get adequate sleep and reduce stress.
- Consider supportive supplements: CLA, green coffee bean extract, Phase 2, and soluble fibre.

OSTEOARTHRITIS

Osteoarthritis (OA), also known as degenerative joint disease, is the most common form of arthritis, affecting 3 million (1 in 10) Canadians.

The disease is caused by wear and tear on the joints and deterioration of joint cartilage, which is a gel-like material that covers and protects the ends of bones. OA can affect any moving joint but it most commonly impacts the weight-bearing joints, namely the knees, lumbar spine, and hips.

As the cartilage breaks down, we lose the cushion that it provides between our bones. As a result, the bones start to rub against each other, causing a grinding or clicking of the joints. The condition may go unnoticed for a long time. Cartilage doesn't contain free nerve endings so there may not be pain until it is considerably advanced.

As the condition progresses, bone damage, inflammation, and pain may occur. Oxidative stress is recognized as a factor in contributing to cartilage destruction and inflammation. As the disease progresses, the pain can become severe and affect one's mobility and quality of life.

SIGNS & SYMPTOMS

The disease can affect any joint, but it is most common in weight-bearing joints such as the knees, hips, ankles, fingers, neck, and spine, and it causes the following:

- Grinding or clicking in the joints

- Growths (spurs)

- Joint stiffness and pain in the morning or after exercise

- Pain

- Red, warm, swollen joints

- Reduced mobility

In some people, the symptoms remain mild or even go away at times. In others the condition progresses as the joint deteriorates and inflammation sets in. Cold weather and humidity can worsen the symptoms.

RISK FACTORS

- Age: It is more common in those over the age of 45, but can occur at any age.

- Family history: Inheriting abnormal joint or cartilage structure

- Obesity: Excess weight puts stress on joints, especially hips and knees. Fat tissue also releases inflammatory compounds, which worsen the problem.

- Injury: Joint damage due to an accident, sports, or occupation (i.e., carpet laying)

- Having another form of arthritis, such as rheumatoid

DOCTOR'S ORDERS

There are various drugs that doctors use to manage the symptoms of OA. The first-line approach is typically the use of analgesics, such as acetaminophen (Tylenol), which can help reduce pain (but not the inflammation). Use of high doses over a long time can cause liver damage and liver failure. Codeine is a narcotic used for severe pain. Side effects include drowsiness, constipation, and addiction.

Non-steroidal anti-inflammatory drugs (NSAIDs), such as ibuprofen (Advil/Motrin), naproxen (Aleve), indomethacin (Indocid), and celecoxib (Celebrex), help reduce pain and inflammation. While they are effective, they do not prevent joint damage, and there is evidence that they can actually accelerate cartilage breakdown. There are numerous serious side effects, including stomach ulcers and bleeding, diarrhea, stomach pain, kidney and liver problems, and worsening of heart failure.

Corticosteroids, such as cortisone, are injected into the joint to relieve severe inflammation. Prednisone is taken orally. These drugs are used only for severe cases and for the short term because they can damage cartilage and remove minerals from the bone, further weakening the joint.

Visco supplementation involves a clear gel-like substance that is injected into the joint to lubricate the cartilage, which helps to reduce pain and improve mobility.

Arthroscopic procedures to remove loose bone fragments or a joint replacement (with a plastic, ceramic, or metal joint) may be done for severe cases.

HOMEOPATHIC RECOMMENDATIONS

Aconitum napellus: This remedy may be helpful for pain and inflammation that comes on suddenly after exposure to cold wind and weather. If the individual also reports feeling fearful, panicked, or agitated, this remedy may be of further benefit.

Belladonna: Sudden flare-ups of arthritis with a sensation of heat and throbbing pain indicate a need for this remedy.

Ledum palustre: Indicated for pain and inflammation that often begins in the toes and spreads up through the ankles and knees. The joints may make cracking sounds and may be very swollen.

SHERRY'S NATURAL PRESCRIPTION

Dietary Recommendations

Foods to include:

- Asparagus, cabbage, garlic, and onions contain sulphur, which is beneficial for the joints.

- Cold-water fish, olive oil, chia seed, flaxseed, and hemp are rich in essential fatty acids and can help reduce inflammation.

- Ginger contains anti-inflammatory and antioxidant compounds. Fresh ginger root contains more beneficial compounds compared to dried ginger powder.

- Green tea: Several studies have found that the antioxidants in green tea (catechins) can reduce chronic joint inflammation and slow cartilage breakdown.

- Pineapple contains the enzyme bromelain, which can help reduce inflammation.

Foods to avoid:

- Nightshade vegetables (potatoes, tomatoes, peppers, eggplant) contain a substance called solanine, which can trigger pain and inflammation; preliminary studies have found benefits in avoiding these foods.

- Processed, fast, and deep-fried foods contain trans fatty acids, which trigger inflammation.

- Red meat, full-fat dairy, and deep-fried foods contain saturated fat, which triggers inflammation.

- Sugar, refined carbohydrates, and alcohol can worsen inflammation.

Lifestyle Suggestions

- Acupuncture offers short-term benefits for pain relief.

- Apply ice or heat packs to the affected joints. Heat relaxes aching muscles and reduces joint pain. Cold helps to reduce inflammation and pain.

- Assistive devices, such as canes, walkers, and joint supports, reduce joint strain.

- Avoid activities that put excess strain on the joints (running, jumping, kneeling, or standing for long periods). Take a load off and rest when doing heavy or repeated tasks such as gardening, shovelling snow, or doing housework.

- Exercise helps reduce pain and prevent further joint damage; strengthens muscles and bones, which will help improve mobility and function; and also helps with weight management. Do a combination of light strength-training exercises for the muscles, low-impact cardiovascular activities to improve blood flow and circulation, and stretching to maintain flexibility and range of motion.

- Light massage with botanical oils (camphor, eucalyptus, pine needle, or rosemary) can help reduce pain and promote relaxation. Topical creams with capsaicin, a hot pepper extract, can reduce pain.

Top Recommended Supplements

Boswellia: A tree resin used in traditional Indian medicine; studies show that it reduces pain and inflammation and improves joint function. Dosage: 100–200 mg daily. Look for products that contain Aflapin, a researched form of Boswellia.

Chondroitin: A component of human cartilage, bone, and tendon. It enhances the shock-absorbing properties of collagen, stimulates cartilage repair, and blocks enzymes that break down cartilage. Studies have shown that it reduces pain and inflammation, improves joint function, and reduces the need for NSAIDs. It may also slow the progression of OA. Chondroitin is often combined with glucosamine. It may take several months to work. Dosage: 1,200 mg daily.

Glucosamine: A major component of joint cartilage that provides building blocks for growth, repair, and maintenance of cartilage. Supplements stimulate cartilage cells to make proteoglycans and collagen, which are essential for joint health. Glucosamine also helps cartilage absorb water to keep joints lubricated, and it has anti-inflammatory properties. Regular use may reduce symptoms and slow the progression of OA. Numerous studies have found glucosamine comparable to NSAIDs, yet better tolerated. It may take six to eight weeks to notice benefits. Avoid if allergic to shellfish. Supplements are available as a glucosamine hydrochloride or glucosamine sulphate; studies have found the sulphate form superior for improving osteoarthritis. Dosage: 1,500 mg daily.

S-adenosylmethionine (SAMe): A nutrient involved in cartilage formation and repair. It reduces pain and inflammation and stimulates cartilage formation. Numerous studies have found it equally effective as NSAIDs with no major side effects, but it may take four weeks to notice benefits. Dosage: 400–1,200 mg daily.

Complementary Supplements

BioCell Collagen: A patented formula that provides collagen, chondroitin, and hyaluronic acid. Research suggests it can strengthen cartilage and joint structure, lubricate joints, and promote healthy connective tissue. Dosage: 2,000 mg twice daily.

Bromelain: An enzyme with anti-inflammatory activity that improves joint mobility. It is well tolerated; however, it may thin the blood, so use cautiously along with blood-thinning medications. Dosage: 90 mg three times daily or 2,000–6,000 MCU daily.

Celadrin: A blend of fatty acids that reduces inflammation and pain, lubricates joints, and promotes healing. Three small studies have shown benefits for reducing joint pain and inflammation and improving mobility. Celadrin is available in capsules and cream. Dosage: 1,500 mg daily; apply cream twice daily.

Curcumin: An antioxidant that has been shown in studies to have anti-inflammatory effects comparable to cortisone. Dosage: 400 mg three times daily.

Essential fatty acids: Both the omega-3s (fish oil) and omega-6s (borage, primrose oil) help to reduce pain and inflammation and lubricate the joints. Dosage: 2–4 g daily.

Natural Eggshell Membrane (NEM): A proprietary product made from eggshell membrane that contains compounds naturally occurring in the joint such as chondroitin and hyaluronic acid, along with collagen and other beneficial proteins that are important for joint health. Studies show supplements can reduce pain and stiffness and improve joint health and flexibility. Benefits are usually noticed within 10 days. Dosage: 500 mg once daily.

FINAL THOUGHTS

To reduce the pain and inflammation associated with OA and protect your joints, consider the following:

- Eat more fish, flaxseed, olive oil, and pineapple, and drink green tea.
- Minimize red meat, dairy, sugar, and refined/processed foods; avoid nightshade foods.
- Do light strength training and cardiovascular and stretching activities regularly to improve joint function and mobility and to reduce pain.
- Try acupuncture, massage, and heat to reduce pain.
- Consider supplements of boswellia, glucosamine/chondroitin, or SAMe as a first-line approach.

OSTEOPOROSIS

Osteoporosis, which means "porous bones," is a disease that thins and weakens the bones to the point where they can easily fracture or break. Approximately 1.4 million Canadians suffer with the disease, with an estimated annual cost of $1.9 billion. Osteoporosis was once seen primarily as a woman's disease, and although it is still much more common in women, rates in men are on the rise and about one-third of those with osteoporosis are men.

Bone is living tissue that consists of a matrix of protein fibres (collagen), hardened with calcium, phosphorus, magnesium, zinc, copper, and other minerals. An interconnecting structure gives bone its strength: On the outside there is a tough, dense rind of cortical bone, and on the inside there is spongy-looking trabecular bone.

Bone cells called osteoclasts are constantly breaking down old bone at the same time that other cells, called osteoblasts, are building new bone. The activity of these cells is regulated primarily by the hormones estrogen, testosterone, and parathyroid hormone.

Peak bone mass is achieved between the ages of 16 and 20 for women and ages 20 to 25 for men. Until about age 30, there is a balance in activity of osteoclasts and osteoblasts. After that point, bone loss begins for both women and men, and more bone is broken down than is replaced. In women, the rate of loss accelerates for several years after menopause, and then slows again. In men, as testosterone levels wane bone loss occurs, although it is a slower process than what occurs in women.

Many factors contribute to and accelerate bone loss, including hormonal imbalance, nutrient deficiencies, lack of weight-bearing activity, oxidative stress, inflammation, elevated blood sugar, and the use of certain medications.

The trabecular bone normally looks like a honeycomb, but in those with osteoporosis the spaces in that honeycomb grow larger because more bone is destroyed than replaced. This makes the bones weaker and more susceptible to fractures. According to Osteoporosis Canada, at least one in three women and one in five men will suffer from an osteoporotic fracture during their lifetime.

Osteoporosis is largely preventable through a proper diet and lifestyle. Since bone health affects our mobility and ability to carry out daily activities, it is important to learn how to prevent osteoporosis and maintain strong, healthy bones throughout life.

SIGNS & SYMPTOMS

Osteoporosis is referred to as the silent thief because bone loss can occur slowly for many years without symptoms until a sudden strain, bump, or fall causes a bone fracture. It most commonly affects bones in the hip, spine, or wrist. Once the bones have become weakened, osteoporosis may cause back pain, collapsed vertebrae, loss of height, and spinal deformities.

RISK FACTORS

- Age: Those 65 years of age or older are at greatest risk due to lower levels of estrogen and testosterone and exposure to inflammation and oxidative stress.

- Body frame: Those with small, thin bones are at greater risk.

- Eating disorders: Anorexia, bulimia

- Ethnicity: Caucasian or Asian

- Family history

- Gender: Women are more susceptible than men; women with late puberty or early menopause are at greatest risk due to lower lifetime estrogen exposure

- High alcohol consumption: More than two drinks per day

- Medical conditions that affect calcium absorption, such as celiac and Crohn's disease and hyperthyroidism

- Nutritional deficiencies: Low calcium and vitamin D intake; high caffeine intake (more than four cups of coffee per day)

- Osteopenia (mild bone loss)

- Prescription medications: Prolonged use of steroids (prednisone) and use of diuretics, anticonvulsants, and drugs that reduce androgens (testosterone) such as Lupron increase risk. The blood thinner warfarin (Coumadin) may block the beneficial effects of vitamin K on the bone and can lead to decreased bone mineralization in some people.

- Sedentary lifestyle: Lack of weight-bearing activity

- Smoking

Mounting research suggests that the following factors may also increase the risk of osteoporosis:

- Uncontrolled high blood sugar: Leads to formation of advanced glycation end-products, or AGEs, that impair mineralization and increase the number of osteoclasts (cells that break down bones)

- Vitamin K deficiency: Impairs proper bone formation

- Heart disease: There is a correlation between osteoporosis, bone fractures, and heart disease. These diseases share some common risk factors such as inflammation and oxidative stress.

- Obesity: It was once thought that carrying extra weight would be protective against osteoporosis because of greater strain on the bones; however, recent research suggests that conditions common among those who are obese, including insulin resistance, high blood pressure, high triglycerides, and low HDL (good) cholesterol, are risk factors for low bone mineral density.

DOCTOR'S ORDERS

Canadian guidelines recommend that adults over the age of 50 be assessed for osteoporosis and fracture risk. Screening involves a physical exam, medical history, and various blood tests, including 25-hydroxyvitamin D. In those considered at risk for osteoporosis or fracture, a DEXA-scan (dual-energy X-ray absorptiometry) to measure bone mineral density (BMD) is recommended. The results are reported as a number, which tells us how far off our BMD is from a healthy adult without osteoporosis. A result of –2.5 SD (standard deviation) or greater indicates osteoporosis. A result between –1 SD and –2.5 SD means there is some bone loss, a condition called osteopenia, which often leads to osteoporosis.

Proper nutrition and exercise are essential for osteoporosis prevention. For those with osteoporosis or at high risk of fracture, drug therapy may be recommended to either slow the rate of bone loss or promote bone development. There are a variety of medications that doctors prescribe, including:

Hormones: Hormone replacement therapy (estrogen and progestins) was widely used for osteoporosis prevention until several large studies revealed that the serious health risks (such as heart attack, stroke, and breast cancer) outweighed the benefits. However, these drugs are still prescribed under certain circumstances, at the lowest dose and over the short term (less than five years).

Selective estrogen receptor modifiers (SERMs): Drugs such as raloxifene (Evista) mimic the beneficial effects of estrogen on the bones and help to build bone density and reduce fracture risk. Side effects include increased risk of blood clots, hot flashes, and leg cramps.

Bisphosphonates: These drugs, which stay in the bone a very long time (10 years), help increase bone density by inhibiting the action of osteoclast cells. Studies show they can help reduce fracture risk. Side effects include upset stomach; bone, joint, and muscle pain. They are generally not recommended for long-term use because prolonged treatment (greater than five years) may increase the risk of esophageal cancer and atypical fractures. Examples include alendronate (Fosamax), etidronate (Didrocal), risedronate (Actonel), and zoledronic acid (Aclasta), which is given by injection just once a year.

Calcitonin: A hormone naturally produced by the thyroid gland. It slows the activity of the osteoclasts and helps maintain and slightly increase bone density. It also helps prevent fractures of the spine. A synthetic form of calcitonin (Miacalcin NS) is used in a nasal spray. The only side effect is nasal irritation and dryness.

Bone metabolism regulators: The only drug in this class is denosumab (Prolia), a human monoclonal antibody that inhibits osteoclast formation and reduces fracture risk. This drug is given by injection twice a year. Side effects include pain in the muscles, itching, redness and/or dryness of the skin, and increased risk of cellulitis (skin infection).

Bone formation agents: Parathyroid hormone and its analogue, a new drug called teriparatide (Forteo), work by activating the osteoblast cells so that new bone is formed faster than the old bone is broken down. This drug effectively increases bone density and reduces fracture risk. It is taken as a daily subcutaneous (under the skin) injection. Side effects include nausea, dizziness, and leg cramps.

HOMEOPATHIC RECOMMENDATIONS

Symphytum: When osteoporosis is confirmed, fractures often occur from mild trauma. This remedy can help in strengthening and healing bones when new fractures occur, and also helps when pain persists in old, healed fractures.

SHERRY'S NATURAL PRESCRIPTION

Dietary Recommendations

Foods to include:

• Calcium-rich foods are essential to build and maintain strong bones. Examples include dairy, canned fish with bones (salmon and sardines), dark-green vegetables (kale, kelp, collards, broccoli, and Brussels sprouts), calcium-fortified orange juice, and soy milk. Some research suggests that people who get their calcium from plant sources have lower rates of osteoporosis. Green vegetables are also a good source of vitamin K.

• Vegetables and fruits are rich in antioxidants and minerals that support bone health. Recent research suggests that polyphenols (plant pigments) in fruits, vegetables, green tea, and red wine have a positive effect on bone-building cells.

• Lycopene, a carotenoid in tomatoes and tomato products, is an antioxidant that may offer some bone-preserving benefits.

• Magnesium is also necessary for bone formation and may be deficient in those with osteoporosis. Food sources include leafy green vegetables, whole grains, nuts, seeds, meat, milk, soybeans, tofu, legumes, and figs.

• Soy foods (tofu, soy milk, miso, soy beans, soy powders, and soy bars) can play a role in the prevention of osteoporosis. Soy contains isoflavones, which are plant-based estrogens that protect against bone loss. A total daily dose of about 54–110 mg isoflavones can help prevent loss of bone mineral content and reduce markers of bone resorption.

• Vitamin D aids in the absorption of calcium. Food sources include fortified milk products and breakfast cereals, fatty fish, and egg yolks.

• Yogurt contains friendly bacteria necessary to convert vitamin K to its active form, which helps in calcium absorption.

Foods to avoid:

• Caffeine (more than three cups coffee per day) or sodium can increase calcium loss through urination, accelerating bone deterioration.

• Don't drink tea with meals because the tannins can reduce calcium absorption.

• Fast food and processed foods are acidifying and can promote bone loss.

• Minimize alcohol (less than two drinks per day).

Lifestyle Suggestions

• Weight-bearing activities, which place stress on the bone, help to strengthen bones, prevent bone loss, and improve bone density. Examples include weight lifting, walking, tennis, and dancing. Exercise also increases muscle strength, coordination, and balance, helping to preserve mobility and reduce the risk of injury and fracture.

• Spend 15 minutes outdoors daily. Your body manufactures some vitamin D through sunlight exposure.

• Don't smoke. Smoking increases bone loss, and the risk of osteoporosis.

Top Recommended Supplements

Calcium: Essential for bone health; since it may not be possible to get adequate amounts through diet, supplements may be necessary. Studies show calcium (with vitamin D) can slow bone loss and may slightly improve bone density. Recommended intake for men and women ages 19 to 50 is 1,000 mg daily and 1,200 mg over age 50, through diet and supplements. Many products combine calcium with other nutrients for bone health such as vitamin D, magnesium, silicon, zinc, boron, and vitamin K. To maximize absorption, take no more than 500 mg of elemental calcium at one time and take with meals. Separate calcium-rich foods and supplements by two hours from iron supplements (calcium reduces iron absorption).

Ipriflavone: An isoflavone derivative that is used worldwide for the treatment and prevention of osteoporosis. It prevents bone loss, primarily by reducing bone breakdown. Numerous studies have found that it can slow the progression of osteoporosis and improve bone density. It also reduces bone pain caused by osteoporosis and fractures. It is most effective when taken along with calcium. Dosage: 200 mg three times daily.

Vitamin D: Aids in the absorption of calcium. Dosage: The most recent Osteoporosis Canada guidelines recommend that healthy adults at low risk of vitamin D deficiency take 400 to 1,000 IU of vitamin D per day. Adults over the age of 50 should take 800 to 1,000 IU daily. Certain individuals may require even higher amounts, such as those who are taking medications or have medical conditions that impair vitamin D absorption. Dosages up to 2,000 IU are safe and do not require monitoring.

Complementary Supplements

Antioxidants: Oxidative stress is a contributor to bone loss; antioxidant vitamins can play a role in osteoporosis prevention. In particular, vitamins C and E are involved in the production of proteins, development of bone-forming cells, and bone mineralization. Studies have shown that vitamins E and C can protect postmenopausal women against bone loss. Dosages: 600 mg vitamin E and 1,000 mg vitamin C. Other antioxidants that have shown some benefits for bone health include resveratrol and quercetin.

Omega-3 fatty acids: Recent research suggests that the omega-3 fatty acids in fish oils (EPA and DHA) reduce activity of bone-resorbing cells, increase activity of bone-forming cells, and increase calcium absorption and delivery to the bones. Plus they have strong anti-inflammatory and antioxidant effects. Dosage: 3–6 g daily.

Vitamin K: A cofactor required for production of the major bone protein, osteocalcin, which binds to calcium to create healthy bones. A deficiency can impair proper bone formation. Supplements have been shown to help support bone health by reducing bone breakdown. Dosage: 120 mcg daily; higher amounts, such as 1,000–1,500 mcg daily, have been used in research.

FINAL THOUGHTS

Osteoporosis is preventable and is not inevitable with aging. To strengthen your bones and protect yourself against this disease, consider the following:

- Eat a diet that is rich in vegetables, fruits, whole grains, beans, and legumes.
- Get regular weight-bearing exercise.
- Spend at least 15 minutes outdoors.
- Don't smoke, and minimize alcohol and caffeine intake.
- Consider supplementing your diet with bone-building nutrients, such as calcium, ipriflavone, and vitamin D.

OVARIAN CYSTS

Ovarian cysts are fluid-filled sacs that develop within or on the surface of an ovary. The ovaries are two small almond-shaped organs located on each side of a woman's uterus that produce eggs and female hormones.

There are several different types of cysts that can form on the ovaries. Each month, the ovaries grow tiny follicles (sacs) that hold the eggs. When an egg is mature, the follicle breaks open to release the egg and then dissolves. If the follicle doesn't break open to release the egg, it forms a follicular cyst. This type of cyst usually disappears within one to three months.

Another type of cyst, called a corpus luteum cyst, occurs after the egg is released from the follicle. The follicle becomes the corpus luteum. If pregnancy doesn't occur, the corpus luteum normally breaks down and disappears. If this does not happen and fluid builds up in the corpus luteum, it can form a cyst. These cysts can grow to almost 10 cm and may cause bleeding or twist the ovary and cause pain. This type of cyst usually goes away on its own after a few weeks.

Other types of cysts include the following:

Cystadenomas: Cysts that develop from cells on the outer surface of the ovary. They are often filled with a watery fluid or thick, sticky gel and can become large and painful.

Dermoid cyst: Ovarian cells are able to make hair, teeth, and other tissues. An abnormal growth of these cells can form a cyst. These cysts typically affect younger women.

Endometriomas: A type of cyst that develops in women with endometriosis, a condition where tissue from the lining of the uterus grows outside of the uterus. The tissue may attach to the ovary and form a cyst, which can be painful.

Polycystic ovarian syndrome: Multiple cysts appear on the ovaries due to a hormonal imbalance and high insulin levels. This topic is covered separately in this book.

Many women have ovarian cysts at some time during their lives, and most ovarian cysts are benign (non-cancerous) and disappear without treatment. However, some cysts can rupture and cause serious symptoms and consequences. For this reason, knowing the signs and symptoms and having regular pelvic exams is important to preserving ovarian health. Strategies to improve hormone balance may be helpful in preventing development of ovarian cysts.

SIGNS & SYMPTOMS

Some women have few or no symptoms, while others experience the following:

• Abdominal fullness or heaviness

• Menstrual irregularities (heavy bleeding or abnormal cycles)

• Nausea, vomiting, or pelvic tenderness

- Pelvic pain that may radiate down the back and thighs. Cysts that are large, break open, or become twisted are more likely to cause pain.

- Pelvic pain during intercourse

- Pressure on the rectum or bladder

Most ovarian cysts are benign (non-cancerous) and go away within a few months. If you develop sudden and severe abdominal or pelvic pain along with fever or vomiting, seek immediate medical attention.

RISK FACTORS

- Age: Women of childbearing age are at greatest risk.
- Hormonal imbalances (high estrogen levels)
- Fertility treatments (drugs taken to stimulate ovulation can lead to cysts)
- Race: Caucasian and Hispanic women are at increased risk.

DOCTOR'S ORDERS

The treatment of ovarian cysts depends on the size and type of cyst, symptoms, and the woman's age. Follicular and corpus luteum cysts are usually just monitored by the doctor and go away on their own. Oral contraceptives or progesterone cream are sometimes given to women who get frequent cysts as a way of controlling hormone levels and preventing cyst growth. Procedures to drain a cyst or surgery are usually considered as a last resort for women with malignant cysts, those who have very large cysts that do not go away, and those with severe symptoms or infertility.

SHERRY'S NATURAL PRESCRIPTION

Dietary Recommendations

Foods to include:

- Beets, carrots, artichokes, and lemons contain nutrients that support liver health, aiding the detoxification of estrogen.

- Fibre may help the body eliminate excess hormones. Boost intake of fruits, vegetables, and whole grains. Aim for 21–38 g daily.

- Broccoli, cauliflower, Brussels sprouts, and cabbage contain a compound called indole-3-carbinol, which can help the body detoxify estrogen.

- Flaxseed, soy, beans, and legumes contain phytoestrogens, which may help reduce the impact of other hormones.

- Choose organic foods as much as possible to avoid ingestion of estrogen-like compounds.

- Drink plenty of water.

Foods to avoid:

- Meat contains saturated fat, hormones, and chemicals that can affect ovarian health and trigger inflammation. Choose organic and free-range meats to avoid ingestion of hormones.

- Minimize caffeine (coffee, tea, chocolate), as it may worsen menstrual irregularities.

Lifestyle Suggestions

- Get regular pelvic examinations. Report any unusual symptoms or changes in your menstrual cycle to your doctor.

- Castor oil packs can help reduce pain and inflammation.

- Reduce stress. Try meditation, breathing exercises, or yoga.

- Exercise regularly to reduce stress levels and improve circulation and overall well-being. Aim for 30 minutes to one hour daily.

Top Recommended Supplements

There is limited research on supplements for the prevention or treatment of ovarian cysts. The supplements outlined here may help minimize symptoms and support hormone balance and liver health.

Calcium D-glucarate: Helps the liver detoxify and eliminate excess hormones, particularly estrogen. Dosage: 150–300 mg daily.

Chasteberry: Balances estrogen-to-progesterone ratio and may help normalize ovulation. Dosage: 150–300 mg daily.

Indole-3-carbinol: A compound found naturally in cruciferous vegetables that aids in detoxification of estrogen, protects liver function, and may protect against hormonal cancers. Dosage: 400 mg daily.

Complementary Supplements

Gamma linoleic acid (GLA): Products containing GLA, such as evening primrose oil and borage oil, may help reduce pain and inflammation. Dosage: 3,000 mg daily.

Milk thistle: Supports liver function and aids detoxification. Dosage: 50–100 mg daily.

FINAL THOUGHTS

To manage ovarian cysts and protect ovarian health, consider the following:

- Get regular pelvic exams and report any changes to your doctor.
- Boost intake of fibre and eat more eggplant, flaxseed, and beans.
- Minimize saturated fat (meat/dairy).
- Get regular exercise and reduce stress levels.
- Consider supplements of indole-3-carbinol, calcium D-glucarate, and chasteberry.

PARASITES

Our bodies are filled with billions of microorganisms. Some are harmless and even beneficial for health, and others can cause illness and disease. A parasite is an organism that lives on or in a host organism and gets its food from or at the expense of its host.

There are two main classes of parasites that can cause intestinal disease in humans:

Helminths: Derived from the Greek word for "worms," these large, multicellular organisms are generally visible to the naked eye. They can be either free-living or parasitic in nature. In their adult form, helminths cannot multiply in humans. The three main groups of helminths that are human parasites are flatworms (tapeworms), thorny-headed worms, and roundworms (hookworms and pinworms).

Protozoa: Microscopic, one-celled organisms that can be free-living or parasitic in nature. They can multiply in humans, which contributes to their survival and also permits serious infections to develop from just a single organism. The most common protozoa that infect humans are *giardia* and *Cryptosporidium.*

Parasites get into the body from consumption of contaminated food or water. When the organisms are swallowed, they move into the intestine, where they can reproduce and cause disease. You can also contract parasites from intimate contact (oral–anal) with someone who has them.

In some people, intestinal parasites do not cause any symptoms or the symptoms may be mild. In others they can cause horrible gastrointestinal problems, weight loss, irritability, and more. Parasites can be eliminated with medication or natural supplements. There are also a variety of lifestyle measures that can reduce your risk of contracting parasites.

SIGNS & SYMPTOMS

- Abdominal cramping and pain
- Bloody stools; mucus in stool
- Coughing
- Diarrhea and foul-smelling stools
- Fatigue
- Fever
- Gas and bloating
- Irritability and restlessness
- Itching in the rectal area
- Loss of appetite
- Vomiting
- Weight loss

Parasites

- Age: Children are more commonly infected.
- Consuming contaminated water or food
- Contact with infected animals
- Dysbiosis (imbalanced gut flora)
- Ingestion of undercooked meat or food containing parasites
- International travel
- Poor hygiene
- Sexual or intimate contact with someone who has parasites
- Weakened immune system (e.g., HIV)

DOCTOR'S ORDERS

If you suspect you have a parasite, see your doctor for proper diagnosis. Fecal testing (examination of your stool) can identify both helminths and protozoa. It is important to do stool tests before taking any antidiarrheal drugs or antibiotics. Typically three to five stool samples are needed to find the parasite.

The treatment will depend on the particular parasite that you have. Mebendazole (Vermox) is used for roundworm, hookworms, and pinworms. Metronidazole (Flagyl) is used for giardiasis.

SHERRY'S NATURAL PRESCRIPTION

It is critical to see your doctor for proper diagnosis and treatment. Natural products, while helpful, are not as effective and take longer to work compared to prescription drugs.

Dietary Recommendations

Foods to include:

- Boost intake of fibre, which helps improve elimination. Eat more whole grains, vegetables, and beans.
- Drink lots of purified water to prevent dehydration, which often occurs with persistent diarrhea.
- Eat more raw garlic, pumpkin seeds, pomegranates, beets, and carrots, all of which have antiparasitic properties.

Foods to avoid:

- Refined carbohydrates and sugars impair immune function.
- Spicy foods, dairy, alcohol, and caffeine can worsen gastrointestinal symptoms.

Lifestyle Suggestions

To reduce the risk of contracting parasites, consider these tips:

- Wash your hands after using the toilet, changing diapers, or handling animals, or before eating or preparing food. Use soap and water and don't forget to scrub under your nails.

• Drink purified or bottled water, especially when travelling to developing countries. When travelling, also avoid ice and fruits that cannot be peeled.

• When camping, boil stream water for at least 10 minutes. Untreated stream water is almost invariably contaminated with giardia, even in North America.

• Avoid rare meats and undercooked poultry and avoid foods prepared by street vendors as sanitation (hand washing) is often lacking.

• When swimming in pools, lakes, or streams keep your mouth and eyes closed and try not to swallow water.

• Practise safe sex. Use condoms and avoid oral–anal sex without protection.

Top Recommended Supplements

Probiotics: Beneficial bacteria such as *Lactobacillus* and *Bifidobacteria* can help in the prevention and treatment of parasites by maintaining healthy gut flora and reducing overgrowth of parasites and other pathogens. Probiotics can also help shorten episodes of diarrhea. Probiotic supplements are particularly important to take prior to and during travel to developing countries. Dosage: One to three capsules daily with meals. For infants/children look for *Lactobacillus reuteri* (BioGaia), which is available in drops and chewable tablets.

Propolis: A resinous substance collected by bees from the leaf buds and bark of trees. It has antimicrobial properties and may help protect against parasitic intestinal infections. Preliminary research found that propolis extract was helpful in eliminating giardiasis in adults and children. Dosage: 30 drops four times daily.

Herbal products such as black walnut, wormwood, oil of oregano, and ginger have antiparasitic properties. Consult with a natural health care provider for advice and dosage guidelines because there are a variety of side effects and precautions associated with the use of these products.

Complementary Supplements

Berberine: A compound found in many plants, such as Oregon grape and goldenseal. Preliminary studies have shown that berberine can be used successfully to treat giardia infections. Dosage: 200 mg three times daily for adults. Not recommended for children.

Digestive enzymes: Aid digestion and make your intestinal tract less hospitable to parasites. Dosage: Take before meals.

FINAL THOUGHTS

To manage a parasitic infection, consider the following:

• See your doctor for proper diagnosis and discuss the benefits and risks of drug therapy.
• Boost intake of fibre, drink lots of purified water, and eat more raw garlic, pumpkin seeds, pomegranates, beets, and carrots.
• Minimize sugar, refined starches, dairy, spicy food, caffeine, and alcohol.
• Wash your hands after using the toilet and before touching food, and practise safe sex to avoid spreading the parasites.
• Probiotics can help in the prevention and treatment of parasites. Discuss the role of herbal products with your health care provider.

PARKINSON'S DISEASE

Parkinson's disease is a progressive nervous system disorder that affects muscle movement. The disease causes degenerative changes in an area of the brain called the substantia nigra. Nerve cells in this area are responsible for producing the neurotransmitter dopamine. As these nerve cells become damaged and die, there is insufficient dopamine to relay messages between nerve and muscle cells, and it becomes progressively more difficult for the body to move smoothly. This causes tremors and shaking, which interfere with normal activities such as walking, sitting, and standing.

In Canada, about one out of every 100 adults has Parkinson's disease. Parkinson's most often affects older adults, and as Canada's population continues to age, the incidence of Parkinson's disease is expected to rise.

Researchers are working to understand the underlying causes of Parkinson's. Everyone loses some dopamine-producing neurons with age, but those with Parkinson's lose around 60 percent or more of the neurons in the substantia nigra. Scientists believe that a combination of factors is involved, including genetics, inflammation, oxidative stress, nutrient deficiencies, and environment.

Parkinson's disease is treatable. Over the years there have been great advances in science that have improved quality of life for those with Parkinson's.

SIGNS & SYMPTOMS

In the early stages, symptoms may be subtle, such as mild tremor in the fingers, fatigue, or difficulty sleeping. As the disease progresses, it may cause the following:

- Dementia: Some people with Parkinson's develop impaired mental function, which affects their ability to think, reason, and remember.

- Difficulty swallowing

- Impaired balance and coordination

- Impaired speech: The voice becomes monotone and soft and speech is slower.

- Loss of automatic movements: The face becomes less expressive; some people lose the ability to blink, smile, make hand gestures, and move their arms while walking.

- Rigid, stiff muscles; often occurs in the limbs and neck

- Slowed movement: A slow, shuffling walk with an unsteady gait and stooped posture; leg muscles may freeze up, making it difficult to walk and move.

- Tremors: Often starts in the hands and fingers; sometimes hand tremors cause a back-and-forth rubbing of the thumb and forefinger known as "pill-rolling"; tremors may also develop in the legs; tremors are often worse under stress.

RISK FACTORS

- Age: The risk increases with age. Parkinson's is usually diagnosed after the age of 60; however, 1 in 20 are diagnosed under age 40. It is thought that genetic or environmental factors over time lead to neural damage.

- Environmental factors: Several studies have shown that exposure to pesticides and herbicides substantially increases risk. Farmers, those handling these chemicals, and those who drink well water are at higher risk. Heavy metal toxicity also increases risk.

- Family history: Having one or more close relatives with Parkinson's increases risk.

- Free radicals: Some research suggests that Parkinson's may be caused by unstable oxygen molecules that cause cell damage.

- Gender: Men are at greater risk.

DRUG-INDUCED PARKINSON'S

Several drugs, when used chronically or in excessive dosages, can cause symptoms of Parkinson's disease. Examples include haloperidol (Haldol) and chlorpromazine (Thorazine), which are used to treat psychiatric disorders; drugs used to treat nausea, such as metoclopramide (Reglan); and the epilepsy drug valproate (Depakene). Once these drugs are stopped, the symptoms disappear.

DOCTOR'S ORDERS

Drug therapy is used to boost dopamine levels, and this can dramatically improve symptoms. However, with chronic use the benefits often diminish and it may be necessary to adjust the dosage, switch medications, or take multiple medications. Some of the most common medications used include the following:

Amantadine: An antiviral that reduces the side effects that are sometimes caused by taking levodopa for a long time. Amantadine is sometimes used alone or, in the early stages of the disease, along with levodopa.

Anticholinergics: An older class of drugs used before the discovery of levodopa. They help control tremor in the early stages of the disease but are only mildly beneficial and cause side effects such as dry mouth, nausea, confusion, hallucinations, and urine retention. Examples: trihexphenidyl and benztropine (Cogentin).

COMT inhibitors: Prolong the effect of Sinemet by blocking an enzyme (Catechol-O-methyltransferase) that breaks down dopamine. The only drug in this class approved for use in Canada is entacapone (Comtan).

Dopamine agonists: Drugs that mimic the effects of dopamine in the brain. They are often used for young adults or those in early stages, along with Sinemet. Examples include bromocriptine (Parlodel), pramipexole (Mirapex), and ropinirole (Requip).

Side effects include involuntary movements, hallucinations, drowsiness, and the risk of inflammatory reactions in the heart and lungs.

MAO-B inhibitors: These drugs help prevent the breakdown of dopamine by inhibiting the enzyme monoamine oxidase B (MAO-B), which is responsible for breaking down dopamine. Drugs in this class include selegiline (Deprenyl), which has been around since the 1960s, and the new drug rasagiline (Azilect). Side effects are uncommon, but may include nausea, headaches, or dyskinesias (involuntary movements). When added to Sinemet, there is a risk of hallucinations. These medications can't be used in combination with most antidepressants or certain narcotics, due to potentially serious reactions.

Sinemet: A combination of levodopa and carbidopa. Levodopa is a natural substance found in plants and animals that is converted into dopamine by nerve cells in the brain. Carbidopa enhances the amount of levodopa that gets into the brain and helps reduce the side effects of therapy. Side effects include involuntary movements, hallucinations, and low blood pressure when standing.

There are a variety of experimental procedures under development, such as stem cell transplants and tissue grafts.

SHERRY'S NATURAL PRESCRIPTION

Dietary Recommendations

Foods to include:

- Boost fibre intake to prevent constipation. Eat more fruits, vegetables, whole grains, nuts, and seeds. Fruits and vegetables also provide antioxidants that help to neutralize damaging free radicals. Eat organic as much as possible to avoid ingesting toxic pesticides.

- Coffee contains antioxidants that protect brain cells, and this can be helpful for those with Parkinson's disease. Coffee extracts have been shown to inhibit MAO-A and -B enzymes, thus preventing the breakdown of dopamine (similarly to some drugs). Studies have also found that those who consume large amounts of coffee are much less likely to develop Parkinson's disease.

- Green tea contains a range of antioxidants, including EGCG, which is neuroprotective. Studies have found a correlation between tea consumption and a lower incidence of dementia and Parkinson's. There is also preliminary evidence that green tea may prevent the breakdown of dopamine, leaving more available in the brain.

- Eat small, frequent meals. Chew food slowly to make it easier to swallow.

- Keep protein intake at breakfast and lunch low and have a high-protein dinner. Good protein sources include wild fish, organic poultry, eggs, nuts, and seeds. The absorption of levodopa and its ability to reach the brain cells is hindered by consumption of certain dietary proteins. Several studies have shown that you can enhance the action of levodopa and improve the symptoms of Parkinson's by consuming most of your day's protein requirement at dinner, while keeping the protein content of breakfast and lunch extremely low (less than 10 g). Consult with a dietitian for advice on planning meals.

- Healthy fats such as olive oil and flaxseed oil and wheat germ contain vitamin E, which is a potent antioxidant, and essential fatty acids that help reduce inflammation. Palm fruit oil contains tocotrienols (a potent form of vitamin E), which is neuroprotective.

- Yogurt, kefir, and fermented dairy contain beneficial bacteria that can aid digestion, support immune function, and help in the absorption of nutrients.

Foods to avoid:

- Avoid processed and fast foods and artificial sweeteners, which contain chemicals that may have a negative effect on brain function.

- Diets high in saturated fat (meat and full-fat dairy) may increase the risk of Parkinson's due to increased formation of free radicals in the brain and oxidative damage to the nerve cells in the substantia nigra. Saturated fat can also trigger inflammation. Minimize saturated fat to less than 10 percent of total calories.

- Eating large amounts of fava beans (broad beans) can boost the action of levodopa and can possibly lead to overdose. Speak with a dietitian before adding fava beans to your diet if you are taking levodopa.

- Minimize or avoid alcohol, as it can impair brain function.

Lifestyle Suggestions

- Exercise can help improve mobility, range of motion, and muscle tone and strength. Tai chi is particularly helpful. Weight-bearing activities (walking, dancing) can help strengthen the bones, which helps in the prevention of osteoporosis. Wear proper footwear and consult with a physical therapist or personal trainer to get advice on exercises that can improve balance, coordination, and strength.

- Spend 15 minutes outdoors to allow your skin to make vitamin D, which can help protect against osteoporosis and improve Parkinson's symptoms.

- Manage stress with yoga, breathing techniques, or meditation.

- A speech pathologist can help improve problems with speaking and swallowing.

- Get adequate sleep. The medications may make you tired, so it is important to rest as needed.

- Take measures to reduce the risk of falls (remove throw rugs, keep walking areas clear, and use handrails on stairs and grab bars around the tub and toilet).

Top Recommended Supplements

CDP-choline (citicoline): A substance that occurs naturally in the body. It increases the amount of dopamine in the brain. Studies have shown it can improve symptoms and enhance the efficacy of levodopa. Dosage: 400 mg three times daily. This is a specialty supplement that is available through natural health care practitioners.

Coenzyme Q10: An antioxidant that is involved in energy production in the cells. People with Parkinson's tend to have low Q10 levels, and several studies have shown that supplements can slow the progression of the disease and may also help reduce symptoms. Dosage: 1,200 mg daily. Lower dosages have been used, but with less benefit.

NADH: Nicotinamide adenine dinucleotide hydrogen is the active form of vitamin B3, a cofactor that works with enzymes in the body to produce energy. It is also involved in the production of levodopa and has antioxidant properties. Preliminary studies using high doses of NADH for Parkinson's disease have shown reduced symptoms and improved brain function. Dosage: 5 mg twice daily.

Complementary Supplements

Amino acids: L-tyrosine, methionine, and acetyl-L-carnitine may help in the management of Parkinson's by nourishing the cells that produce dopamine. Preliminary studies with methionine and L-carnitine have shown benefits for reducing symptoms. L-tyrosine should not be taken with L-dopa as it may interfere with the transport of L-dopa to the brain. Consult with your health care provider before supplementing with amino acids.

Creatine: An amino acid–like compound that plays an important role in cellular energy. Preliminary research suggests it is neuroprotective and may help prevent or slow the progression of Parkinson's. Dosage: 10 grams daily. A loading dose of creatine— 20 grams per day for 6 days followed by 2 grams daily for 6 months, and then 4 grams daily for 18 months—has also been used.

Ginkgo biloba: An antioxidant that improves blood flow to the brain. Many studies have shown that it can improve memory and cognitive function in the elderly. Dosage: 120–240 mg daily, standardized to 6 percent terpene lactones and 24 percent flavone glycosides. It may take six weeks to notice benefits.

Vitamin B6: May improve Parkinson's symptoms and enhance the effectiveness of Sinemet. Do not take if you are taking levodopa alone as this can increase the conversion of levodopa to dopamine outside the brain. Dosage: 50–100 mg daily. Take as part of a B-complex.

Vitamins C and E: Antioxidants that protect against free radical damage in the brain, including key dopamine-producing brain cells. In one study, people with early Parkinson's given a dosage of 750 mg vitamin C and 800 IU vitamin E four times daily were able to delay the need for drug therapy by an average of about two and a half years, compared with those not taking the vitamins.

Vitamin D: Research suggests that inadequate vitamin D levels can lead to a chronic loss of dopaminergic neurons in the brain. Vitamin D has been shown to exert a protective effect on the brain through antioxidant activities, regulation of calcium levels, detoxification, modulation of the immune system, and enhanced conduction of electricity through neurons. Studies have also found that higher vitamin D levels are associated with lower risk of Parkinson's. Dosage: 800–2,000 IU daily.

FINAL THOUGHTS

To improve the management of Parkinson's, consider the following:

- Boost intake of fibre (whole grains, fruits, and vegetables) along with healthy fats and green tea. Speak with a dietitian about consuming your daily protein in the evening.
- Minimize or avoid saturated fat, alcohol, processed and fast foods, and artificial sweeteners.
- Exercise regularly to improve strength, coordination, and balance. Work with a trainer or physical therapist.
- Get adequate sleep and manage your stress.
- Consider supplements of CDP-choline, coenzyme Q10, and NADH.

P

Parkinson's Disease

POLYCYSTIC OVARIAN SYNDROME

Polycystic ovarian syndrome (PCOS) is a disorder characterized by hormonal imbalance (excess male hormones), irregular menstrual periods, acne, excess hair growth, insulin resistance, and obesity. Originally it was thought that women with PCOS had to have multiple cysts on their ovaries (hence the name of the condition); however, not all women will have cysts. While the condition is more common in those who are overweight or obese, it can also occur in women with a normal body weight. PCOS is the most common hormonal disorder among women of reproductive age, affecting an estimated 5 to 10 percent.

In PCOS, the body produces an excess amount of androgens, and the ratio of luteinizing hormone to follicle-stimulating hormone is abnormally high. Ovulation occurs less frequently, or the ovaries don't release eggs at all. In the absence of ovulation, the menstrual cycle is irregular or absent, and cysts containing the immature eggs may form on the ovaries. This causes the ovaries to enlarge and secrete higher amounts of male hormones (androgens).

Research suggests that PCOS may result from a combination of obesity and insulin resistance, which boosts male hormone production, leading to menstrual cycle disturbances, acne, and coarse hair growth. Genetic factors may also be at play since this occurs more commonly in those with a family history.

Early diagnosis and treatment of PCOS is important to improving quality of life and reducing the risk of long-term complications, such as diabetes and heart disease.

PCOS AND INSULIN RESISTANCE

Insulin resistance is a common feature of both PCOS and metabolic syndrome. Metabolic syndrome is a cluster of symptoms (abdominal obesity, high cholesterol and triglyceride levels, and insulin resistance) that greatly increases the risk of heart disease and diabetes. Researchers at Virginia Commonwealth University found that metabolic syndrome is twice as prevalent in women with PCOS compared to those without this hormonal disorder.

SIGNS & SYMPTOMS

- Acne, oily skin, or dandruff
- Hormonal imbalances: Elevated testosterone, androstenedione, DHEA, estrogen, and insulin
- Enlarged ovaries with cysts
- Increased hair growth on the face, chest, stomach, back, thumbs, or toes (hirsutism), and thinning or male pattern baldness on the head
- Infertility

- Irregular or absent menstrual periods

- Overweight or obesity (particularly around the waist)

- Patches of thickened and dark brown or black skin on the neck, arms, breasts, or thighs

- Pelvic pain

- Skin tags, or tiny excess flaps of skin in the armpits or neck area

Note: PCOS increases the risk of developing type 2 diabetes, high blood pressure, increased triglyceride levels, decreased high-density lipoprotein (HDL) cholesterol, and cardiovascular disease. Women with PCOS are also at risk of abnormal uterine bleeding and endometrial cancer because the uterus is exposed to higher amounts of estrogen.

RISK FACTORS

- Family history/genetics

- High insulin levels

- Obesity

- Race (women of Mediterranean descent are at greater risk)

Other risk factors that may play a role in the development of PCOS include early puberty; chronic inflammation; exposure to endocrine-disrupting chemicals (xenoestrogens); autoimmune disorders, especially those involving the ovaries, pancreas, thyroid and adrenal glands; and the use of medications that increase prolactin production.

DOCTOR'S ORDERS

Healthy eating and regular exercise are critical to reduce the risk of diabetes and heart disease. There are several medications that doctors prescribe to address the symptoms of infertility, hirsutism, and acne.

For those not trying to become pregnant, low-dose oral contraceptives are used to regulate the menstrual cycle, decrease androgen production, improve acne, reduce hair growth, and reduce the risk of endometrial cancer. However, recent research suggests that taking the pill may worsen PCOS symptoms when a woman stops taking it. Oral or topical progesterone for 10 to 14 days each month is sometimes used to regulate the menstrual cycle. Spironolactone is a drug used to decrease androgens and reduce hair growth and acne. Other, non-drug methods of hair removal include electrolysis, laser, sugaring, and waxing.

Drugs such as metformin (Glucophage) are used to improve insulin sensitivity, reduce androgen levels, and improve ovulation. For women trying to conceive, fertility drugs such as clomiphene and gonadotropin shots are used to stimulate ovulation. About 30 to 70 percent of women with PCOS on clomiphene will conceive; however, use of this drug carries the risk of multiple births.

P

Polycystic Ovarian Syndrome

SHERRY'S NATURAL PRESCRIPTION

Dietary Recommendations

Foods to include:

• Small frequent meals with high-fibre, low-glycemic vegetables, whole grains, lean protein, and healthy fats can help to improve blood sugar and insulin levels. Refer to Appendix B for more information on the glycemic index.

• Broccoli, cabbage, cauliflower, kale, and Brussels sprouts contain compounds called glucosinolates that help the body detoxify and eliminate hormones. To get the most nutrients and benefits, eat raw, organic vegetables.

• Cinnamon can improve insulin sensitivity. Add ½ tsp daily to cereals, breakfast shakes, or other foods.

• Green tea contains various antioxidants, in particular epigallocatechin gallate (EGCG), which can help improve glucose metabolism, reduce inflammation, and boost metabolism.

• Flaxseed, soy, beans, and legumes contain phytoestrogens, which may help reduce the impact of other hormones.

• The omega-3 fatty acids in fish help reduce inflammation, balance hormones, and reduce triglycerides.

• Choose organic foods as much as possible.

• Drink plenty of water.

Foods to avoid:

• Sugar (candy, soft drinks, juices, and sweets) and refined starches (white flour products) cause blood sugar imbalances and trigger high insulin.

• Meat and dairy products may contain saturated fat, hormones, and chemicals that can worsen PCOS and trigger inflammation.

• Minimize alcohol and caffeine products, as they may interfere with hormone function.

Lifestyle Suggestions

• Exercise regularly, which will help with weight loss, which in turn can reduce both insulin and androgen levels and may restore ovulation. Aim for 30 minutes to one hour daily.

• Reduce stress, as stress can worsen insulin response. Try meditation, breathing exercises, or yoga.

• Follow a good skin care regime. Wash your face morning and night using skin care products containing tea tree oil (10 to 15 percent) to help reduce acne and oily skin. Minimize wearing cosmetics, and use products designed for oily skin.

Top Recommended Supplements

D-chiro-inositol (Chirositol): A form of inositol that has been shown in research to improve glucose metabolism and insulin sensitivity, reduce testosterone levels, and improve ovulatory function and fertility in those with PCOS. It also has a positive effect on blood pressure and triglyceride levels. Dosage: 600–1,200 mg daily.

N-acetylcysteine (NAC): A form of the amino acid cysteine that also has antioxidant activity. Studies have shown that it can improve insulin sensitivity and fertility, particularly in those who have not responded to fertility treatments. Dosage: 1.2 g daily.

Complementary Supplements

Calcium D-glucarate: Helps the liver detoxify and eliminate excess hormones, particularly estrogen. Dosage: 150–300 mg daily.

Chasteberry: Balances the estrogen-to-progesterone ratio and may help normalize ovulation. Dosage: 150–300 mg daily.

Chromium: Helps improve glucose tolerance and insulin sensitivity. Preliminary research suggests benefits for those with PCOS. Dosage: 200 mcg chromium picolinate daily.

Indole-3-carbinol: A compound found naturally in cruciferous vegetables. Although not specifically studied for PCOS, it aids in detoxification of estrogen, protects liver function, and may protect against hormonal cancers. Dosage: 400 mg daily.

Lipoic acid: Helps improve blood glucose control, insulin sensitivity, blood pressure, and lipid levels. Preliminary research found that it improved insulin sensitivity and triglycerides in those with PCOS. Dosage: 1,200 mg daily.

Magnesium: Helps improve glucose uptake and insulin secretion in those with type 2 diabetes. Many women with PCOS have low magnesium levels, which can contribute to the progression of insulin resistance to type 2 diabetes and heart disease. Dosage: 300–600 mg daily.

FINAL THOUGHTS

To manage PCOS and prevent further health risks, consider the following:

- Boost intake of fibre-rich vegetables, whole grains, nuts, and seeds.
- Minimize refined starches and sugars.
- Get regular exercise.
- Reduce stress levels.
- Consider supplements of Chirositol and NAC along with the supportive nutrients.

P

Polycystic Ovarian Syndrome

PREMENSTRUAL SYNDROME (PMS)

Premenstrual syndrome (PMS) is a group of symptoms linked to the menstrual cycle. It is one of the most common conditions affecting women of childbearing age. Approximately 85 percent of women have one or more symptoms of PMS.

Years ago, the symptoms of PMS were dismissed as being psychological. Today, however, it is recognized there are a number of factors involved in causing the notorious symptoms, including hormonal and biochemical imbalances, diet, and environment.

During the menstrual cycle a woman's levels of estrogen and progesterone naturally fluctuate as the body prepares for a possible pregnancy. In the first half of the cycle, estrogen levels rise, causing the uterine lining to thicken in preparation for egg implantation. After the egg is released (ovulation), progesterone levels rise dramatically and then decline if pregnancy does not occur during this luteal phase, or second half, of the cycle. Women who suffer with PMS have hormonal imbalances during this phase: progesterone deficiency and estrogen dominance. As noted below, there is evidence that women with severe PMS have lower levels of certain neurotransmitters (chemical messengers) in the brain that regulate mood, appetite, and sleep. Research also suggests that alterations in prostaglandins (fatty acids that act as chemical messengers) lead to the cramping and pain that women experience.

While the symptoms of PMS can be distressing, there are a number of lifestyle measures and natural products that can greatly improve both the physical and emotional symptoms.

SIGNS & SYMPTOMS

The symptoms of PMS often start a few days to a week before the menstrual cycle and then disappear after menstruation. They vary greatly among women in both severity and the number of symptoms experienced. Common signs and symptoms include the following:

- Breast swelling and tenderness
- Changes in appetite or food cravings
- Crying spells
- Depression and anxiety
- Fatigue
- Headache
- Insomnia
- Lower abdominal bloating and pain
- Mood swings and irritability
- Weight gain from fluid retention

PREMENSTRUAL DYSPHORIC DISORDER

Premenstrual dysphoric disorder (PMDD) is a severe and debilitating form of PMS that affects about 10 percent of menstruating women. Symptoms include severe depression, feelings of hopelessness, anger, anxiety, low self-esteem, difficulty concentrating, irritability, and tension. The symptoms of PMDD typically begin a week before a period.

RISK FACTORS

- Biochemical imbalance: Low levels of serotonin, a brain chemical that regulates emotional well-being, and reduced sensitivity to gamma-aminobutyric acid (a neurotransmitter associated with relaxation)

- Depression

- Exposure to environmental toxins and estrogens (xenoestrogens)

- Hormonal imbalance (low thyroid or progesterone levels)

- Nutrient deficiencies in B-vitamins, magnesium, or essential fatty acids

- Poor diet: Eating foods high in sugar or saturated fat, or drinking too much alcohol

- Poor liver function

- Seasonal affective disorder

- Stress

Note: Hormonal imbalances are often difficult to determine through blood tests alone. Saliva testing offers certain advantages and is discussed in Appendix E.

DOCTOR'S ORDERS

There are several medications that doctors prescribe for PMS. Non-steroidal anti-inflammatory drugs (NSAIDs) like ibuprofen (Advil or Motrin) are used to relieve cramping and pain. Oral contraceptives are sometimes given for those with severe PMS symptoms and heavy bleeding. Antidepressants such as paroxetine (Paxil), fluoxetine (Prozac), or sertraline (Zoloft) are given to those with severe depressive symptoms. All of these drugs have serious side effects and should be used only for the short term and under doctor supervision.

SHERRY'S NATURAL PRESCRIPTION

Dietary Recommendations

Eating small, frequent meals will help to stabilize blood sugar levels, which will have a positive impact on mood and energy levels.

Foods to include:

- Several studies have shown that diets low in fat or high in fibre can help reduce PMS symptoms, so eat more vegetables, fruits, whole grains, nuts, seeds, and fish. These foods are also good sources of vitamins, minerals, and essential fatty acids, which may be depleted in those with PMS.

• Cruciferous vegetables (broccoli, cauliflower, and cabbage) contain indole-3-carbinol, which helps to balance estrogen levels.

• A diet rich in calcium and vitamin D may reduce the risk of PMS. Research has found that women who consumed an average of 1,200 mg of calcium and 400 IU of vitamin D daily (from food) were less likely to suffer from PMS. Foods rich in calcium include dairy, dark leafy greens, sardines, soybeans, and fortified cereals, soy milk, and juice. Foods rich in vitamin D include milk, eggs, and fortified cereals and juice.

• Fish provides omega-3 fatty acids, which reduce inflammation and support emotional health. Salmon is a particularly good source of omega-3s, along with vitamin D.

• Turkey and salmon contain the amino acid tryptophan, which elevates serotonin production.

Foods to avoid:

• Sugar and refined carbohydrates can cause mood swings, irritability, and worsened PMS symptoms.

• Caffeine has been found in studies to worsen PMS symptoms.

• Processed/fast foods often contain chemicals that may upset neurotransmitter levels and mood.

• Alcohol is a nervous system depressant and can affect hormone metabolism. It should be minimized or avoided completely.

Lifestyle Suggestions

• Regular exercise can reduce several symptoms of PMS (breast tenderness, fluid retention, depression, and stress). Aim for 30 minutes to one hour of moderate-intensity activity daily, such as brisk walking, cycling, or swimming.

• Acupuncture may offer benefits for PMS by stimulating the production of neurotransmitters that regulate mood.

• Massage, yoga, and reflexology help relieve stress and tension, and promote relaxation.

Top Recommended Supplements

Calcium: Studies have found that calcium can significantly reduce mood swings, pain, bloating, depression, back pain, and food cravings. Dosage: 1,000–1,200 mg daily. Take along with vitamin D (800–1,000 IU) and magnesium, as noted below.

Chasteberry: An herb that is widely used in Europe. It helps balance hormone levels and reduces symptoms of irritability, depression, headaches, and breast tenderness. Dosage: 150–300 mg daily.

L-tryptophan: A precursor to the neurotransmitter serotonin. Studies show that it can help improve mood and depression. Available by prescription only in Canada. Dosage: 2–6 g daily during the second half of the menstrual cycle. 5-HTP, which is the direct precursor to serotonin, may also offer benefits for PMS. Although it has not been specifically studied for PMS, research on depression has found significant benefits with better tolerability than other prescription antidepressants. Dosage: 50–200 mg daily.

Complementary Supplements

Gamma-linoleic acid (GLA): A fatty acid found in evening primrose, borage seed, and black currant oils. Levels of GLA are abnormal among women with PMS, and supplementing may offer benefits. Some studies with evening primrose oil have found benefits for emotional symptoms and breast tenderness. Dosage: 3–4 g daily.

Ginkgo biloba: Preliminary research has found that it can alleviate emotional symptoms and breast pain. Dosage: 80 mg twice daily.

L-theanine: An amino acid that promotes calming and relaxation and improves sleep quality. Look for the clinically studied form Suntheanine. Dosage: 100–200 mg at bedtime.

Magnesium: Some research suggests that it may help emotional symptoms and headaches. Combining magnesium with vitamin B6 may improve results. Dosage: 100–200 mg twice daily with meals.

Vitamin B6: Has been widely used for PMS, although studies have yielded mixed results. It may work best in those with a deficiency of B6 or when used along with magnesium. Dosage: Take 50–100 mg as part of a B-complex product.

FINAL THOUGHTS

There is good evidence that lifestyle adjustments and supplements can help alleviate the symptoms and improve quality of life. Here are the main points to keep in mind:

- Boost intake of cruciferous vegetables, fish, whole grains, nuts, and seeds.
- Minimize sugar, caffeine, processed foods, and alcohol.
- Exercise every day and get adequate sleep.
- Reduce stress with meditation, acupuncture, or yoga.
- Consider supplements of chasteberry, calcium, vitamin D, and tryptophan (or 5-HTP).

P

Premenstrual Syndrome (PMS)

PROSTATE ENLARGEMENT (BENIGN PROSTATIC HYPERPLASIA)

Benign prostatic hyperplasia (BPH) is a non-malignant enlargement of the prostate gland, which is located just below a man's bladder, surrounding the urethra (the tube that drains urine from the bladder). This gland produces seminal fluid, which nourishes and transports sperm. About half of men at age 50 have prostate enlargement and up to 90 percent of men in their seventies and eighties are affected.

At birth, the gland is about the size of a pea. In a man, it is the size of a walnut and stays this size until his late forties when it undergoes a growth phase. The cells in the gland begin to reproduce more quickly, which causes the gland to enlarge. As it enlarges, it compresses the urethra and partially blocks the flow of urine. Prostate enlargement is not related to prostate cancer, nor does it indicate that a man will get prostate cancer, but it can cause distressing urinary symptoms, such as difficulty in starting or stopping a stream of urine and the need to void frequently.

The cause of prostate enlargement is believed to be hormonal changes associated with aging. As men age, testosterone levels decline and estrogen levels increase. Levels of another hormone called dihydrotestosterone (DHT) increase. These changes are implicated in triggering growth of the prostate, so treatments for BPH are geared toward correcting the hormonal imbalances. There are a number of medications that are effective, but they can cause unpleasant side effects. Vitamin and herbal supplements can also help.

SIGNS & SYMPTOMS

- Blood in the urine

- Difficulty in starting or stopping urination

- Dribbling

- Inability to empty the bladder completely

- Increased frequency of urination

- Increased nighttime urination

- Recurring urinary tract infections

- Weak urine stream

Note: The signs and symptoms of prostate enlargement vary greatly among men. Only about half of men with prostate enlargement experience urinary symptoms that become troubling enough for them to seek medical treatment.

- Age: It is most common in men over the age of 60.

- Diet: High intake of saturated fat and low intake of fibre

- Ethnicity: It is more common in North American and Australian men and less common in Asian men.

- Family history

DOCTOR'S ORDERS

The treatment of BPH depends on the severity of the symptoms. If there are little to no symptoms, your doctor may just monitor your situation to see if it changes. Those with bothersome symptoms may be prescribed medications.

Commonly used medications include alpha blockers, such as terazosin (Hytrin), tamsulosin (Flomax), doxazosin (Cardura), alfuzosin (Xatral), and silodosin (Rapaflo), which relax the muscles at the neck of the bladder, making it easier to urinate. These drugs work quickly (within a day or two), but side effects include low blood pressure, lightheadedness, dizziness, and retrograde ejaculation (semen goes back to the bladder rather than out of the penis).

The 5-alpha-reductase inhibitors, finasteride (Proscar) and dutasteride (Avodart), work by inhibiting an enzyme that converts testosterone to DHT, thus helping to shrink the prostate gland. These drugs take longer to work (about three months) and side effects include impotence, reduced sexual desire (low libido), and retrograde ejaculation.

Another approach to management of BPH is heat therapy to destroy the excessive prostate tissue. Examples include microwave heat, radio waves, electric currents, or laser. Heat therapy works better than drugs, with fewer side effects, but it does require a brief hospital stay and a few days' recovery.

Various surgical procedures can be done to remove the excess prostate tissue and improve symptoms. Surgery is reserved for those with severe symptoms and complications, such as frequent infections, bleeding, and kidney damage. Risks of surgery include impotence, retrograde ejaculation, and incontinence.

CAUTION

Over-the-counter decongestants, such as pseudoephedrine (Sudafed), which is found in cold remedies, can worsen BPH symptoms because they cause the band of muscles that control urine flow from your urethra (urethral sphincter) to tighten, making urination more difficult. Antihistamines can also worsen symptoms by causing urinary retention. Ask your pharmacist for help when looking for a cold or allergy product.

SHERRY'S NATURAL PRESCRIPTION

Dietary Recommendations

Foods to include:

- Drink plenty of water to keep fluid moving through your urinary tract.

- Fish, chia seed, and flaxseed contain beneficial fatty acids that reduce inflammation.

- Foods rich in soy, like tofu, contain substances (isoflavones) that may protect the prostate.

- Pumpkin seeds contain zinc, an essential nutrient for the prostate.

- Tomatoes contain lycopene, a nutrient that has protective effects on the prostate. Cooked tomato products, such as tomato sauce and ketchup, actually contain more lycopene than fresh tomatoes.

Foods to avoid:

- Alcohol increases urine production and irritates your bladder.

- Caffeine will increase urine production, cause bladder irritation, and aggravate your symptoms.

- Saturated fat (red meat and dairy) can worsen symptoms.

- Sugar hampers immune function and may increase the risk of bladder infections. Limit candy, soft drinks, and sweets.

- Limit drinking after 7 p.m. to reduce your need to go to the bathroom during the night.

Lifestyle Suggestions

- Get regular checkups with your doctor. A symptom questionnaire, digital rectal exam, and PSA test (see below) are helpful in detecting an enlarged prostate.

- Exercise regularly. Studies show that men who are active have fewer symptoms of BPH.

- Empty your bladder regularly.

....

PSA TEST

Have your doctor do a PSA test. PSA stands for prostate-specific antigen, which is naturally produced in your prostate gland to help liquefy semen, and a small amount circulates in your blood. Having higher than normal levels in your blood could indicate BPH, prostate cancer, or prostatitis (infection or inflammation of the prostate).

....

Top Recommended Supplements

Beta-sitosterol: A cholesterol-like compound found in many plants. It reduces inflammation, and several studies have shown that it can improve urinary flow and BPH symptoms. Dosage: 60–130 mg daily. It may take four weeks to notice benefits.

Saw palmetto: An extract from saw palmetto berries, it is believed to work by inhibiting 5-alpha-reductase, the enzyme that converts testosterone to DHT. Numerous studies have shown that it can significantly improve urinary flow rate, reduce nighttime wakening, and improve most other measures of prostate disease. Studies have compared saw palmetto to the drugs Proscar and Flomax and found it equally effective, only better tolerated. Dosage: 160 mg twice a day of an extract standardized to contain 85 to 95 percent fatty acids and sterols.

Complementary Supplements

Nettle: Contains compounds that inhibit the binding of DHT to prostate cells. It has been studied alone and in combination with saw palmetto and pygeum and found to be beneficial. Dosage: 120 mg twice daily.

Pumpkin seed oil: Contains various compounds such as zinc, fatty acids, and plant sterols that support the health of the bladder and urethra. Preliminary research found that pumpkin seed oil with saw palmetto was beneficial for reducing symptoms of BPH. Dosage: 160 mg three times daily with meals.

Pygeum: An extract from the bark of the African tree; contains compounds that have anti-inflammatory and diuretic effects, and also inhibits prostate growth factors. Studies show that it can reduce symptoms such as nighttime urination, urinary frequency, and residual urine volume. It is sometimes combined with saw palmetto. Dosage: 50 mg twice daily.

FINAL THOUGHTS

To manage the symptoms of BPH, consider the following:

- Eat more tomato products, pumpkin seeds, soy, fish, and flaxseed.
- Avoid or minimize saturated fat, alcohol, caffeine, and sugar.
- Get regular exercise.
- Empty your bladder regularly.
- Consider supplements of beta-sitosterol and/or saw palmetto.

PSORIASIS

Psoriasis is a common and recurring condition that affects the life cycle of skin cells. Normally, it takes about a month for our skin cells to move from the lowest skin layer (where they're produced) to the outermost layer (where they die and flake off). In people with psoriasis, the entire life cycle takes only days. With rapid cell growth, the skin cells build up, forming thick, silvery scales and itchy, dry, red patches that are sometimes painful. This is considered a chronic condition as there are persistent periods of remission and then flare-ups.

It is thought that psoriasis is caused by a disorder of the immune system. Specifically, researchers believe that overactive T cells (a type of white blood cell) attack healthy skin cells, causing an increased production of skin cells and other immune responses that lead to an ongoing cycle of rapid skin turnover. Dead skin and white blood cells can't slough off quickly enough and build up in thick, scaly patches on the skin's surface. Researchers are not sure what causes the immune system to malfunction, but it is believed to be a combination of genetic and environmental factors. Certain factors can trigger or worsen psoriasis, such as a skin injury (a cut, bug bite, or severe sunburn), infection, extreme cold weather, smoking, heavy alcohol consumption, and use of certain medications such as lithium, beta-blockers, or anti-malaria drugs.

Psoriasis affects nearly 1 million Canadians. While it can be an uncomfortable and embarrassing condition to deal with, there are a number of medical treatments and natural approaches that can help improve the symptoms and quality of life for those suffering with this condition.

SIGNS & SYMPTOMS

- Bleeding, itching, burning, and soreness of the skin

- Dry, red patches of skin covered with silvery scales

- Pus-filled blisters

- Small scaly spots

- Swollen and stiff joints

- Thickened, pitted, or ridged nails

Note: The signs and symptoms vary in severity from person to person. Psoriasis most commonly affects areas of the body that are exposed to friction, irritation, or injury, such as the knees, elbows, feet, lower back, and scalp. Psoriasis can affect fingernails and toenails, causing pitting, abnormal nail growth, and discoloration. Severe cases may cause the nail to crumble. It can also affect the armpits and groin (called inverse psoriasis) or the joints (called psoriatic arthritis).

- Family history: About one in three people with psoriasis has a close relative with it.

- Immune system disorders, such as HIV or diabetes

- Obesity increases risk of inverse psoriasis (psoriasis in armpits, groin, and skin folds, and under breasts).

- Stress hampers immune function and increases risk of psoriasis.

- Smoking increases the risk of psoriasis and also makes the disease more severe.

DOCTOR'S ORDERS

The goal of treatment is to interrupt the cycle that causes an increased production of skin cells, thereby reducing inflammation and plaque formation, and to remove scales.

Topical products are helpful for mild to moderate psoriasis. They work on reducing inflammation and itching. Examples include the following:

- Corticosteroids: Hydrocortisone, betamethasone, mometasone (Elocom). Side effects include burning, itching, and thinning of the skin.
- Retinoids: Tazarotene (Tazorac). Side effects include skin irritation and sun sensitivity.
- Vitamin D analogues: Calcipotriene (Dovonex). These synthetic forms of vitamin D slow down the growth of skin cells. Side effects include skin irritation.
- Calcineurin inhibitors: Tacrolimus (Prograf) and pimecrolimus (Elidel). These products are not approved for use in psoriasis, but they have been shown to be beneficial in research and they are often prescribed. They work by reducing the activation of T cells, which reduces inflammation and plaque buildup. The most common side effect is skin irritation. They are not recommended for long-term or continuous use because of increased risk of skin cancer and lymphoma.
- Immunomodulator drugs or biologics are the newest class of drugs, and they work by interrupting the immune process that drives psoriasis. These drugs are typically only used in those who don't respond to other therapies. Examples include alefacept (Amevive), etanercept (Enbrel), infliximab (Remicade), and ustekinumab (Stelara). These drugs are given by injection.

Creams, ointments, and scalp treatments containing anthralin, coal tar, or salicylic acid are available over the counter or in specially made compounds in the pharmacy. Anthralin is a drug that has been used for decades for psoriasis. It helps reduce inflammation and remove scales, and makes the skin smoother. Side effects include skin irritation, and it stains the skin and anything it comes in contact with yellow/brown. Coal tar has also been used for a long time. It reduces scaling, itching, and inflammation, and it can also stain anything it comes in contact with. Salicylic acid helps slough off dead skin cells and reduces scaling.

Light therapy (phototherapy) involves the use of natural or artificial light. Light causes the activated T cells in the skin to die, thus slowing down skin cell turnover. Risks include skin irritation, sunburn, and increased risk of skin cancer.

Oral medication, such as retinoids (vitamin A derivatives), work by reducing the production of skin cells. Methotrexate helps psoriasis by decreasing the production of skin cells, suppressing inflammation, and reducing the release of histamine. There are also immune suppressants (azathioprine and cyclosporine) that are used for more severe cases. All of these drugs carry the risk of serious side effects, and some can deplete nutrients in the body (for example, methotrexate depletes folic acid), so it is important to discuss the benefits versus the risks with your doctor.

HOMEOPATHIC RECOMMENDATIONS

Graphites: Skin that is tough or leathery with cracks and soreness can benefit from this remedy.

Petroleum: This remedy helps people whose psoriasis is especially aggravated by stressful and emotional experiences.

Sulphur: This remedy may help psoriasis that is intensely burning, itching, with inflamed eruptions that worsen when warm. Affected areas often look bright red and irritated, with scaling skin that gets inflamed from scratching.

SHERRY'S NATURAL PRESCRIPTION

Dietary Recommendations

Foods to include:

- Essential fatty acids help to reduce inflammation. Eat more cold-water fish (salmon, herring, mackerel, and trout). Choose wild (not farmed) fish to avoid ingestion of toxic chemicals. Flaxseed and chia seed are also good sources of EFAs.

- Fibre-rich foods (whole grains, vegetables, and fruits) aid detoxification.

- Orange, yellow, and green vegetables contain vitamin A, which may be deficient in those with psoriasis.

- Pumpkin seeds provide zinc, which is often deficient in those with psoriasis.

- Yogurt contains beneficial bacteria that support gut health and immune function.

Foods to avoid:

- Alcohol can cause flare-ups and also decrease the effectiveness of treatments.

- Gluten, a protein in wheat, rye, and barley, can be a trigger for some people.

- Saturated fat (red meat and full-fat dairy products) may worsen inflammation.

To determine if food sensitivities are triggering your psoriasis, try an elimination diet (see Appendix D).

Lifestyle Suggestions

- Work on identifying and avoiding/minimizing your triggers. Stress, smoking, cold weather, and food sensitivities are common triggers.

- Bathe daily in warm water to remove scales and calm inflamed skin. Add mineral or sea salts, bath oil (lavender), or oatmeal to the water and soak for at least 15 minutes. Avoid hot water and harsh soaps, which can make your symptoms worse.

- Apply a moisturizer after bathing and reapply as needed. Use a heavy cream or an ointment as they will keep the skin hydrated longer than lotions. Products containing calendula, lavender, and avocado are soothing to the skin.

- Do not scratch, pick, or rub at the lesions; this will only make it worse.

- Acupuncture may be helpful.

- Spend some time in the sun. The body produces vitamin D when skin is exposed to sunlight, and vitamin D can improve skin lesions. However, too much sun can worsen the problem. Try 10 to 15 minutes in direct sunlight. When spending a longer time outdoors, apply a sunscreen to areas not affected with psoriasis to protect against sunburn.

Top Recommended Products

Fish oils: Contain omega-3 fatty acids that help reduce inflammation and skin lesions. Dosage: Choose a product with a high EPA concentration. One study found benefits with 3.6 g of EPA daily. Some research has also found benefits with applying fish oils (10 percent concentration) directly to the psoriatic lesions twice daily.

Oregon grape: Contains compounds that slow the rate of abnormal cell growth and reduce inflammation. Several studies have shown benefits for reducing symptoms, but it does not appear to be as effective as prescription creams. Dosage: Apply a cream containing 10 percent Oregon grape extract three times daily to the affected areas.

Complementary Products

Aloe vera: Helps to reduce inflammation and has antibacterial and antifungal properties. Some research has shown that it can reduce psoriasis symptoms. Dosage: Apply a cream that contains 0.5 percent aloe three to four times daily.

Capsaicin: An extract from cayenne pepper. Creams made from capsaicin are used to treat a number of pain-related conditions. Some research found that capsaicin cream may be helpful for psoriasis. Wash hands after application; avoid contact with eyes.

Celadrin: A blend of fatty acids that reduces inflammation, redness, and pain. Preliminary research suggests benefits for psoriasis. Dosage: Apply cream twice daily.

Probiotics: Support digestive health and immune function. Preliminary research on a specific probiotic, *Bifidobacterium infantis* 35624 (Align), found that it reduced markers of inflammation in those with psoriasis. Dosage: Take as directed.

FINAL THOUGHTS

To improve the management of psoriasis, consider the following:

- Eat more cold-water fish, pumpkin seeds, colourful vegetables, and whole grains.
- Avoid alcohol and minimize saturated fat intake.
- Reduce stress and don't smoke.
- Spend 10 to 15 minutes daily outdoors in the sun.
- Consider fish oil supplements and Oregon grape cream to reduce inflammation.

RESTLESS LEG SYNDROME

Restless leg syndrome (RLS) is a neurological or nervous system disorder causing discomfort and abnormal sensations throughout the legs and sometimes into the pelvis and arms. For some, the sensations may feel as though insects are creeping on or in their legs. People with RLS feel a strong urge to move, stretch, flex, or shake their limbs to ease the discomfort. This restlessness may prevent them from sitting comfortably for extended periods of time. Symptoms of RLS often worsen in the evening, causing serious disruptions to sleep.

Restless leg syndrome is very common—between 2 to 15 percent of people around the world suffer from this condition. Over 80 percent of people with RLS also experience uncontrollable movements of the arms or legs during sleep, a phenomenon called periodic limb movements in sleep (PLMS), which usually occur every minute or so throughout the night.

RLS may occur spontaneously (referred to as idiopathic) or may be triggered by an existing health condition, such as peripheral neuropathy or damage to the nerves in the hands and feet that is often due to chronic diseases such as diabetes and alcoholism. An imbalance of the brain chemical dopamine, which sends messages to control muscle movement, may be involved. Genetic factors may also play a role. Researchers have identified sites on the chromosomes where genes for RLS may be present. However, for many cases there is no known cause.

SIGNS & SYMPTOMS

- Abnormal sensations deep in the legs or arms (creeping, crawling, gnawing feelings)
- Itching, twitching, burning, throbbing, tugging, tingling, pins and needles, and pain
- Movement may help relieve symptoms temporarily

Note: The symptoms of RLS are worse in the evenings when a person is inactive, such as sitting or lying down or sleeping.

RISK FACTORS

- Age: More common in older adults, although it can occur at any age
- Chronic disease such as diabetes, kidney disease, high blood pressure, vascular disease, and Parkinson's disease
- Heredity: About 50 percent of people with RLS report a family member with the same condition.
- Lack of exercise
- Medications (drugs used for nausea, depression, mood disorders, and seizures)
- Nervous system disorders
- Nutritional deficiencies, particularly low levels of iron, calcium, or magnesium

- Obesity
- Poor diet, such as high intake of caffeine, alcohol, or sugar
- Pregnancy (particularly the third trimester) and hormonal changes
- Smoking
- Stress

DOCTOR'S ORDERS

Many people do not go to the doctor for RLS until their symptoms have become intolerable, often due to insomnia. Consult with your doctor if you have experienced the symptoms of RLS for more than a week.

RLS is often a sign of an existing health problem, so the standard treatment is to first identify and then treat the underlying cause. This may involve blood tests or a general examination regarding overall health, diet, lifestyle, and prescription drug use. If an underlying cause, such as nutritional deficiencies, is identified and treated, the symptoms of RLS may decrease or disappear altogether.

To counter mild symptoms, a doctor may recommend lifestyle approaches as noted below, and, for severe cases, medication.

There are four types of prescription medications that are used:

Anticonvulsants, like gabapentin (Neurontin), help ease the abnormal sensations.

Dopaminergic drugs boost dopamine levels, which help the central nervous system function better and reduce leg movements. Examples include pramipexole (Mirapex) and ropinirole (Requip).

Muscle relaxants and sedatives help promote relaxation and sleep, but they also cause drowsiness the next day and are addictive. Examples are clonazepam (Rivotril), lorazepam (Ativan), and temazepam (Restoril).

Opioids are narcotic pain killers, such as codeine and oxycodone (Percocet).
All of these medications have potential side effects and drug interactions. Make sure to discuss the benefits and risks with your doctor.

HOMEOPATHIC RECOMMENDATIONS

Zincum metallicum: This remedy relieves fidgety, restless legs, especially if drinking alcohol aggravates the condition.

SHERRY'S NATURAL PRESCRIPTION

There are a variety of natural strategies that can be effective in managing the symptoms of RLS.

Dietary Recommendations

Foods to include:

- Eat small, frequent meals to keep blood sugar levels stabilized as hypoglycemia (low blood sugar) can trigger RLS.

- Whole grains, fruits, vegetables, nuts, and seeds contain essential vitamins and minerals that are needed to support the nerves and muscles. Choose low-glycemic foods to prevent blood sugar fluctuations (see Appendix B).

Foods to avoid:

- Alcohol and caffeine can aggravate RLS symptoms. Minimize caffeine-containing products (including chocolate, coffee, tea, and soft drinks) for a few weeks to see if this helps.

- Refined starches (white bread) and sugar (soft drinks and candy) can cause blood sugar fluctuations, which can worsen RLS.

Lifestyle Suggestions

- Get regular exercise. Aim for 30 minutes to one hour daily. This will help reduce stress and improve sleep at night. Do not overdo it, because vigorous exercise can exacerbate the symptoms of RLS.

- Do not sit for extended periods of time. Take regular stretching breaks when seated at a desk or in a car.

- Lose excess weight, which may cause or worsen RLS.

- Reduce your stress load. Try acupuncture, meditation, massage, or yoga.

- Don't smoke, as smoking can trigger or worsen symptoms.

- Get adequate sleep. Fatigue can worsen symptoms. Aim for seven to nine hours of sleep per night and establish good sleep hygiene habits (make your bedroom quiet and comfortable, do relaxing activities in the evening, and go to bed and get up at the same time every day).

- To manage symptoms, try warm or cold packs, or alternating therapies to reduce the sensations.

Top Recommended Supplements

Iron: A deficiency in iron (even mild) can cause RLS. According to some reports, 25 percent of people with RLS have an iron deficiency. Studies have shown that when iron deficiency is the cause of RLS, supplementing can reduce the severity of the symptoms. Do not take iron supplements unless you have low iron levels (ask your doctor to check this) because too much iron can cause side effects. Dosage: Consult with your health care provider for dosage guidelines.

Magnesium: Helps to promote muscle relaxation and also improves sleep in those with RLS, according to preliminary research. Dosage: 300 mg at bedtime. Take along with 500 mg calcium to avoid loose stools. Calcium is also important for proper muscle and nerve function.

Multivitamin/mineral complex: Ensures that your body is getting all essential nutrients. Low levels of B-vitamins (especially B1, B6, B12, and folic acid) can impair muscle function and nerve health. B12 deficiency can cause peripheral neuropathy, which can trigger RLS. Dosage: Take daily.

Complementary Supplements

Melatonin: A hormone that is naturally secreted by the brain in response to darkness and regulates sleep/wake cycles. Supplements reduce the time needed to fall asleep, reduce nighttime wakening, and improve sleep quality. Melatonin has not been studied particularly for its effects on RLS, but it may be helpful for managing insomnia. Dosage: 3–6 mg one hour before bed.

Valerian: An herb that is widely used for insomnia; it improves many aspects of sleep and is non-addictive. It also helps reduce stress and anxiety, and preliminary research found it beneficial for RLS symptoms. Some formulas combine valerian with hops, passionflower, and other herbs that promote relaxation. Dosage: 600 mg half an hour to one hour before bed, or 2 mL of a tincture.

FINAL THOUGHTS

To relieve the discomfort of RLS, consider the following:

- Eat small, frequent meals with lots of whole grains, vegetables, and fruit. Reduce or eliminate caffeine, sugar, and alcohol.
- Don't smoke.
- Get regular exercise and avoid sitting for extended periods of time without stretching.
- Consider taking iron (if deficient), magnesium, and a multivitamin.
- Consider taking melatonin or valerian to improve sleep.

ROSACEA

Rosacea is a type of inflammatory skin condition that causes flushing, red splotches, lesions or bumps, and broken blood vessels across the cheeks, chin, forehead, and nose. Rosacea is often mistakenly referred to as "adult acne" or "acne rosacea" because it afflicts adults. While rosacea may resemble acne in that the outbreaks can come and go, triggered by a variety of lifestyle factors, unlike acne, rosacea outbreaks do not cause blackheads or whiteheads, and may often be accompanied by burning, stinging, or chapped, dry skin. Rosacea is also associated with several eye conditions, including swollen, burning, itchy eyes called ocular rosacea. Some estimates suggest that up to 2 million Canadians suffer from various degrees of rosacea. Since this condition has a traumatic impact on sufferers, it is critical to find ways to control the symptoms and reduce outbreaks.

DON'T IGNORE ROSACEA

If left untreated, advanced cases of rosacea may cause a condition called rhinophyma in which the skin thickens unnaturally. While rare, rhinophyma may cause large warty growths to appear around the nose, and the skin to take on a wax-like appearance.

SIGNS & SYMPTOMS

- Burning, stinging, dry skin
- Facial flushing, with persistent redness (though cheeks are not warm to the touch)
- Itchy, sore eyes
- Red, inflamed pimples or bumps (erythema)
- Swollen nose (mostly in men)
- Visible red veins on the face and blood vessel lines

RISK FACTORS

- Age: Affects adults between the ages of 20 and 60
- Gender: Women are more commonly affected
- Having fair skin
- Heredity
- Hormonal changes (pregnancy and menopause)

Factors that may trigger or worsen rosacea include use of birth control pills or drugs that affect blood vessels (vasodilators); caffeine; alcohol; hot or spicy foods or drinks; exposure to sun, wind, or cold temperatures; emotional stress; vigorous exercise; and hot baths or saunas.

DOCTOR'S ORDERS

There is no cure for rosacea, but medications are often prescribed to help control symptoms and prevent the skin condition from progressing. For mild rosacea, doctors often recommend topical antibiotic creams. For more severe cases, antibiotic pills may be prescribed in combination with antibiotic creams.

Azelaic acid cream (Finacea) is a new product available in Canada for the treatment of rosacea. This acid is found naturally in wheat, rye, and barley and has antimicrobial effects. Studies have found that it can reduce rosacea symptoms. One study that compared it to metronidazole (a commonly used antibiotic) found that azelaic acid provided better results for improving skin redness and pimples.

For advanced cases of rosacea, cosmetic surgery such as laser surgery or dermabrasion may be recommended. Dermabrasion is a cosmetic procedure that "sands" or "finishes" the top layer of the skin, giving it a smoother appearance.

Do not use over-the-counter products formulated for treating common (teenage) acne as the main ingredients (salicylic acid and benzyol peroxide) can worsen rosacea.

SHERRY'S NATURAL PRESCRIPTION

Dietary Recommendations

Foods to include:

- Drink at least eight glasses of filtered water daily.

- Eat a fibre-rich diet (whole grains, vegetables, and fruits) to support the body's natural elimination and detoxification process. These foods also contain vital nutrients (vitamin C, B-vitamins, and zinc) for skin health.

- Essential fatty acids help reduce inflammation. Eat three or more servings per week of cold-water fish, along with flaxseed, chia seed, and other nuts and seeds.

- Green tea is a potent antioxidant and detoxifier. Drink green tea instead of coffee or black teas. A green food supplement may support improved digestion and detoxification.

- Yogurt and kefir with active cultures provide beneficial bacteria that support digestion and immune health and may offer benefits for reducing inflammation. It is particularly important to eat these foods if you are using antibiotics such as metronidazole, which can deplete the beneficial bacteria.

Foods to avoid:

- Avoid hot, spicy foods and beverages, as they can worsen symptoms.

- Minimize salt and alcohol intake, which can dilate blood vessels and worsen symptoms.

- Reduce stimulants in your diet, such as chocolate and coffee.

- Saturated fats (red meat and dairy) can worsen inflammation. Keep a food journal to determine potential triggers.

Lifestyle Suggestions

- Reduce stress; try stress-reduction techniques like massage.

- Avoid washing with hot water or using scrub brushes or face cloths.

- Use a gentle cleanser and moisturizer daily. Look for products that contain soothing ingredients such as aloe vera, burdock, calendula, chamomile, rosehips, and vitamin E. Look for the words "safe for sensitive skin" or "hypoallergenic."

- Avoid extended sunlight exposure as the sun is a common trigger. Use sunscreen with at least SPF 30 when going outdoors, and wear a wide-brimmed hat.

- Consider stress-reduction therapies such as massage, yoga, or meditation. Exercise is also a great way to reduce stress and boost confidence.

- Avoid smoking and second-hand smoke as nicotine damages blood vessels.

Top Recommended Supplements

Golden chamomile cream: Also known as *Chrysanthellum indicum*, it helps reduce redness and inflammation. In a large clinical study, application of this cream twice daily significantly improved rosacea symptoms. Look for a product that contains a 1 percent concentration, and apply twice daily.

Green tea: Has antioxidant and anti-inflammatory properties. Some research has shown that green tea cream can reduce redness and pustules. Look for a product that contains 2 percent polyphenone and apply twice daily.

Complementary Supplements

Digestive enzymes: It is thought that some people with rosacea have digestive problems and low stomach acid. Preliminary research has found benefits with digestive enzymes supplements. Dosage: One or two capsules with each meal.

Cetylated fatty acids: Help to reduce inflammation. One preliminary study of a topical product called Celadrin found that it reduced inflammation and redness. Oral supplements of fish oils, borage, or evening primrose may also be helpful. Dosage: Follow label directions.

Zinc: Those with rosacea may be deficient in zinc; one study found significant benefits with supplements. Dosage: 23 mg three times daily; this is a higher than usual dosage and should be taken along with copper to avoid copper depletion. Consult with your health care provider for guidance.

R

Rosacea

FINAL THOUGHTS

To manage rosacea, consider the following:

- Identify triggers of your outbreaks and reduce exposure to those triggers.
- Eat lots of fibre-rich foods such as fruits, vegetables, legumes, nuts and seeds, whole grains, fish, and flaxseed.
- Reduce stress and minimize sun exposure (wear sunscreen).
- Use a gentle facial cleanser that contains soothing ingredients such as aloe vera, calendula, and rosehips.
- Use a topical cream containing golden chamomile or green tea regularly.

SEASONAL AFFECTIVE DISORDER (SAD)

Seasonal affective disorder (SAD) is a form of depression that follows the seasons, where there are recurrent and cyclic bouts of depression and increased need for sleep. It typically occurs during the winter months and goes away during the spring and summer, although a small number of people experience depression during the summer.

Approximately 4 percent of Canadians suffer from SAD, while another 15 percent may experience mild winter blues. Although the exact cause is unknown, it is thought that a disruption in the circadian rhythm (our sleep–wake cycle) is at the root of the problem. Our circadian rhythm is controlled by the rise and fall of various hormones, most notably melatonin. Melatonin is a hormone secreted by the pineal gland when photoreceptors in the eye sense darkness. Melatonin makes us feel sleepy and helps keep us asleep. Levels of melatonin wane toward morning when we wake up.

Several factors may lead to alterations in our circadian rhythm, including increased melatonin secretion during the darker winter months, which causes increased sleepiness and difficulty waking in the morning. Elevated levels of inflammatory chemicals released by the body during the winter months may lead to a serotonin deficiency, which cause depression. There is also evidence that those with SAD have lower levels of the neurotransmitters serotonin, acetylcholine, and dopamine for unknown reasons.

Fortunately, there are a number of lifestyle measures and supplements that can improve emotional well-being and reduce SAD symptoms.

SIGNS & SYMPTOMS

- Cravings for carbohydrates (sweets and starchy foods)
- Depression
- Difficulty concentrating
- Fatigue and increased need for sleep
- Feelings of hopelessness and sadness
- Increased appetite and weight gain
- Irritability and anxiety
- Loss of interest in sex
- Social withdrawal
- Thoughts of suicide

DOCTOR'S ORDERS

Medical treatment of SAD involves light therapy and/or medication. Light therapy should be tried first, as it is highly effective—80 percent of people experience improvement. A specially made light box providing full-spectrum light is used for 30 to 60 minutes. Benefits may be noticed in as little as a few days to a week. Light therapy should be used daily during the fall and winter until symptoms subside and enough daylight is available.

If light therapy doesn't help, doctors may recommend medication. Antidepressant drugs that raise serotonin or dopamine levels can help alleviate symptoms. Examples include paroxetine (Paxil), fluoxetine (Prozac), sertraline (Zoloft), and bupropion (Wellbutrin). These drugs cause a number of side effects such as increased appetite and weight gain, fatigue, nausea, sexual dysfunction, and anxiety.

SHERRY'S NATURAL PRESCRIPTION

Dietary Recommendations

Foods to include:

- Vegetables, fruits, whole grains, nuts, and seeds provide vitamins, minerals, and essential fatty acids, which may be depleted in those with depression.

- Turkey, chicken, tuna, salmon, legumes, nuts, and seeds contain the amino acid tryptophan, which elevates serotonin production.

- Fish is also a good source of omega-3 fatty acids, which are important for emotional well-being. Flaxseed and chia seed provide plant sources of omega-3s.

- Eat small, frequent meals to maintain energy levels and mood.

Foods to avoid:

- Sugar and refined carbohydrates may temporarily elevate your mood, but the effect is short term and these foods cause blood sugar imbalances, mood swings, and irritability.

- Caffeine is a stimulant that offers a temporary rush of energy followed by fatigue and irritability, plus it depletes nutrients from your body. Have no more than one cup of coffee per day and minimize other caffeinated beverages such as soft drinks.

- Processed and fast foods often contain chemicals and preservatives that may upset brain chemistry.

- Alcohol is a depressant and should be minimized or avoided completely.

Lifestyle Suggestions

- Exercise regularly; engage in fall/winter activities outside to maximize available sunshine. With proper winter clothing, walking, skating, and skiing can be a great way to get exercise and sunshine, plus exercise is a natural mood elevator, improves sleep, and helps combat stress.

- Increase the amount of light in your environment—sit near a window, open blinds, and trim any trees that block your exposure to the sun.

- Try light therapy. Specially made light boxes or light visors are available that provide broad spectrum light. These are used for 30 minutes to several hours each day. Benefits may be noticed in as little as a few days. However, it may take a week or longer to get the full effect. Light therapy should be used regularly during the fall and winter months until symptoms subside and enough daylight is available.

- Acupuncture has been found to be beneficial for depression. It may work by stimulating the production of neurotransmitters.

- Massage and reflexology relieve stress and tension, and promote relaxation.

- Counselling or psychotherapy can help provide coping techniques and strategies.

Top Recommended Supplements

5-hydroxytryptophan (5-HTP): A substance used by the body to create serotonin. Research shows benefits for depression and improving quality of sleep. It may cause nausea, which can be minimized by taking an enteric-coated product. Dosage: 100–200 mg three times daily.

S-adenosylmethionine (SAMe): Supports the production of neurotransmitters (serotonin, dopamine, and norepinephrine); is shown to be beneficial for depression. SAMe is well tolerated, has benefits for joint and liver health, and a quick onset of action (two weeks). Dosage: 400–1,600 mg daily on an empty stomach; start with a low dose and gradually increase if needed.

....

AVOID EXCESS SEROTONIN

Be cautious about combining products that elevate serotonin, such as SSRI or MAO-I drugs, St. John's wort, SAMe, and 5-HTP together. This should be done only under the supervision of a health care professional, as excess serotonin can cause serotonin syndrome. Symptoms include confusion, anxiety, racing heart, nausea, and muscle spasms.

....

Complementary Supplements

B-complex: B-vitamins (such as B12 and folic acid) may be deficient in those with SAD. Folic acid works with SAMe to boost neurotransmitter levels. Several studies have found benefits. Dosage: Take 400–1,000 mcg of folic acid along with 50–100 mg of other B-vitamins daily to support brain function.

Fish oils: Rich in omega-3 fatty acids, which are essential for the nervous system and neurotransmitter function. Levels may be depleted in those with depression. Studies show benefits for depression, especially for those not getting an adequate response to antidepressant drugs. Dosage: 3–9 g daily.

Magnesium: A deficiency may contribute to alterations in the circadian rhythm and low levels of serotonin. Dosage: 150–00 mg at bedtime.

Vitamin D: Vitamin D is produced by the body in response to sun exposure, and levels may be depleted in those with SAD. Preliminary studies have found that supplements can minimize symptoms of SAD in those with low levels of vitamin D. Dosage: 400–1,000 IU daily.

St. John's wort: Several studies have found it effective for mild to moderate depression and SAD. Dosage: 300 mg three times daily.

Note: St. John's wort can interact with many medications, and it should be used cautiously along with light therapy because it can cause light sensitivity, skin rash, and eye damage.

FINAL THOUGHTS

To improve mood and reduce the symptoms of SAD, consider the following:

- Minimize sugar, refined/processed foods, caffeine, and alcohol.
- Eat more tryptophan-containing foods.
- Exercise regularly to reduce stress and improve mood and sleep.
- Maximize your exposure to natural light and try light therapy.
- Consider supplements of SAMe or 5-HTP. Fish oils, B-vitamins, magnesium, and vitamin D can play an important supportive role.

S

Seasonal Affective Disorder (SAD)

SINUSITIS

Sinusitis is an inflammation of the sinuses, the air-filled hollow cavities around your nose and nasal passages. Sinusitis develops when the mucous membranes of your upper respiratory tract (nose, pharynx, sinuses, and throat) become inflamed. The swelling obstructs the sinus openings and prevents mucus from draining normally. This creates a moist environment that can breed infection. It also makes it difficult to breathe and causes pain around the nose, eyes, and forehead.

Sinusitis can be either acute (short term) or chronic. Acute sinusitis often develops as a result of the common cold virus. Most colds resolve within a week or two, but nearly 2 percent develop into acute sinusitis. A virus can damage the tissues in the sinuses and then bacteria can invade, creating an infection. Acute sinusitis can also result from a fungal infection, especially in those with diabetes or compromised immune function.

Sinusitis is considered chronic when it lasts longer than 12 weeks. Chronic sinusitis can result from a weakened immune system, which leads to recurrent respiratory infections and chronic inflammation of the sinuses. Nasal polyps, a deviated septum, smoking, allergies, and exposure to irritants can also cause chronic sinusitis.

There are many things that can be done from a dietary and lifestyle perspective to prevent and manage sinusitis. Nutritional supplements can also play a role in helping to speed healing and reduce inflammation.

SIGNS & SYMPTOMS

- Bad breath

- Cough

- Difficulty breathing through your nose

- Fatigue

- Fever

- Nasal congestion and greenish-yellow discharge

- Nausea

- Pain under the eyes or around the nose, cheeks, jaw, or forehead

- Redness of the skin over the sinus caused by increased blood flow to the capillaries

- Reduced sense of smell or taste

Note: If untreated, sinusitis may trigger asthma attacks and cause visual impairment. If it is severe and untreated, it can also lead to meningitis.

- Allergies trigger inflammation that may block your sinuses.

- Dental infection (abscessed tooth)

- Deviated septum (alterations in the wall between the nostrils)

- Having a respiratory infection such as a cold or flu

- Having cystic fibrosis, gastroesophageal reflux disease, or a weakened immune system (e.g., HIV)

- Nasal polyps

- Smoking or exposure to air pollution

DOCTOR'S ORDERS

See your doctor for proper diagnosis because sinusitis and migraines can cause similar symptoms (pain in the area around the sinuses and causing your eyes to tear) and both can be triggered by weather. They differ in the origin of the problem. Sinus pain (headache) is due to inflammation or infection of the sinuses, while migraines cause inflammation of nerves and blood vessels in the head. When the trigeminal nerve is affected, it sends signals to the sinus region, causing sinus pain.

Most cases of sinusitis subside within a week or two and rarely require antibiotics. If your doctor suspects you have a bacterial infection, then an antibiotic may be necessary. If allergies are suspected, you may be referred to an allergist to identify your triggers and develop a treatment strategy.

Corticosteroids may be prescribed to treat the inflammation. They are available as tablets and sprays. Oral tablets such as prednisone are used for more serious cases and only on a short-term basis, because they can cause a range of side effects including weight gain, thinning of the bones, mood swings, high blood pressure, and acne. Sprays are less likely to cause these side effects and include such products as beclomethasone (Beconase), mometasone (Nasonex), budesonide (Rhinocort), and fluticasone (Flonase). They are also more rapidly acting.

Over-the-counter nasal decongestants, such as pseudoephedrine (Sudafed) tablets and oxymetazoline (Dristan) spray, can help relieve congestion and nasal stuffiness. Both oral and nasal decongestants can cause racing heart, increased blood pressure, and insomnia, and they can interact with certain medications. They should not be used for longer than three days because of the risk of rebound congestion. Saline nasal sprays are a safer alternative. They lubricate the nasal passages and reduce stuffiness without the side effects of the decongestants. If necessary, pain relievers such as acetaminophen (Tylenol) or ibuprofen (Motrin) can be taken.

SHERRY'S NATURAL PRESCRIPTION

Dietary Recommendations

Foods to include:

- Drink plenty of fluids (water, juice, and herbal tea) to dilute mucus secretions and promote drainage. Look for herbal teas that contain marshmallow, licorice, and slippery elm.

- Eat foods fortified with Wellmune, a natural ingredient that activates immune cells and enhances immune function. It can help with prevention and recovery. It is found in various juices, cookies, bars, and soups. It is safe for children as well as adults.

- Elderberry is antiviral and can help improve the immune response to infection. This is available in pure juice form, teas, and supplements (Sambucol).

- Fish and flaxseed contain essential fatty acids that help reduce inflammation.

- Fruits and vegetables (especially berries, citrus, garlic, onions, and ginger) provide important nutrients and compounds that support immune function.

- Green tea contains antioxidants that help support the immune system. There is some evidence that chicken soup can help reduce symptoms (congestion and sore throat) and speed healing.

- Horseradish helps break up mucus. Have ½ tsp to 1 tsp of the freshly grated root three times per day.

Foods to avoid:

- Alcohol can worsen swelling in the sinuses.

- Cow's-milk dairy products may worsen mucus secretions in those with a dairy sensitivity.

- Minimize salt as it can be dehydrating.

- Sugar can hamper immune function.

Many people with chronic sinusitis have food allergies. If you suspect food allergies, try an elimination diet (see Appendix D) to determine which foods are triggering your symptoms.

Lifestyle Suggestions

- Nasal irrigation, such as using a Neti pot or nasal wash, can help clear mucus from your nasal passages, relieve congestion and dryness, and improve breathing. Make a salt-water solution by mixing 1 tsp salt with 500 mL (16 ounces) purified lukewarm water. Lean forward over a sink and slowly pour the solution into one nostril and let it run out the other nostril. This can be repeated a few times daily. You can also use a nasal wash solution with essential oils such as menthol, eucalyptol, thymol, camphor, wintergreen, spearmint, and/or pine. Nasal irrigation can help relieve congestion and soothe and lubricate the nasal passages.

- Try a therapeutic steam inhalation by leaning over a bowl of hot water with a few drops of eucalyptus oil.

- Don't smoke, and avoid second-hand smoke as tobacco is very irritating to the nasal passages and causes inflammation.

- Minimize exposure to pollution and known allergens and irritants, such as perfumes, chemicals, and preservatives.

- Use an air purifier in your home and a humidifier if the air is dry.

- Apply warm compresses around your nose, cheeks, and eyes to ease pain.

- Acupuncture and craniosacral therapy are helpful in clearing the sinuses and relieving nasal congestion and pressure.

Top Recommended Supplements

American ginseng: Helps support immune function. Studies conducted with a particular extract of North American ginseng (COLD-FX), standardized to polysaccharides, have shown that it can reduce the frequency, severity, and duration of colds and flu. It may help prevent respiratory infections from leading to sinusitis. Dosage: 200–300 mg twice daily.

Bromelain: An enzyme derived from pineapple, which has anti-inflammatory properties and has been shown in studies to reduce symptoms of sinusitis. Dosage: 250–500 mg three times daily between meals.

Echinacea: Helps support immune function, and studies show that it can reduce the severity and frequency of cold symptoms. It may also help prevent a cold from developing into sinusitis. Look for *Echinacea purpurea*. Dosage: 300–600 mg capsules twice daily or 2–4 mL tincture four to six times daily at the first sign of a cold for seven to ten days. Some products combine echinacea with astragalus, which also has antiviral and antibacterial properties.

Complementary Supplements

Aged garlic extract: Contains antioxidant compounds that help support immune function. When taken regularly, it may help prevent colds and bacterial infections. Dosage: 600 mg daily.

Fish oils: Contain essential fatty acids that help reduce inflammation. One study in children found that daily fish oil supplements reduced the risk of recurrent respiratory tract infections. Dosage: Children should take 15 mg EPA plus DHA per pound of body weight per day; adults should take 1–3 g EPA plus DHA daily.

N-acetylcysteine (NAC): An amino acid derivative that helps break up mucus and clear the sinuses. Dosage: 300–600 mg daily.

Vitamin C: Supports immune function and helps prevent oxidative damage to the lungs. Studies have shown that it can reduce the severity and duration of the common cold, which may reduce the likelihood of complications like sinusitis. Dosage: 500 mg daily.

FINAL THOUGHTS

To improve healing of sinusitis and prevent it from occurring, consider the following:

- Eat more fruits, vegetables, fish, onions, garlic, ginger, and horseradish.
- Drink lots of fluids, especially water and herbal teas.
- Avoid smoking and being around smoke and other irritants.
- Try nasal irrigation to clear the sinuses, ease congestion, and make breathing easier.
- Bromelain can help reduce inflammation and symptoms. Echinacea and COLD-FX may help to shorten the duration of a cold, and COLD-FX can be taken to prevent a cold from becoming sinusitis.

Sinusitis

STRESS

Stress has become an all too familiar complaint today, hence the commonly heard phrase "stressed out." While we think of stress as an outside force, it is actually how we react internally to external stimuli, whether it is family pressures, deadlines at work, or being stuck in traffic.

Nearly half of all adults suffer adverse health effects from stress, and stress-related ailments account for between 75 and 90 percent of all visits to the doctor.

This innate mechanism was designed to help us cope with short bursts of stress, such as that caused by the attack of a predator. Our bodies have not adapted to handle the chronic stress that is so common today, which leads to damage and destruction throughout the body.

According to Dr. Hans Selye, a Canadian endocrinologist and the first person to coin the term *stress*, the physical experience of continuous stress has three stages: alarm, resistance, and exhaustion. In the alarm stage, the sympathetic nervous system activates our biologically programmed fight-or-flight mode. The stress hormones catecholamines (adrenaline and noradrenaline) and glucocorticoids (cortisol) are released. Secreted by the adrenal glands, these hormones prepare the body to fight. When this occurs, the body enters a catabolic state; that is, it begins to break down fuels (fats, stored sugar) to provide energy. Our senses are heightened and heart rate, blood pressure, blood volume, and pulmonary (lung) tone increase to enhance the function of the heart and lungs. When the perceived threat or danger is gone, the parasympathetic system activates the relaxation response.

More recently stress experts have modified the name of this stage to the flight-fight-freeze response, recognizing that some people will freeze in a state of alarm, like a deer in headlights. The freeze response can occur when a person feels like there is no chance of survival or escape and they freeze as a mechanism of self-preservation. The same neurotransmitters and hormones that help the body relax are also dumped into the bloodstream in huge amounts when the freeze response kicks in.

At the resistance stage, the body works to heal itself by adapting resistance mechanisms to counter the negative effects of stress. More cortisol is released to stimulate the conversion of protein, fat, and carbohydrates into energy in an attempt to help the body cope. If this stage continues, the elevated cortisol levels can wreak havoc on various body systems and cause a person to feel tired but wired and anxious, and to have difficulty sleeping.

If the stress continues, we may eventually fall into the exhaustion stage, where the adrenal glands can no longer respond to the stress. Cortisol levels drop, mental and physical fatigue (burn out) sets in, and stress-related disorders may surface.

Numerous studies have linked chronic stress to a number of serious health conditions. Stress promotes inflammation and clotting, raises blood pressure and cholesterol levels, and is a well-established risk factor for heart attacks and stroke. Chronic stress is associated with insulin resistance and diabetes. Stress is also linked to various forms of cancer, anxiety, depression, memory loss, insomnia, muscle tension, obesity, fatigue, low libido, hypothyroidism, erectile dysfunction, and menstrual cycle disturbances.

It is absolutely critical to find positive ways to handle stress. There are a variety of lifestyle, nutritional, and supplemental approaches that can help, which are discussed in this section.

SIGNS & SYMPTOMS

- Changes in appetite and weight
- Decreased concentration, memory problems
- Depression, mood swings
- Digestive problems (upset stomach, ulcers, colitis, constipation, and diarrhea)
- Exacerbation of asthma or arthritis
- Fatigue
- Headaches
- High blood pressure
- Hormonal imbalances (cortisol, DHEA, thyroid, estrogen, and testosterone)
- Infertility
- Insomnia
- Loss of libido (low sex drive)
- Muscle tension
- Nervousness, anxiety, irritability
- Skin disorders (rash, hives)
- Weakened immune system and increased risk of infection

RISK FACTORS

Almost any aspect of life, from the weather to work, traffic, and family relationships, can cause stress depending on how you respond to these events. Even small things such as spilling your morning coffee or being low on gas might trigger stress. Here are some of the most common triggers for stress:

- Being the victim of a crime or being in an accident
- Family demands and disagreements
- Financial concerns and taxes
- Holidays and special events
- Home-related concerns such as renovations, buying or selling, and moving
- Illness or death of a loved one
- Unexpected events or events we cannot control
- Work, new work, or loss of work

DOCTOR'S ORDERS

Doctors frequently see patients only after the negative effects of prolonged stress have started. As a result, they are often left to treat the visible complaint, such as insomnia, blood pressure, ulcers, or depression. In most cases, these secondary health concerns are treated with prescription medications, but healthy eating, sleep, and stress management should be the central focus. As well, it is important that hormone levels be checked to see if there are any abnormalities in cortisol, DHEA, or thyroid and sex hormones. For example, chronic stress and high cortisol levels can lead to low DHEA levels, which can lead to a variety of physical and emotional symptoms. Hormone levels need to be addressed as part of a comprehensive strategy.

In some cases drugs are necessary to treat the consequences of stress, such as depression or anxiety. The main class of drugs used to treat anxiety and stress include the benzodiazepines, namely, alprazolam (Xanax), clonazepam (Rivotril), diazepam (Valium), and lorazepam (Ativan). These drugs work quickly (within 30 to 60 minutes) to ease anxiety and promote relaxation, but they are addictive and have numerous side effects, including drowsiness, loss of coordination, dizziness, and impaired memory. These drugs can also cause tolerance (meaning you need higher dosages to get the same effect). Antidepressants are sometimes prescribed for stress when it occurs with depression or anxiety. Examples include fluoxetine (Prozac), sertraline (Zoloft), and citalopram (Celexa). Side effects of these drugs include sleep disturbances, weight gain, and sexual dysfunction. In some cases, they can worsen anxiety.

People suffering from chronic stress may also want to seek the help of a mental health professional to identify and resolve issues in their life or to provide support for coping.

SHERRY'S NATURAL PRESCRIPTION

Dietary Recommendations

Foods to include:

- Drink lots of purified water and calming herbal teas containing chamomile, lemon balm, and passionflower.

- Start your day with a proper breakfast to fuel your body with energy and provide essential nutrients to be able to cope with stress. Good choices include oatmeal, eggs, berries, and yogurt.

- Eat small, frequent meals with low-glycemic carbohydrates such as whole grains, legumes, and fruits and vegetables and healthy fats (olive, palm fruit, chia seed, avocado, fish). These foods provide the body with good sources of energy and essential nutrients, such as minerals, B-vitamins, and essential fatty acids that are needed to help the body deal with stress.

- Ensure adequate protein intake. Protein provides sustained energy and is required for muscle repair and growth. Choose lean poultry, fish, beans, legumes, nuts, and seeds (chia and flaxseed).

Foods to avoid:

- Caffeine and alcohol can trigger cortisol release and worsen stress and mood. Wean off caffeine slowly to avoid withdrawal symptoms, which can worsen anxiety. Avoid soft drinks, which are high in caffeine, sugar, and artificial chemicals. Limit alcohol to one to two drinks per day.

- Fast foods and processed foods (snack foods) are high in saturated fat and sugar and low in nutritional value. These foods can trigger anxiety and mood swings.

- Sugary foods cause fluctuations in blood sugar, which may cause mood swings and worsen stress. Cut down on candy, baked goods, condiments, and snack foods.

Lifestyle Suggestions

- Develop a positive attitude toward life's many challenges and work on managing anger and hostility. Practise controlling or redirecting your frustrations into something positive.

- Train your mind to react differently to current triggers.

- Learn to be more flexible and let go of things you cannot control.

- Develop strategies to deal with stressful situations or avoid the things that cause the most stress. (For example, listen to music, news, or an audio book while driving; bring a book to the doctor's office and read while you are waiting.)

- Proper time management and organizational skills help prevent stressful situations from occurring.

- Embrace friends and family. Studies show that close friendships contribute to less stress and a longer life.

- Get regular exercise. Exercise releases nervous energy and induces a calming effect. You can do vigorous exercise such as running or calming exercises such as yoga.

- Get adequate sleep at night. Sleep allows the body to recuperate and regenerate. When we are tired, we are more susceptible to stress.

- Deep breathing calms the body and slows the heart rate. Consider meditation or acupuncture to promote calming.

- Massage helps loosen muscle tension caused by stress and improves circulation.

- Don't smoke. Many smokers light up when they are stressed, but smoking actually worsens stress and causes nervous system damage.

Top Recommended Supplements

Multivitamin/mineral complex: Several studies have shown that a daily supplement of B-vitamins, vitamin C, and minerals can improve the effects of chronic stress, reducing fatigue and anxiety and improving concentration, mood, and overall well-being. These nutrients are essential for nervous system and adrenal function; a deficiency can cause anxiety and worsen the response to stress.

Lactium: A milk protein that contains bioactive peptide with antistress properties. Several studies have shown that lactium can help reduce the physical and mental effects and symptoms of stress. Dosage: 150 mg twice daily as needed.

Stress

Suntheanine: A patented extract of the amino acid L-theanine. It promotes calming and relaxation without drowsiness or addiction. It also helps improve sleep quality. Dosage: 50–200 mg daily.

Complementary Supplements

Panax ginseng: An adaptogenic herb that helps reduce the response to stress. It also supports physical and mental performance, immune function, and adrenal gland function, all of which can be hampered by stress. Dosage: 100–200 mg daily.

Relora: A combination of magnolia and phellodendron, which reduces stress without causing drowsiness. It is non-addictive. Dosage: 250 mg three times daily.

Rhodiola: An adaptogenic herb (increases the body's resistance to stress). Research suggests it can help reduce fatigue and improve mental alertness when under stress. Dosage: 100–200 mg daily.

Tongkat ali: Also known as *Eurycoma longifolia*. Several clinical studies on a patented form of this plant, Physta, show that it can boost DHEA levels, normalize cortisol levels, and increase energy and vitality. Dosage: 200–600 mg daily.

Valerian: An herb with relaxing and calming properties. It causes drowsiness, so it can be helpful for those with insomnia due to stress. Dosage: 300–500 mg of an extract an hour before bed.

Vitamin C: Helps the adrenal glands deal with the stress response. It also helps in the production of important neurotransmitters that are required for mood and proper sleep, and it provides support for cardiovascular and immune function. Dosage: 500 mg twice daily.

FINAL THOUGHTS

To better manage stress and reduce its adverse health effects, consider the following:

- Eat a healthy diet that is rich in vegetables, fruits, legumes, nuts, and seeds, and choose lean protein and healthy fats.
- Reduce or eliminate processed fast foods, caffeine, refined starches, sugar, alcohol, and tobacco.
- Identify your stress triggers and work on strategies to cope more effectively. Try yoga, tai chi, meditation, massage, or acupuncture to promote relaxation.
- Get regular exercise and adequate sleep.
- Consider taking B-vitamins, calcium, magnesium, Lactium, and Suntheanine.

STROKE

A stroke, which is also called a brain attack, is sudden loss of brain function that develops when an artery supplying oxygen-rich blood to the brain becomes blocked or ruptures. Without adequate blood flow, brain cells begin to die within minutes. Areas of the brain commonly affected by stroke are those that control movement, speech, vision, and sensation. Stroke is a medical emergency that requires immediate treatment to minimize damage to the brain and disability.

There are two types of stroke: ischemic and hemorrhagic. About 80 percent of all strokes are ischemic strokes. They occur when blood clots or other particles block arteries to your brain and cause severely reduced blood flow (ischemia). This deprives your brain cells of oxygen and nutrients, and cells may begin to die within minutes. Hemorrhagic stroke occurs when a blood vessel in your brain leaks or ruptures. This can result from a number of conditions that affect your blood vessels, such as uncontrolled high blood pressure (hypertension) and weak spots in your blood vessel walls (aneurysms).

Stroke is the third leading cause of death in Canada. According to the Heart and Stroke Foundation, 6 percent of all deaths in Canada are due to stroke, and each year nearly 14,000 Canadians die from stroke. The economic impact of stroke can also be devastating. It is estimated that stroke costs the Canadian economy $3.6 billion a year in physician services, hospital costs, lost wages, and decreased productivity.

With recent medical advances and prompt treatment, your chance of surviving a stroke today is much greater than it was a few decades ago. About half of all people who have a stroke recover to some degree, although about one-third of first strokes are fatal, so prevention and early detection/treatment are critical. The various factors known to increase your risk of stroke are outlined below. Many of them are lifestyle related and within your control.

SIGNS & SYMPTOMS

- Confusion or memory loss
- Problems with spatial orientation or perception
- Sudden difficulty speaking, seeing clearly, or understanding speech
- Sudden dizziness and loss of balance and coordination
- Sudden massive headache, which may be accompanied by a stiff neck, facial pain, and pain around the eyes
- Sudden numbness, weakness, or paralysis of your face, arm, or leg, which often occurs on one side of your body
- Women may experience unique symptoms such as hiccups, nausea, chest pain, shortness of breath, and palpitations.

Unfortunately, some people have no warning signs of a stroke and it happens suddenly. Some people may have a mini-stroke called a transient ischemic attack (TIA) before a major stroke. A TIA is a temporary interruption of blood flow to a part of your brain. It causes the same signs and symptoms as a stroke, but it lasts for a short time (a few minutes to several hours) and then disappears. A TIA represents a serious risk that a full-blown stroke may follow.

- Age: More common in older adults (over the age of 55).

- Alcohol: Excessive intake of alcohol (more than two drinks per day for women and three for men) can increase risk.

- Diabetes is a major risk factor for stroke because it increases the risk of high blood pressure and atherosclerosis; diabetes also interferes with your body's ability to break down blood clots, increasing your risk of ischemic stroke.

- Estrogen therapy: Taking birth control pills or estrogen therapy for menopause increases your risk; the risk is higher for smokers and those over the age of 35.

- Family history: Having a parent or sibling who had a stroke or TIA.

- Gender: Strokes affect men and women about equally, but women are more likely to die of stroke than are men.

- Heart disease: Having congestive heart failure, a previous heart attack, an infection of a heart valve (endocarditis), an abnormal heart rhythm (atrial fibrillation), aortic or mitral valve disease, valve replacement, or a hole in the upper chambers of the heart will increase risk.

- High blood pressure weakens and damages blood vessels in and around your brain, leaving them vulnerable to atherosclerosis and hemorrhage.

- High LDL cholesterol and triglycerides increase your risk of atherosclerosis; in contrast, high levels of HDL (good) cholesterol reduce your risk of atherosclerosis by removing cholesterol from your body through your liver.

- Inactivity doubles the risk for stroke.

- Obesity increases the risk of high blood pressure, heart disease, atherosclerosis, and diabetes, all of which increase your risk of a stroke.

- Personal history: Having one TIA or stroke increases the risk of another one.

- Race: First Nations and those of African or South Asian descent are at greater risk of stroke partly because of a higher prevalence of high blood pressure and diabetes.

- Smoking contributes to plaques in your arteries and makes your heart work harder by increasing your heart rate and blood pressure; it also reduces oxygen delivery to your tissues, including the brain.

- Stress increases blood pressure, cholesterol, and risk of atherosclerosis, all major risk factors for stroke.

- Emerging research suggests that elevated levels of homocysteine, C-reactive protein, and fibrinogen are associated with an increased risk of stroke.

DOCTOR'S ORDERS

Recognizing the early signs and getting immediate medical attention can greatly improve survival and recovery. Treatment depends on the type of stroke.

For immediate treatment of an ischemic stroke (caused by a blood clot), acetyl-salicylic acid (ASA or aspirin) is often given in the emergency room to reduce the risk of having another stroke. A doctor can also administer a clot-busting drug called TPA (tissue plasminogen activator), which breaks up the clot and restores blood flow and oxygen to the brain. This drug can improve your chances of a full recovery, but it is most effective when given within three hours of initial symptoms. This drug does not work for hemorrhagic stroke, and can actually worsen the problem. Recent research suggests that TPA may still be helpful if given within four and a half hours of a stroke, but the fact remains that the sooner a person gets treatment the better the outcome.

If you have had a stroke or are at risk of ischemic stroke, your doctor may prescribe anticoagulant or antiplatelet drugs to be taken regularly.

Antiplatelet drugs, such as aspirin, clopidogrel (Plavix), or ticlopidine (Ticlid), help prevent platelets from sticking together and therefore prevent blood clots from forming. The most commonly used and affordable antiplatelet drug is aspirin.

The most recent guidelines issued by the Canadian Cardiovascular Society recommend that those who have had a heart attack or stroke take low dose (81 mg) ASA for life to reduce the risk of another episode. ASA is *not* recommended as a primary prevention therapy for people who have not had a heart attack, stroke, or other vascular disease, even if they have diabetes or other risk factors. Not everyone can take aspirin because of allergies and side effects, which include a risk of bleeding and upset stomach, so check with your doctor before taking this drug.

Anticoagulant drugs such as warfarin (Coumadin) and heparin are blood thinners that prevent new blood clots from forming and keep existing blood clots from getting larger. They work by interfering with certain parts of the blood needed to form clots. They are usually prescribed for people with an irregular heartbeat (atrial fibrillation), which can cause blood clots to travel from the heart to the brain. They are commonly used in people who have had a stroke to help prevent stroke from recurring.

There are procedures that can open up an artery narrowed by plaque. A carotid endarterectomy involves an incision in your neck to expose your carotid artery and remove the plaques. Angioplasty is another option. This involves inserting a balloon-tipped catheter into the obstructed artery to open it up.

Those with high blood pressure or cholesterol will be given medications to manage these conditions. Refer to those sections of this book for more information.

Surgical procedures can be done for the treatment and prevention of hemorrhagic stroke to remove blood that has pooled in the brain, repair broken blood vessels, or remove plaque from inside the carotid artery. Aneurysm clipping involves placing a tiny clamp at the base of the aneurysm to keep it from bursting. This can also prevent re-bleeding of an aneurysm that has recently hemorrhaged. There are other procedures that can seal off or remove the aneurysm.

THE FIVE WARNING SIGNS

Stroke is a medical emergency. It is important to recognize the warning signs and call 9–1–1 immediately. These signs include the following:

1. Weakness: Sudden loss of strength or sudden numbness in the face, arm, or leg, even if temporary.

2. Trouble speaking: Sudden difficulty speaking or understanding or sudden confusion, even if temporary.

3. Vision problems: Sudden trouble with vision, even if temporary.

4. Headache: Sudden severe and unusual headache.

5. Dizziness: Sudden loss of balance, especially with any of the above signs.

(Source: Heart and Stroke Foundation of Canada)

SHERRY'S NATURAL PRESCRIPTION

Stroke is a medical emergency that requires immediate medical treatment. The strategies outlined here can aid recovery and help prevent stroke. Do not stop taking any medication unless advised by your doctor.

Dietary Recommendations

Foods to include:

- Boost fibre intake by eating lots of whole grains, vegetables, fruits, beans, nuts, and seeds, which will help lower cholesterol levels, improve blood sugar control (essential to prevent diabetes), and help with weight management. Colourful fruits and vegetables contain a range of antioxidants that help reduce inflammation, promote relaxation of blood vessels, lower cholesterol levels, and reduce blood clot formation. Apples, oranges, tomatoes, and bananas are a particularly good source of potassium, which can help lower blood pressure.

- Coffee contains antioxidants that offer a number of benefits: they are protective to blood vessels, reduce inflammation, and improve insulin sensitivity. Recent research in women suggests that moderate coffee consumption can decrease stroke risk. Those who have high blood pressure or are sensitive to caffeine should consult with their doctor prior to adjusting caffeine intake.

- Cold-water fish contain beneficial omega-3 fatty acids, which help reduce cholesterol, inhibit blood clot formation, and reduce the risk of heart disease. Try to eat three servings per week of fresh cold-water fish such as salmon, trout, herring, mackerel, and tuna. To reduce consumption of toxins, choose wild (not farmed) fish. Plant sources of omega-3s include chia seed and flaxseed.

- Garlic helps reduce cholesterol and thin the blood (prevent clots), and has antioxidant properties. Try to eat one or more cloves daily.

- Green tea contains antioxidants that have modest effects in lowering blood pressure and cholesterol. Preliminary research also suggests that the antioxidant catechins in green tea may help limit damage caused by ischemic stroke.

- Non-hydrogenated margarines, salad dressings, and spreads that contain plant sterols (plant substances) can help lower cholesterol.

- Nuts (almonds and walnuts) help lower cholesterol levels. Nuts contain fibre and nutrients such as vitamin E, alpha-linolenic acid, magnesium, potassium, and arginine, which are important for heart health. Although nuts are high in calories, some studies have found that increasing nut consumption by several hundred calories per day does not cause weight gain.

- Oat bran is rich in a soluble fibre called beta glucan, which has been shown to lower cholesterol levels. A typical dose of oat bran is 5–10 g taken with each meal. Beta glucan is also available in supplement form. The recommended intake is 10–15 g of beta glucan per day.

- Olive oil contains monounsaturated fat that can help reduce blood clots and lower LDL cholesterol. Olive oil is best to add to foods after they are cooked or to use in salad dressings; it is not heat stable and not recommended for cooking.

- Palm fruit oil is rich in polyunsaturated fatty acids, tocotrienols (a potent form of vitamin E), and other antioxidants that can help raise HDL (good) cholesterol levels. Preliminary research also suggests the tocotrienols in Malaysian palm fruit oil may help prevent brain cell death after stroke. Palm fruit oil is available in specialty grocery stores. It is heat resistant, so ideal to use when cooking. It is also an added ingredient in many commercial foods such as peanut butter and margarine spreads.

- Phytosterols (plant sterols) are plant compounds that are effective in lowering LDL cholesterol levels. They are thought to work by attaching to cholesterol in the digestive tract and carrying it out of the body. They also remove cholesterol from substances made in the liver. They are naturally present in small amounts in fruits, vegetables, nuts, seeds, and legumes. Manufacturers are now adding plant sterols to a variety of foods, such as orange juice (Minute Maid Heart Wise with CoroWise plant sterols), margarine (Becel pro.activ), and yogurt (Danacol).

- Soy products (tofu, soybeans, miso, and soy protein powder) can help lower cholesterol and triglyceride levels. Substituting as little as 20 g per day of soy protein for animal protein can significantly lower cholesterol.

- Yogurt and fermented milk products can help lower cholesterol.

Foods to avoid:

- Foods high in cholesterol such as organ meats, egg yolks, shrimp, squid, fatty meats, and whole milk products may have a small effect on raising blood cholesterol levels in those with high blood cholesterol or type 2 diabetes. However, studies have shown that in healthy people with no history of heart disease, diabetes, or high blood cholesterol, eating an average of one egg per day does not increase the long-term risk of heart disease. If your cholesterol levels are normal you may eat up to one egg per day (or seven eggs per week). If you have diabetes or high blood cholesterol, limit your whole eggs to no more than four per week.

- High alcohol intake can increase your blood pressure and triglycerides and contribute to the development of heart disease and stroke. Limit alcohol to no more than two drinks per day or 10 drinks per week for women and three drinks per day or 15 per week for men.

- High-glycemic foods (white bread and refined starches) raise blood sugar levels and increase the risk of diabetes. See Appendix B for more information.

- Salt causes water retention and increases the pressure inside your arteries. Reducing salt intake reduces blood pressure in most people. Aim for no more than 2,500 mg daily. Avoid adding salt to foods and minimize eating processed and fast foods such as deli meats, snacks (chips, pretzels), french fries, and burgers.

- Saturated fat, which is present in animal foods (beef, pork, and dairy) and trans fat, which is found in hydrogenated oils, can raise cholesterol levels. Limit consumption of saturated fat to 10 percent of total calories. Read food labels carefully.

- Trans fatty acids, found in hydrogenated oils, which are present in some margarines, snack foods (chips, microwave popcorn), and deep-fried foods (french fries), can raise cholesterol levels and increase the risk of heart disease and stroke.

....

POTASSIUM LOWERS STROKE RISK

Studies have found an association between diets low in potassium and increased risk of stroke. Conversely, high potassium intakes have been associated with a lower risk of stroke. Some of the protective effects of potassium lie in its ability to lower blood pressure. Foods high in potassium include bananas, potatoes, oranges, raisins, artichokes, avocados, spinach, nuts, seeds, lima beans, cod, chicken, and salmon.

....

Lifestyle Suggestions

• Don't smoke, and avoid second-hand smoke. Smoking contributes to atherosclerosis, increases the risk of blood clots, reduces the oxygen in your blood, increases your blood pressure, and makes your heart work harder. In fact, smoking nearly doubles the risk of ischemic stroke.

• Lose excess weight. Losing even 5 to 10 percent of excess weight can lower cholesterol and blood pressure.

• Exercise regularly. Moderate-intensity activities, such as brisk walking, biking, or swimming, can reduce cholesterol and blood pressure and help with weight management. Aim for one hour daily. Not being active nearly doubles your risk of heart disease and stroke.

• Reduce stress levels. Stress increases the risk of heart disease and stroke. Try meditation, exercise, or yoga to promote calming and relaxation.

• Manage your blood sugar levels. If you have diabetes or are at risk for diabetes, work on improving your blood sugar levels with exercise and a low-glycemic diet.

• See your doctor regularly for checkups and to monitor your blood pressure, cholesterol, and blood sugar. Discuss the results with your doctor.

Top Recommended Supplements

The supplements outlined here can play a role in recovery and prevention, but should never be used in place of medications prescribed by your doctor. For recommendations on managing the risk factors for stroke, such as high blood pressure and cholesterol, refer to those sections of this book.

Citicoline (CDP-choline): A form of the B-vitamin choline that has neuroprotective properties, citicoline prevents brain damage caused by lack of oxygen, helps restore key membrane components called phospholipids, and counteracts the effects of membrane-injuring molecules known as free radicals. Several studies have shown that treatment with choline within 14 days of onset of ischemic or hemorrhagic stroke can significantly reduce death and disability. Dosage: 500–2,000 mg daily. This nutrient is given as a prescription drug in many countries but it is sold in Canada through natural health care practitioners.

Fish oils: Contain beneficial omega-3 fatty acids that can lower triglycerides, modestly raise HDL cholesterol, and reduce inflammation and blood clotting. Studies have shown that fish oils reduce the risk of stroke. Dosage: The typical dosage is 3–9 g total of EPA and DHA daily, although higher amounts have been used in some studies. Look for a product that provides at least 400 mg EPA and 200 mg DHA per dosage.

Policosanol: Several studies have shown that it can significantly reduce blood clotting (comparable to aspirin) and it also lowers cholesterol. Dosage: 20 mg daily. Do not combine with other blood thinners such as aspirin unless advised by your health care provider.

Complementary Supplements

Aged garlic extract (Kyolic): Helps lower total and LDL cholesterol and triglyceride levels, reduces blood clotting, and slows/prevents atherosclerosis. Dosage: 600 mg or more daily.

B-vitamins: Lower levels of homocysteine, an amino acid linked to increased risk of stroke in many studies. Folic acid, vitamin B6, and vitamin B12 can lower homocysteine levels, but studies have not yet demonstrated whether this will result in a decreased risk of stroke. Consider a B-complex or take a multivitamin that provides 50–100 mg of the B-vitamins.

Ginkgo biloba: Inhibits blood clotting and improves blood flow to the brain. It may be helpful for both the prevention and treatment of stroke (improving recovery). Dosage: 120–240 mg daily, standardized to 6 percent terpene lactones and 24 percent flavone glycosides.

Stanols and sterols: Plant substances that have been shown in many studies to lower LDL cholesterol. They are thought to work by attaching to cholesterol in the digestive tract and carrying it out of the body. They also remove cholesterol from substances made in the liver. A sterol ester, called beta-sitosterol, has been shown to decrease cholesterol absorption by about 50 percent. Dosage: Varies depending on the product and potency.

Tocotrienols: A potent form of vitamin E that has been shown to reduce atherosclerosis. Tocotrienols derived from Malaysian palm fruit oil have been shown to help reduce brain cell death after a stroke. Dosage: Follow label instructions.

S

Stroke

FINAL THOUGHTS

To prevent stroke and aid recovery, consider the following:

- Know the warning signs and seek immediate medical attention if you suspect a stroke.
- Eat lots of fruits, vegetables, high-fibre whole grains, beans, nuts, fish, soy, garlic, and yogurt, and drink green tea.
- Minimize intake of alcohol, trans fats, sugar, and salt.
- Get regular exercise, reduce stress, and don't smoke.
- Consider fish oils and policosanol for prevention, and citicoline to improve recovery.

THRUSH (CANDIDIASIS)

Thrush is an overgrowth of the fungus *Candida albicans.* It typically affects the mouth (called oral thrush) or the vagina (called *Candida vulvovaginitis,* or more commonly a yeast infection). This section deals specifically with oral thrush; yeast infections are covered in the section on vaginitis.

We all have a variety of microorganisms in our bodies; some are essential for health and others can become a problem when they grow out of control. This is the case with *Candida albicans.* Levels of this fungus are usually kept under control by our normal bacteria (flora). However, when our normal bacteria are depleted, *Candida* can proliferate, causing thrush, vaginitis, and other problems. Oral thrush can spread throughout the mouth and throat if left unchecked. It may also be passed from an infant to the mother's breasts during breastfeeding.

There are a number of dietary and lifestyle suggestions and supplements that can help prevent thrush and improve healing if you are infected.

SIGNS & SYMPTOMS

- Bad breath

- White lesions or coating on the tongue or the inside cheeks

- Dry mouth

- Inflamed, painful red or white patches in or around the mouth

The lesions can spread into the esophagus, causing difficulty or pain in swallowing and a sensation of food sticking in the throat. In severe cases the infection can spread throughout the body, which is called systemic candidiasis. This may cause fatigue, pain, fever, mood swings, chronic infections, allergies, skin conditions, and digestive problems.

Infants with oral thrush may have difficulty feeding or be irritable or inconsolable. When the mother is infected she may have bright red, shiny, sore, cracked, or painful nipples.

RISK FACTORS

- Age: The very young and the very old are most susceptible.

- Chronic illness such as cancer

- Dry mouth could be caused by a salivary gland disorder, chemotherapy, or radiation, or by use of diuretics, antihistamines, or tranquillizers.

- Immune disorders such as diabetes or HIV/AIDS

- Smoking

- Use of antibiotics, corticosteroids, or birth control pills

- Weakened or underdeveloped immune system function

- Wearing dentures

DOCTOR'S ORDERS

Oral thrush in infants is treated with nystatin (Nilstat), an antifungal liquid medication applied directly to the patches. If diaper rash has also occurred, then an antifungal ointment may be used. In healthy babies, oral thrush may clear up on its own and may be left untreated but carefully watched.

Thrush transferred from a breastfeeding baby to the mother's breasts is often treated with an antifungal ointment. Breastfeeding can continue during treatment.

Adults with oral thrush are usually treated with either a topical or oral antifungal medication (such as nystatin or fluconazole), depending on the extent of the infection.

Systemic candidiasis is more difficult to diagnose, but it may also be life threatening, particularly for people with weakened immune health or illness. Up to 75 percent of people with systemic candidiasis die from complications. As such, if you suspect you may have a *Candida* infection, see your doctor immediately.

SHERRY'S NATURAL PRESCRIPTION

Dietary Recommendations

Foods to include:

- Eat lots of low-starch vegetables (leafy greens, broccoli, celery, cabbage, cauliflower) and yeast-free whole grains (pita bread); asparagus, Jerusalem artichokes, and soybeans contain substances (FOS) that promote the growth of beneficial bacteria.

- Garlic and onions help reduce fungal growth.

- Yogurt with live cultures and other fermented dairy (kefir) provide beneficial bacteria that help to reduce *Candida* overgrowth.

Foods to avoid:

- Alcohol hampers immune function; beer and wine contain yeasts that can be a problem.

- Dairy products and aged cheese can increase the risk of *Candida* in some people.

- Fruit and fruit juices are high in sugar and should be minimized; drink vegetable juices, water, or green tea instead.

- Limit foods that contain sugars (candy, sweets, soft drinks) or yeasts (breads) as these foods can encourage growth of *Candida*. Use xylitol and stevia instead of sugar.

- Nuts and nut butters may contain moulds. Choose fresh cracked or whole nuts.

Note: Food allergies may trigger *Candida* infections. Try an elimination diet (see Appendix D) to determine if you have food allergies.

Lifestyle Suggestions

- Avoid the use of mouthwash or oral sprays that contain alcohol because the alcohol can destroy healthy bacteria in your mouth and cause dry mouth. To alleviate dry mouth use a salt-water or baking soda solution in warm water and do not swallow. For bad breath try an alcohol-free mouthwash with tea tree oil (5 percent concentration or less). Tea tree has antiseptic and antifungal properties and preliminary research suggests it can treat thrush. Use 1 tbsp (15 mL), rinse mouth for 30 to 60 seconds, and then spit out.

- Be on the lookout for signs of oral thrush before breastfeeding.

- Clean bottle nipples and pacifiers regularly using hot, soapy water.

- Clean breasts with warm cloth and apply conditioning lotion or oil to nipples after breast-feeding.

- Don't smoke.

- Practise good oral hygiene; brush and floss twice daily; clean your mouth and dentures; soak dentures in a denture cleaner nightly and rinse well.

Top Recommended Supplements

Aged garlic extract: Supports immune function and has antifungal properties. Studies have shown that it can reduce growth of *Candida albicans*. Dosage: One capsule twice daily. This clinically studied form of garlic is odourless. It is also available in liquid.

Probiotics: *Lactobacillus acidophilus* and *Bifidobacterium* are beneficial bacteria that help prevent overgrowth of *Candida*. It is especially important to take a probiotic after a course of antibiotics. Suggested product: Kyo-Dophilus. For infants and children look for BioGaia, which is available in drops and chewable tablets. Dosage: Take two or three capsules orally daily with meals.

Complementary Treatment

Caprylic acid: A fatty acid derived from coconut oil that has antifungal properties. Dosage: 1,000 mg three times daily. Avoid if you have ulcerative colitis.

Gentian violet: An old remedy for eliminating thrush that is becoming popular again today. It has antifungal properties and works quickly to relieve thrush. Pharmacists can prepare a 1 percent solution of gentian violet. To use, dip a cotton swab in the solution and apply to the affected areas of the mouth and tongue. Use for up to one week. This product can be used on infants, adults, and mother's breasts.

Note: This product will stain fingers and clothing dark purple.

FINAL THOUGHTS

To reduce oral thrush, consider the following:

- Eat fermented dairy products (yogurt), vegetables, garlic, onions, yeast-free breads, and foods containing FOS.
- Avoid sugar, yeast, and alcohol.
- Don't smoke, and avoid alcohol-containing mouthwashes.
- Inspect your infant's mouth (and your breasts) regularly and see your doctor if there are signs of thrush.
- Aged garlic extract and probiotics can help prevent and treat *Candida* infections.

TINNITUS

Tinnitus is the sensation of ringing, buzzing, roaring, or hissing in the ears. According to the Tinnitus Association of Canada, this condition affects about 20 percent of all Canadians. Tinnitus is often associated with hearing loss or noise exposure, although even people with normal hearing develop this problem.

Tinnitus is not a disease, but rather a symptom that can result from a large number of factors including medical conditions, injury, or side effects of medication. Inside the inner ear there are thousands of auditory cells that maintain an electrical charge. There are tiny hairs on these cells that move with the pressure of sound waves. The movement triggers the cells to discharge electricity through the auditory nerve and the brain interprets these signals as sound. If these hairs become bent or broken, they move randomly and the auditory cells send random electrical impulses to the brain as noise. Damage to the auditory cells or hair in the inner ear most often results from exposure to loud noise, a blow to the head, or a whiplash injury. Other risk factors for tinnitus are described below. In some cases the underlying cause of tinnitus is unknown.

Although tinnitus can be distressing, it is rarely a sign of a serious health problem. Identifying and treating the underlying cause is essential. For those with irreversible tinnitus, there are a variety of holistic therapies and lifestyle measures that help reduce the symptoms and improve quality of life.

SIGNS & SYMPTOMS

- Hearing loss

- Ringing, buzzing, roaring, or hissing sounds in the ear when no external sounds are present

The symptoms of tinnitus vary in intensity from mild to severe. The sounds may be heard intermittently or continuously. It may be heard in one ear or both, and it can vary in pitch.

KEEP YOUR EARS CLEAN

A buildup of earwax can reduce your ability to hear outside noises and amplify internal noises. If you produce a lot of earwax, speak to your doctor about having excess wax removed. Do not try to remove it yourself unless advised by your doctor. Using cotton swabs improperly can damage the ear and push the wax deeper into your ear.

440

T

Tinnitus

RISK FACTORS

- Age: Tinnitus is most common in those over 65 and those with age-related hearing loss (presbycusis).

- Arteriovenous malformation (AVM): A condition where there are malformations of capillaries between arteries and veins. This generally occurs in only one ear.

- Blood vessel disease: High blood pressure and atherosclerosis (buildup of cholesterol in the blood vessels of the inner ear) causes loss of elasticity, making blood flow more forcefully and making it more easily heard.

- Buildup of wax in the ear canal can cause tinnitus.

- Ear or sinus infection: Usually this form of tinnitus is temporary and goes away once the infection is healed.

- Exposure to loud noises can cause irreversible damage to hair cells in the inner ear.

- Gender: Tinnitus is more common in men.

- Head or neck trauma

- Insulin resistance: High insulin and blood sugar levels (which precede type 2 diabetes) have been linked to tinnitus in some studies.

- Jaw misalignment or TMJ (problems with the temporomandibular joint)

- Medications: Some drugs are toxic to the ear, such as aminoglycoside antibiotics, the malaria drug quinine, and the cancer drug cisplatin; others cause tinnitus as a side effect, such as aspirin (ASA) and anti-inflammatory drugs (NSAIDs), diuretics (furosemide), erythromycin, gentamicin, vancomycin, and some blood pressure and cholesterol-lowering drugs. This effect can be temporary or permanent.

- Meniere's disease: A condition caused by abnormal inner ear fluid pressure

- Post-traumatic stress disorder

- Structural abnormalities in ear bones or stiffening of the bones in the middle ear

- Tumours or benign growths called acoustic neuromas can put pressure on auditory nerves, causing tinnitus.

DOCTOR'S ORDERS

The treatment of tinnitus depends on the cause. To determine the cause, your doctor may refer you to an otolaryngologist, otherwise known as an ear, nose, and throat specialist. Another specialist, an audiologist, can measure your hearing and fit you with a hearing aid if needed.

The drug gabapentin (Neurontin) has been used with some success in relieving tinnitus. Tricyclic antidepressants, such as amitriptyline and nortriptyline, have also been helpful for some people, but their use is limited by side effects (dry mouth, blurred vision, constipation, and risk of heart problems).

If the problem is due to earwax or a side effect of medication, it may be reversible. Tinnitus that is due to hearing loss or excessive noise exposure cannot be reversed, but there are a variety of lifestyle measures discussed below that can be helpful in coping.

Ask your doctor to measure your homocysteine level. Chronic tinnitus may be associated with an elevation in homocysteine levels.

HOMEOPATHIC RECOMMENDATIONS

Chininum sulphuricum: Buzzing, ringing, and roaring sounds that are loud enough to impair the person's hearing suggest a need for this remedy.

Graphites: This remedy may be beneficial to a person who has tinnitus with associated deafness and reports hearing hissing and clicking sounds or even loud sounds resembling gunshots.

SHERRY'S NATURAL PRESCRIPTION

Dietary Recommendations

Foods to include:

• Fruits and vegetables contain antioxidants that support the health of the blood vessels.

• Whole grains and legumes provide vital fibre, which helps reduce blood cholesterol levels. These foods are also lower in the glycemic index and can help improve blood sugar control and prevent type 2 diabetes. Refer to Appendix B for more information on the glycemic index.

• Drink plenty of water.

Foods to avoid:

• Alcohol increases the force of blood by dilating your blood vessels and causing greater blood flow to the inner ear area.

• Caffeine constricts blood vessels, increasing the speed of blood through your veins and arteries.

• Trans fats and saturated fat elevate cholesterol levels and contribute to atherosclerosis, which can cause or worsen tinnitus.

• High-glycemic foods (processed grains such as white bread and rice) increase insulin levels and can worsen tinnitus.

FOOD FLARES

Many people with tinnitus find that certain foods or drinks will worsen their symptoms. There is no simple test to determine which foods can worsen tinnitus. Keeping a food diary or trying an elimination diet can be helpful in pinpointing foods that trigger tinnitus. Refer to Appendix D for more information on food allergies and the elimination diet.

Lifestyle Suggestions

• Don't smoke: Smoking causes blood vessel damage and can worsen tinnitus.

• Protect your ears: Wear earplugs or earmuffs if you work in a noisy environment or are exposed to loud noise at home.

• Mask the noise: Using a fan or low-volume, soft music can help mask the noise from tinnitus. There are also special devices that emit white noise (low-tone sound that neutralizes other sounds).

• Consider a hearing aid: If you have hearing loss, amplifying outside sounds can make the tinnitus less noticeable.

• Reduce stress levels: Stress can worsen tinnitus. Try breathing techniques, yoga, and massage to promote relaxation.

• Exercise regularly to improve blood flow, reduce stress, and improve blood sugar control.

• Get adequate sleep, which will help with coping and reduce stress.

• Acupuncture and hypnosis may be helpful for reducing tinnitus and promoting relaxation. Biofeedback treatments can also help relieve tinnitus.

Top Recommended Supplements

Ginkgo biloba: Improves circulation to the brain and inner ear. Some studies found reduction in symptoms while others showed no benefit. It appears that ginkgo works for some people and not for others, likely depending on the underlying cause. As well, it may take several weeks to months to detect a benefit. Dosage: 120 mg daily of a product standardized to contain 24 percent flavone glycosides and 6 percent terpene lactones.

Zinc: Highly concentrated in the inner ear; a deficiency of this mineral can cause tinnitus. Some studies have found improvement in symptoms with zinc supplements in those who are deficient in this mineral. Blood tests can detect zinc deficiency. High dosages were used in studies (90–150 mg daily); levels should be monitored by a doctor. It is important to take copper (2 mg) along with zinc because zinc interferes with copper absorption.

Complementary Supplements

Bioflavonoids: Support blood vessel health and improve circulation. There is preliminary research showing benefits with a product called Lipo-Flavonoid Plus, which contains a combination of bioflavonoids and other nutrients and vitamins. It appears to help improve hearing and relieve dizziness and ringing in the ears. Take as directed.

Magnesium: Essential for nerve health and hearing. A deficiency of magnesium can cause blood vessels to constrict, which can reduce circulation to the brain and inner ear. Dosage: 100 mg three times daily with meals.

Melatonin: A hormone secreted by the pineal gland in the brain in response to darkness. It regulates our sleep–wake cycles. Some studies have found that supplements can improve symptoms of tinnitus and also improve sleep quality. Dosage: 3 mg one hour before bed.

Vitamin B12: Essential in the manufacture of myelin, a fatty substance that covers and shields the nerves and allows them to function normally. Some research has found that those who are deficient are at greater risk of developing tinnitus. In studies, B12 injections reduced the severity of symptoms. Sublingual B12, which is better absorbed than oral B12, may offer similar benefits, although it has not been studied. Take B12 along with a B-complex that contains folic acid and vitamins B1, B3, and B6 as these other B-vitamins also play a role in proper nerve function and together they may help reduce tinnitus. Dosage: 5 mg B12 and 50–100 mg of the other B-vitamins daily.

FINAL THOUGHTS

To reduce the symptoms of tinnitus, consider the following:

- Minimize intake of caffeine, alcohol, trans fats, and processed and refined grains.
- Don't smoke, and get regular exercise and adequate sleep.
- Avoid being around loud noise and protect your ears with earplugs or earmuffs.
- Try masking the noise with music or a fan.
- Consider supplements of ginkgo biloba, zinc, or bioflavonoids.

T

Tinnitus

ULCERS (PEPTIC)

Peptic ulcers are sores that develop on the inside lining of the stomach, upper small intestine, or esophagus, causing significant pain and discomfort. Their name is derived from pepsin, an enzyme secreted by glands in the stomach. Along with pepsin, acids are secreted in the stomach to aid digestion. Other glands in the stomach and intestine secrete mucus, which functions to protect the lining of the digestive tract from the corrosive effect of pepsin and acid. If there is damage to the lining of the stomach or intestine and the mucous layer breaks down, an ulcer can develop.

It is estimated that about one in ten Canadians develops an ulcer at some time in his or her life. Ulcers generally affect people over the age of 30, but children can get them as well.

Years ago stress and poor diet were thought to be the cause of ulcers. In recent years, however, it was discovered that infection with a bacterium called *Helicobacter pylori (H. pylori)* is responsible for causing most ulcers. This bacterium lives within the mucous layer that covers and protects the lining of the stomach and small intestine. *H. pylori* is a normal inhabitant of this area and does not always cause problems. However, in certain individuals and under certain conditions, it can disrupt the mucous layer, erode the lining of the digestive tract, and lead to an ulcer.

Stress and diet may still contribute to the problem, causing damage to the lining and making it easier for bacteria to invade and damage the sensitive tissues. Ulcers can also be caused by taking non-steroidal anti-inflammatory drugs (NSAIDs), which erode and inflame the lining of the stomach and intestines.

It is estimated that one in five people under 40 years of age and half of people over 60 are infected with *H. pylori*. It is not known how it spreads, but it may occur with close contact, such as kissing, or through contaminated food and water.

TYPES OF ULCERS

Ulcers have different names, depending on their location:

Duodenal ulcers develop in the duodenum (the first part of the small intestine), which is the most common location.

Esophageal ulcers are located in the lower section of the esophagus and are often associated with chronic gastroesophageal reflux disease (GERD).

Gastric ulcers occur in the stomach.

SIGNS & SYMPTOMS

The most common symptoms is pain in the stomach or chest area, which is often worse when the stomach is empty and at night and is temporarily relieved by eating or taking antacids. The pain can be intermittent.

Other symptoms that occur less often include the following:

- Dark blood in stools

- Loss of appetite

- Nausea or vomiting

- Weight loss

Note: If left untreated, ulcers can lead to serious problems such as bleeding, obstruction of the digestive tract (due to scarring), or serious infection caused by leaking of the intestinal contents into the belly.

Infection with *H. pylori* can also impair absorption of certain nutrients, including iron, vitamin B12, folic acid, alpha-tocopherol, vitamin C, and beta carotene.

RISK FACTORS

In addition to *H. pylori,* other factors that increase the risk of ulcers include the following:

- Alcohol: Irritates and erodes the mucous lining of the stomach and increases the amount of stomach acid that is produced

- Food allergies: May cause damage to the stomach lining, increasing the risk of ulcers

- Medications: NSAIDs (non-steroidal anti-inflammatory drugs) such as ibuprofen (Advil, Motrin), naproxen (Aleve), and diclofenac (Voltaren) and bisphosphonates (drugs used to treat osteoporosis) such as alendronate (Fosamax), risedronate (Actonel), and ibandronate (Boniva)

- Smoking: Nicotine increases the volume and concentration of stomach acid.

- Stress: May aggravate symptoms and delay healing

NON-STEROIDAL ANTI-INFLAMMATORY DRUGS AND ULCERS

Non-steroidal anti-inflammatory drugs inhibit production of an enzyme (cyclo-oxygenase) that produces prostaglandins, hormone-like substances that protect the stomach lining. Without this protection, stomach acid can damage the lining, causing bleeding and ulcers. Examples of these drugs include aspirin, ibuprofen (Motrin and Advil), naproxen (Naprosyn), and indomethacin (Indocid). Taking these drugs with meals may help reduce stomach upset but will not prevent ulcers. Take only when absolutely necessary at the lowest dosage for the shortest period of time.

U

Ulcers (Peptic)

DOCTOR'S ORDERS

For ulcers caused by *H. pylori* bacteria, a 7- to 14-day course of antibiotics is prescribed to kill the bacteria. Antibiotics commonly used include amoxicillin (Amoxil), clarithromycin (Biaxin), or metronidazole (Flagyl). Two of these are typically prescribed along with an acid-blocking drug, such as lansoprazole (Prevacid), to allow the area to heal. Some companies put the three drugs together in one package, such as the Hp-PAC.

Depending on the severity of the ulcer, acid-reducing drugs may be needed for several weeks to months to allow healing. Histamine (H2) blockers reduce the amount of hydrochloric acid released into the stomach. They work by blocking the action of histamine, a substance that signals acid secretion into the stomach. Examples include ranitidine (Zantac), famotidine (Pepcid), and cimetidine (Tagamet).

Proton pump inhibitors shut down the pumps that secrete acid into the stomach. Examples include lansoprazole (Prevacid), esomeprazole (Nexium), or omeprazole (Losec).

Antacids may be used along with the above drugs or alone. They provide rapid relief and work by neutralizing stomach acid. Examples include Tums, Rolaids, and Maalox.

Cytoprotective drugs protect the lining of the stomach and intestine. Examples include sucralfate (Sulcrate) and misoprostol (Cytotec). They may be given to protect the stomach when NSAIDS are being used.

SHERRY'S NATURAL PRESCRIPTION

Ulcers caused by *H. pylori* infection will most likely require medical treatment. The following suggestions may help improve healing and reduce the risk of developing an ulcer.

Dietary Recommendations

Foods to include:

• Broccoli and Brussels sprouts contain a compound called isothiocyanate sulforaphane that helps suppress infection by *H. pylori*. This compound also reduces inflammation.

• Cultured and fermented foods such as kefir and yogurt provide friendly bacteria that help to combat *H. pylori*.

• Cabbage and aloe vera juice may help improve healing.

• Crushed garlic has antibacterial properties.

• Fibre can help reduce recurrence of ulcers. Eat more fruits, vegetables and high-fibre whole grains such as oats and chia seed.

• Foods rich in vitamin K (leafy green vegetables) and zinc (whole grains and seeds) can improve healing.

• Bananas are protective to the stomach.

• Drink herbal teas with marshmallow, slippery elm, and chamomile, which can soothe the irritated lining.

• Cranberry juice can prevent the adhesion of *H. pylori* to the stomach wall. Recent research has found that consuming cranberry juice can reduce levels of *H. pylori*.

Foods to avoid:

• Alcohol, caffeine, and spicy foods can irritate and increase stomach acid.

• Sugar and salt increase stomach acidity and may aggravate symptoms.

Lifestyle Suggestions

• Don't smoke, as nicotine is very irritating to the stomach lining and slows healing.

• Elevate your pillow to prevent stomach acid from flowing up your esophagus.

• Reduce stress by trying massage, yoga, breathing exercises, or meditation.

Top Recommended Supplements

Deglycyrrhizinated licorice (DGL): Soothes inflamed and damaged mucous lining, promotes healing, and may inhibit growth of *H. pylori*. Some research suggests that it might help protect the stomach against NSAID usage. Dosage: 500 mg 15 minutes before meals and at bedtime. Look for a chewable product.

Probiotics: Several studies have found that probiotics (especially those in the *Bifidobacterium* family) can inhibit the growth of *H. pylori*. They also improve the ability of antibiotics to destroy bacteria and reduce antibiotic side effects such as diarrhea and yeast overgrowth. Dosage: One to three capsules daily of a product providing 1 billion live cells per capsule or tablet.

Complementary Supplements

Glutamine: An amino acid that provides energy for the cells that line the intestine and stomach. Levels may be depleted in those with ulcers, and supplementing has been shown to offer some benefits to promote healing. Dosage: 500–1,000 mg three times daily.

Mastic: A gummy extract of a plant *Pistacia lentiscus* that has been found in preliminary research to help eradicate *H. pylori* and heal peptic ulcers. Dosage: 1 g before breakfast and at bedtime.

Neem: Extracts of freeze-dried bark from neem have been found to reduce stomach acid and help promote healing of ulcers in preliminary research. Dosage: 30–60 mg twice daily.

Zinc: Required for tissue repair. Some evidence suggests that it can promote healing of ulcers. Dosage: 25–50 mg daily. Take copper (1–3 mg) to prevent copper deficiency.

U

Ulcers (Peptic)

FINAL THOUGHTS

To reduce your risk of ulcers and improve healing, consider the following:

• Don't smoke, reduce stress, and avoid taking NSAIDs.
• Eat fermented and cultured foods and drink cranberry juice to inhibit *H. pylori*.
• Cabbage, aloe vera juice, and green vegetables promote ulcer healing.
• Probiotic supplements can inhibit *H. pylori*, improve antibiotic treatment of *H. pylori*, and reduce antibiotic side effects.
• Promote healing of an ulcer with zinc, glutamine, and DGL.

VAGINITIS AND YEAST INFECTIONS

Vaginitis is an inflammation of the vagina that can cause discharge, itching, and pain. The condition often results from irritation, infection, or hormonal changes, such as low estrogen levels in menopause.

There are many different types of bacteria and yeast normally present in the vagina. However, when the numbers of these organisms become out of balance, infection can occur, causing vaginitis.

The most common cause of vaginitis is an overgrowth of the naturally occurring yeast *Candida albicans*. An estimated three out of four women will have a yeast infection in their lifetime. A yeast infection isn't considered a sexually transmitted disease because this yeast is naturally occurring in a woman's body, but it can spread from one partner to another.

Bacterial vaginosis is another common cause of vaginitis. There are several bacteria that can cause these infections, most commonly *Gardnerella*. These infections can spread during sexual intercourse, but it also occurs in people who aren't sexually active. .

Trichomoniasis is an infection caused by a parasite, which is commonly transmitted by sexual intercourse.

Vaginitis can also result from reduced estrogen levels after menopause, which causes the vagina to become thinner and drier, which may lead to itching, burning, or pain. Use of vaginal sprays, douches, perfumed soaps, and spermicidal products can also cause vaginal irritation, burning, and itching. Most women will experience vaginitis at some point in their lives, and while it is unpleasant, it can be dealt with effectively with both conventional and natural approaches.

SIGNS & SYMPTOMS

- Change in your normal vaginal discharge and odour. Bacterial vaginosis typically causes a greyish-white, fishy-smelling discharge. Yeast infections cause a thick, white discharge that resembles cottage cheese. *Trichomoniasis* causes a greenish-yellow, sometimes frothy discharge in women while men often have no symptoms.

- Light vaginal bleeding

- Pain during intercourse or urination

- Vaginal itching or irritation

RISK FACTORS

Risk factors vary depending upon the type of vaginitis.

Yeast infections

- Hormonal changes (pregnancy)

- Medications such as antibiotics, steroids, and birth control pills

- Stress, lack of sleep

- Uncontrolled diabetes

- Use of vaginal contraceptives or feminine hygiene products

- Weakened immune system (HIV, chemotherapy, diabetes)

- Wearing damp or tight-fitting clothing

Bacterial vaginosis

- Douching

- Use of an intrauterine device (IUD)

- Women with new or multiple sex partners

Trichomoniasis

- Sexual contact with an infected partner

DOCTOR'S ORDERS

There are various medications for vaginitis, depending on the underlying cause. Bacterial vaginosis is treated with metronidazole (Flagyl) or clindamycin (Dalacin). The latter drug is also used to treat *Trichomoniasis*.

Yeast infections are usually treated with miconazole (Monistat) or clotrimazole (Canesten) creams or vaginal suppositories, or fluconazole (CanesOral), a single dose oral tablet, all of which are available over the counter. Many women prefer the latter option as it is easy and provides rapid relief (usually within 24 hours). However, it is more expensive than the other products.

For women with vaginitis in menopause, doctors sometimes prescribe estrogen vaginal creams or rings, which help to thicken the vaginal area. Some estrogen still gets absorbed into the bloodstream, so these products should not be used by women with a history of breast cancer or who are at high risk.

V

Vaginitis and Yeast Infections

HOMEOPATHIC RECOMMENDATIONS

Kreosotum: This remedy is strongly indicated for vaginitis with watery, thin, unpleasant-smelling, very irritating discharge that makes the vulva swell and itch. Symptoms may be worse in the morning and worse when standing up. Infections are more likely to appear before the menstrual period or during pregnancy.

Natrum muriaticum: Vaginitis that itches and makes the vagina feel dry and irritated, with a discharge resembling egg whites, is likely to respond to this remedy.

Sepia: If yeast infections cause vaginal discharge (that may be more profuse in the morning) that is yellow and causes itchiness, or is white and curd-like, this remedy may be indicated. A woman needing sepia often feels worn down and irritable, with cold extremities and a weak or sagging feeling in the pelvic region.

SHERRY'S NATURAL PRESCRIPTION

Dietary Recommendations

Foods to include:

• Eat natural (organic) yogurt with live cultures daily. Studies have shown that daily consumption of yogurt (one cup per day) can reduce the occurrence of bacterial vaginosis and yeast infections.

• Eat lots of low-starch vegetables (leafy greens, broccoli, celery, cabbage, cauliflower) and yeast-free whole grains (pita bread); asparagus, Jerusalem artichokes, and soybeans contain substances (FOS) that promote the growth of beneficial bacteria.

• Garlic and onions have antifungal properties.

Foods to avoid:

• Alcohol, aged cheese, and fermented foods (vinegar and soy sauce) contain yeast and moulds, which can be a problem.

• Sugar allows yeast to thrive and can increase the likelihood of yeast infections in susceptible women. Cut down on all sugar-containing foods; use xylitol or stevia as sweeteners instead of sugar.

Food allergies are believed to be a contributory factor in some cases of recurrent irritant vaginitis. See Appendix D for more information on food allergies and the elimination diet.

Lifestyle Suggestions

• Wear cotton underwear and change your underwear a few times daily if exercising or perspiring.

• Minimize or avoid wearing pantyhose. Do not wear pants that are tight at the crotch.

• Do not use deodorized products, such as tampons, douches, and feminine deodorant sprays.

• Wash the vaginal area with a mild, unscented soap.

• Douche with 2 tsp of powdered acidophilus in a quart of warm water daily.

Top Recommended Supplements

Aged garlic extract (Kyolic): Supports immune function and has antibacterial and antifungal properties. Studies have shown that it can reduce *Candida albicans.* Dosage: Two capsules twice daily.

Lactobacillus acidophilus: A type of friendly bacteria (probiotic) that is part of the normal vaginal flora and helps prevent overgrowth of *Candida.* Many supplements contain another probiotic called *Bifidobacterium.* Dosage: Two or three capsules daily of a product that provides at least 1 billion viable cells per capsule, such as Kyo-Dophilus. Capsules can also be inserted vaginally at bedtime.

Complementary Supplements

Boric acid: A substance with antiseptic and antifungal properties. One study found significant benefits with the use of 600 mg boric acid capsules inserted into the vagina twice per day for two to four weeks. It is available at compounding pharmacies. Boric acid suppositories should not be used during pregnancy, and it is very toxic if taken orally.

Tea tree oil: Has antibacterial and antifungal properties. Studies have found topically applied tea tree oil helpful for *Trichomoniasis, Candida albicans,* and other vaginal infections. This should only be done under a doctor's supervision. Tea tree oil must be diluted to a 5 percent solution or less when used as a douche.

Vitamin C: Helps support immune function. One study found vitamin C vaginal tablets helpful for vaginitis. Dosage: 250 mg vaginally or 1,000 mg orally daily.

Vitamin E: When used orally or vaginally it may help relieve itching and irritation and soothe the delicate vaginal tissue. Dosage: 400 IU orally, or apply the oil topically.

FINAL THOUGHTS

To reduce the risk and promote healing of vaginitis, consider the following:

- Eat yogurt with live cultures daily; reduce intake of sugar, alcohol, and fermented foods.
- Wear cotton underwear and loose-fitting pants.
- Avoid using deodorized feminine hygiene products.
- Take a probiotic supplement and aged garlic extract daily.
- Consider supplements of vitamins C and E.

VARICOSE VEINS

Varicose veins are dilated, bulging, discoloured veins that you can clearly see through the skin. It is estimated that at least 15 percent of the adult population in Canada suffers from varicose veins.

The heart pumps oxygenated blood from the lungs through the arteries to the cells throughout the body. Oxygen exchange takes place and blood returns up to the heart through the veins. Tiny one-way valves inside our veins function as trapdoors, opening and closing with each muscle contraction to prevent the backflow of blood.

Varicose veins result from damage to the valves or vein walls, leading to pooling of blood, vein swelling, and increased venous pressure. Spider veins are a similar condition that affects the smaller veins. These veins spread out on the surface of the skin in a web-like fashion, hence their name.

A number of factors can lead to varicose veins, primarily lifestyle factors. Not surprisingly, the incidence of varicose veins is higher in developed (Western) countries due to lifestyle factors such as poor diet (low fibre intake), lack of activity, and obesity. Making positive lifestyle changes can dramatically help in the prevention and management of varicose veins.

SIGNS & SYMPTOMS

- Cramping

- Fatigue

- Heavy aching in the legs

- Itching and burning

- Swelling of leg or ankle

- Tenderness and pain

Note: If left untreated, varicose veins can worsen over time and cause skin changes such as rash, redness, and sores. Varicose veins are not life threatening; however, they can increase the risk of developing a blood clot, which is a serious concern.

RISK FACTORS

- Age: Most common in those over the age of 50 (but can occur earlier)

- Diet: A low-fibre diet and constipation can contribute to varicose veins.

- Family history

- Gender: Women are affected approximately four times more often than men.

- Lifestyle/occupation: Prolonged sitting or standing with little activity causes pooling of blood and damage to the valves.

- Obesity: Weight gain can increase venous pressure and cause the veins to enlarge.

- Pregnancy: Hormonal changes can weaken vein walls, weight gain increases venous pressure, veins enlarge from increased blood volume, and the growing uterus can compress the veins and increase pressure.

Other factors that may contribute to or worsen varicose veins include exposure to excessive heat and use of birth control pills or hormone replacement therapy (estrogen).

DOCTOR'S ORDERS

Depending on the severity, one of the following medical treatments may be recommended:

Ablation/sclerotherapy/laser: These procedures destroy the affected vein. Blood is rerouted through other veins and the damaged vein is absorbed by the body.

Bypass: An artificial or transplanted vein is connected to the damaged vein to help improve blood flow.

Compression stockings: These specially designed stockings provide firm support to improve blood flow back to the heart and prevent swelling in the legs. They are available for both men and women and are custom ordered.

Stripping: This is a surgical procedure to remove the damaged vein.

HOMEOPATHIC RECOMMENDATIONS

Carbo vegetabilis: When varicose veins are accompanied by general poor circulation with icy coldness of the extremities, and a bruised or marbled look, use Carbo veg. The person's legs feel weak and heavy, and often itch and burn.

Hamamelis: This remedy can help when varicose veins are large and sore, and very weak and easily damaged, with a tendency to bleed. The pain is described as a bruise or sometimes a stinging sensation. The muscles of the legs feel tired.

Combination recommendation: Endangitin R63 by Reckeweg

SHERRY'S NATURAL PRESCRIPTION

Dietary Recommendations

Foods to include:

- A high-fibre diet is essential to prevent constipation and straining. Aim for 21–38 g of fibre daily. The best food sources are fruits, vegetables, whole grains (oats and bran), legumes, nuts, and seeds (chia seed, flaxseed, and sunflower seeds).

- Berries and grapes provide flavonoids, which strengthen the walls of the veins and help circulation.

- Buckwheat contains rutin, a flavonoid that is beneficial for vein health.

- Fish, nuts, and seeds contain essential fatty acids, which help reduce inflammation, prevent clotting, and improve circulation.

Foods to avoid:

- Saturated fats (animal fats) and trans fats (fast food and processed food) can impede circulation in both the veins and arteries, cause free radical damage, and trigger inflammation.

- Sodium can increase fluid retention and swelling. Reduce intake from foods such as soft drinks, chips, crackers, and deli meats.

- Minimize caffeine and alcohol, as they are dehydrating and may worsen symptoms.

Lifestyle Suggestions

- Exercise regularly. Activities that involve movement of the calf muscle will help pump blood back to the heart. Try walking, cycling, and swimming.

- Avoid standing or sitting in the same spot for a long time. Move around, flex your ankles, circle your foot, do calf raises, and shift your body weight.

- Lose excess weight, which will reduce pressure on your legs.

- Avoid excessive heat on your legs (sunbathing and hot baths), which can cause the veins to dilate, thus worsening the problem.

- Elevate your legs when sitting and resting. Don't cross your legs, which hampers circulation and can worsen leg aching.

- Minimize or avoid wearing high heels and tight shoes, as they impair circulation.

- Don't wear tight clothing, especially around the waist.

- Avoid constipation and straining on the toilet as this can increase vein pressure.

- Don't smoke, as smoking damages the veins and blood vessels, increases blood pressure, and impairs circulation.

Top Recommended Supplements

Diosmin: A flavonoid that improves the tone and strength of the blood vessels, reduces swelling, fights free radical damage, and stimulates lymphatic flow. Over 30 clinical studies have found it effective for improving vein disorders. Diosmin has a quick onset of action (one to two weeks) and is not associated with any side effects or drug interactions. Dosage: 600 mg once daily. Look for a product standardized to 95 percent diosmin and 5 percent hesperidin.

Horse chestnut seed extract: Promotes circulation, improves vein wall tone, and relieves swelling. It offers modest benefits and may take six to eight weeks to notice results. It may cause nausea and upset stomach and can enhance the effect of blood-thinning medications. Avoid it if you have kidney or liver disease. Dosage: 300 mg twice daily, standardized to 50 mg of aescin.

Pine bark extract: A flavonoid that contains a type of bioflavonoid called oligomeric proanthocyanidin complexes (OPCs) that offers antioxidant activity, strengthens capillaries, improves circulation, and supports the integrity of collagen and elastin (proteins in connective tissue that support organs, joints, blood vessels, and muscles). Studies have shown that OPCs can improve varicose veins and reduce symptoms of swelling, pain, and heaviness. Grape seed extract also contains OPCs and has been found beneficial for varicose veins. Dosage: 100–300 mg daily; no known side effects or drug interactions.

Complementary Supplements

Antioxidants: Help improve circulation and vein health. In addition to diosmin and pine bark, other antioxidants to consider are vitamins C and E, bilberry, and grape seed extract.

Butcher's broom: Improves the strength and tone of the veins, acts as a mild diuretic, and has mild anti-inflammatory effects. Dosage: 100 mg three times daily.

FINAL THOUGHTS

To improve vein health, consider the following:

- Boost intake of fibre and antioxidant-rich foods, and reduce your intake of saturated fats, processed foods, and sodium.
- Exercise regularly, elevate your feet when resting, and avoid standing or sitting in the same spot.
- Don't smoke.
- Wear compression stockings.
- Consider a supplement of diosmin, horse chestnut, or pine bark.

WARTS

Warts are small growths that occur in the skin, most commonly on the fingers, hands, or feet, caused by infection with the human papillomavirus (HPV). There are over 100 different types of HPVs. The most common types of warts are common warts, which appear on the fingers and hands; plantar warts, which grow on the soles of the feet; flat warts, which appear on the face; and genital warts, which appear in the genital or rectal area.

The HPV virus is highly contagious and is transmitted by direct contact with someone who is infected or by touching an object used by someone who has the virus. It is estimated that about 95 percent of Canadians have been exposed to HPV by the time they become adults, but not everyone who comes in contact with the virus will develop warts. This is largely dependent upon the health of your immune system. Those with a compromised immune system are also at greater risk of contracting the virus. As well, if you have a cut or break in your skin it is easier for the virus to enter your body. When the virus infects healthy skin cells, it triggers the skin cells to grow, resulting in warts.

Warts are typically harmless and go away with time, but those that occur in the cervical area are more serious and require medical treatment because they can lead to cervical cancer.

SIGNS & SYMPTOMS

- Warts appear as small fleshy bumps in the skin. They are rough to the touch and can occur in groups.
- Common warts and are usually grey in colour.
- Plantar warts are brown and scaly and can be itchy.
- Flat warts are skin-coloured.
- Genital warts are finger-like growths that are skin-coloured.
- Some warts may have tiny black dots, which are clotted blood vessels.

RISK FACTORS

- Children and young adults and those with a weakened immune system (such as those with HIV/AIDS or those who've had organ transplants) are at greater risk.

DOCTOR'S ORDERS

In most cases warts will go away with time, although they can spread and it may take two years or longer for them to go away without treatment. Warts can be unsightly and uncomfortable, and thus people often opt for treatments to get rid of warts.

There are a variety of medicated creams, liquids, and patches available over the counter that can help eliminate warts. Products such as Compound W, Clear Away, Duoplant, and Soluver Plus contain salicylic acid in varying amounts. Salicylic acid doesn't kill the virus, but it changes the environment so the virus can't survive. These products are highly effective in getting rid of common warts, with an average cure rate of 75 percent. Plantar warts are harder to get rid of and often require a stronger concentration of salicylic acid. The drawback of using these products is that you have to use them daily, for six to eight weeks, to get rid of the warts. If the medication touches the skin around the wart it can cause redness and irritation. To speed healing, soak the wart in warm water for at least 10 minutes, use an emery board or pumice stone to scrape off the dead skin, and then apply the medication.

For the treatment of stubborn and persistent warts (particularly genital warts), medications such as imiquimod or podophyllin may be prescribed.

Other treatment options that your doctor may recommend, depending on the location and severity of the infection, include the following:

- **Cryotherapy** involves using liquid nitrogen to destroy the skin cells affected by HPV by freezing the wart. This method causes temporary pain and a blister to form under the wart, and then the dead tissue sloughs off a week or so later. Cryotherapy is effective, although a second treatment may be required. There are over-the-counter cryotherapy products that have a lower-level freezing effect and often require a few repeat applications.
- **Laser therapy** uses the heat of a laser beam to destroy the infected skin cells. This method also causes pain and blistering, and requires healing time. Laser therapy is about as effective as cryotherapy, but it is usually more expensive. It is often reserved for severe cases and for removal of genital warts.
- **Surgery** can be done to cut away and remove the wart tissue. This method is effective; however, it is painful, requires more healing time, and often leaves a scar.

W

Warts

SHERRY'S NATURAL PRESCRIPTION

Dietary Recommendations

There are no specific foods that can eliminate warts; however, foods that support healthy immune function may help with prevention and support healing.

Foods to include:

- Foods high in zinc (such as oysters, crab, wheat germ, pumpkin and sesame seeds, chickpeas, and peanuts) support immune system function.

- Fruits and vegetables contain important antioxidants, vitamins, and minerals that support a healthy immune system. Choose those that are brightly coloured, such as kale, spinach, bell peppers, berries, cherries, and tomatoes.

- Garlic has antiviral activity. Fresh garlic applied directly to the wart has been shown to help speed healing (see next page).

- Green tea is rich in antioxidants and compounds with antiviral activity.

- Yogurt contains beneficial bacteria that support immune system health.

Foods to avoid:

- Alcohol can suppress immune function, and some research suggests that drinking more than two drinks per day can increase the risk of developing genital warts.

- Fast foods and processed foods are often loaded with unhealthy fats and sugar, which can compromise immune function.

Lifestyle Suggestions

- Do not pick warts; this can cause them to spread. Also, do not try to cut away the wart by yourself. You can use an emery board or pumice stone to slough off the dead skin, but more aggressive approaches can cause damage to the skin and scarring and should only be done by a health care professional.

- For plantar warts, wear comfortable and breathable shoes. You can get cushions to prevent irritation from your shoes.

- There is some evidence that applying duct tape to warts can speed healing. It is thought that the tape causes a local inflammatory reaction that stimulates the immune system to eradicate the wart. Apply the tape daily. Between tape changes soak the wart in warm water and slough off dead skin with emery board or pumice stone.

- Topical products containing herbs such as tea tree, neem, aloe, bloodroot, and colloidal silver are also thought to have antiviral activity.

TO PREVENT WARTS

- Don't walk barefoot in public areas, such as swimming pools and gyms. Always wear sandals or shoes. If you have warts, this will also prevent spreading the infection to others.

- Don't bite or pick at your fingernails or cuticles. Warts are more likely to occur in skin that has been broken.

- Don't share personal care objects, like nail files, with others.

- To avoid contracting genital warts, use a condom.

Top Recommended Supplements/Treatments

Garlic: Studies have shown topically applied garlic to be effective at clearing common warts. It is thought to work by stimulating an immune reaction. Slice a clove of garlic, apply it directly to the wart, and cover with a bandage. Do this at bedtime and remove in the morning. It may take several weeks for the wart to go away.

Zinc: Has antiviral properties and can boost immune function. Research has found that people with persistent warts have low blood levels of zinc. In one study of people with multiple recurring warts, supplementing with zinc resulted in complete disappearance of warts in 87 percent of people treated. Dosage: 50 mg daily (higher dosages have been used in clinical research).

Complementary Supplements

Reishi mushroom: Has antiviral and immune-boosting activity. Dosage: 150—300 mg two to three times daily.

Olive leaf extract: Has antiviral and immune-supportive activity. Dosage: 250—500 mg one to three times daily.

FINAL THOUGHTS

To speed healing of warts, consider the following:

- Eat nutrient-rich vegetables, fruits, garlic, green tea, and yogurt to support immune system health.
- Avoid alcohol, processed food, and fast food.
- Do not pick warts; use a pumice stone to file off dead skin.
- Try topically applied duct tape and/or garlic.
- Oral supplements of zinc may speed healing.

W

Warts

XEROSTOMIA

Xerostomia, known commonly as dry mouth, is a condition where there is not enough saliva to keep the mouth moist. This is a very common condition, particularly among the elderly. Dry mouth can also result from side effects of medications or as a result of certain medical conditions, such as Sjogren's syndrome. It can also be a temporary condition and can occur, for example, when you are nervous or stressed or have eaten certain foods. Dry mouth is not only uncomfortable, but it is associated with other health problems.

Saliva is necessary to maintain the pH (acid–base balance) of the mouth, and it provides a reservoir of the minerals calcium and phosphate, which are important for healthy dental enamel. Saliva also contains enzymes and substances that protect the mouth from bacteria that cause cavities.

Without the protective effects of saliva, a person becomes more susceptible to halitosis (bad breath), tooth decay, and gum disease. There can also be difficulty chewing, swallowing, and talking.

There are a number of ways to help alleviate dry mouth, from dietary approaches to supplements and medications.

SIGNS & SYMPTOMS

- Dry mouth and tongue
- Sore throat
- Thickened saliva
- Bad breath
- Altered sense of taste
- Cracked lips
- Sores or split skin at corners of mouth
- Thrush or ulcers in mouth
- Cavities and gum disease

RISK FACTORS

- Age: Saliva flow declines with age. Older individuals are also more likely to take medications that cause dry mouth. About 30 percent of those over age 65 are affected by xerostomia.
- Use of medications that cause dry mouth as a side effect, such as antihistamines, antidepressants, anti-anxiety drugs, chemotherapy, diuretics, Parkinson's disease medications, and drugs used for treating urinary incontinence
- Use of illicit drugs such as methamphetamine. This is often referred to as "meth mouth."

- Health conditions such as Sjogren's syndrome, diabetes, Parkinson's disease, Alzheimer's disease, and stroke

- Damage to nerves in the head and neck area

- Radiation therapy to head and neck may damage the salivary glands, reducing saliva production.

- Snoring and mouth breathing

- Smoking damages the mouth and dries it out.

DOCTOR'S ORDERS

It is important to determine and manage the underlying cause of dry mouth. For example, if dry mouth is a side effect of your medication, your doctor may change the medication or adjust the dosage. If it is due to factors beyond your control, such as a health condition or aging, then your doctor will recommend measures to help manage the condition. There are saliva substitutes available over the counter, such as Biotene Oral Balance, Salivart, Salix, and Optimoist. A medication called pilocarpine, which helps stimulate the salivary glands to make more saliva, can be prescribed. Side effects include sweating, chills, dizziness, and rhinitis (stuffy/runny nose). Cevimeline (Evoxac) is another prescription medication that is helpful, with fewer side effects compared to pilocarpine.

SHERRY'S NATURAL PRESCRIPTION

Dietary Recommendations

Foods to include:

- Drink lots of water, especially during meals to aid swallowing and improve taste perception. Suck on ice chips throughout the day to keep your mouth moist.

- Chamomile, ginger, and green tea can help stimulate saliva.

- Eat fruits and vegetables with high water content, such as celery, leafy greens, melon, and berries.

- Yogurt contains beneficial bacteria, and can help ward off bacteria that cause bad breath and gum disease.

Foods to avoid:

- Alcohol and caffeine are drying to the mouth.

- Spicy and acidic foods (tomatoes, citrus) can irritate the mouth.

- Sugary foods, such as candy and other sweets, can increase the risk of cavities.

Lifestyle Suggestions

- Breathe through your nose, not your mouth.

- Add moisture to your room with a cool mist vaporizer.

- Chew sugar-free gum sweetened with xylitol. Xylitol helps in the prevention of cavities. Try CulturedCare Probiotic gum, which contains beneficial bacteria (*Streptococcus salivarius K12*) and xylitol to control bacteria that causes bad breath and gum disease.

- Brush your teeth at least twice a day with fluoride toothpaste, and floss daily.

- Avoid mouthwashes that contain alcohol. Instead, use a product formulated for dry mouth, such as Biotene mouthwash.

- Use a dry mouth spray, such as Moi-Stir, Thayer's Dry Mouth spray, or TheraBreath Oral Rinse.

- Don't smoke.

Top Recommended Supplements

Probiotics: Provide beneficial bacteria that can help ward off bacteria that cause bad breath and gum disease and help prevent thrush. Look for a product that contains *Streptococcus salivarius K12*, which has been found in research to be beneficial for oral health, and for reducing bad breath and thrush. Dosage: Take as directed.

Complementary Supplements

Slippery elm: Contains mucilage, a substance that helps coat and soothe the mouth and throat. Try Thayer's Dry Mouth lozenges, which contain slippery elm and apple pectin.

Prickly ash: Used historically to stimulate the flow of saliva and reduce oral irritation. Try 10 to 20 drops of prickly ash tincture in 1/4 cup of water. Swish around mouth and swallow; repeat a few times daily.

FINAL THOUGHTS

To manage dry mouth, consider the following:

- Drink lots of water, especially during and between meals.
- Avoid alcohol, caffeine, and spicy and sugary foods.
- Brush your teeth and floss daily, and use a mouthwash formulated for dry mouth.
- Suck on lozenges that contain slippery elm; try CulturedCare Probiotic gum.
- Take a probiotic with *Streptococcus salivarius K12*.

ZOSTER (SHINGLES)

Shingles, known medically as herpes zoster, is a viral infection that causes a painful rash and blisters. Shingles is caused by the *varicella zoster* virus, the same virus that causes chicken pox. About 95 percent of North American children will contract chicken pox before the age of 18. After you get chicken pox, the virus lies dormant in your nerves and years later it may reactivate as shingles. About one in ten healthy adults who have had chicken pox eventually develop shingles. With shingles, the virus travels along a nerve pathway to your skin, causing rash, blistering, and pain. It typically affects the torso, but it can also affect an area around the eyes, face, or cheeks.

While it can be painful, in most cases shingles clears up in a few weeks. However, about one in five people develop a complication from damaged nerve fibres called postherpetic neuralgia, which causes skin pain and sensitivity that can last for several months.

The best way to help prevent a shingles outbreak is to manage stress levels and follow a healthy lifestyle. Once the virus is reactivated, there are some medical treatments and supplements that can help speed recovery and ease symptoms.

THE HERPES FAMILY

Varicella zoster is part of a group of viruses called herpes viruses, which includes the viruses that cause cold sores, genital herpes, and chicken pox/shingles. While the symptoms among these viruses vary widely, they all can lie dormant in your nervous system for years after an initial infection and then be reactivated and cause infection.

SIGNS & SYMPTOMS

- Clear, fluid-filled blisters

- Fever, chills, and headache

- Pain, burning, tingling, itching, numbness, or extreme sensitivity in a certain area of the body

- Red rash

- Upset stomach

Note: Shingles can lead to other complications, such as postherpetic neuralgia (nerve pain), inflammation of the brain (encephalitis), and other neurological problems. If shingles occurs on your face, it can cause hearing problems, temporary or permanent blindness, and loss of facial movement (paralysis), which is rare. The blisters can also get infected if they are picked or not properly treated.

CHICKEN POX VS. SHINGLES

While chicken pox and shingles are caused by the same virus, chicken pox often strikes in childhood and shingles in adulthood. They both can cause itching, but chicken pox causes intense itching and the blisters can affect the entire body whereas shingles typically affects only one area. Shingles is also more painful.

RISK FACTORS

- Age: Most commonly occurs after the age of 50
- Previous infection with chicken pox
- Weakened immune system caused by stress or illness (HIV, diabetes)

SHINGLES IS CONTAGIOUS

A person with shingles can pass the *varicella zoster* virus to anyone who hasn't had chicken pox before. This usually occurs through direct contact with the blisters or open sores of the shingles rash. Once infected, the person will develop chicken pox (not shingles). Until the blisters scab over, those with shingles should avoid contact with anyone who has a weak immune system (HIV, diabetes), anyone who has never had chicken pox, newborn babies, and pregnant women (chicken pox infection can be dangerous for a developing baby).

DOCTOR'S ORDERS

In most cases shingles usually heals within three to five weeks. If the infection is caught early (within the first 48 to 72 hours), there are antiviral medications that can speed healing and reduce the risk of complications. These drugs include acyclovir (Zovirax), valacyclovir (Valtrex), and famciclovir (Famvir).

The drug cimetidine (Tagamet) can help reduce the severity and duration of an outbreak. It works by temporarily inhibiting T-suppressor cells (cells that reduce immune function). This drug is available over the counter and is primarily marketed for heartburn and ulcers. Because of its effects on the immune system, it should not be used by anyone who has an autoimmune disease or who has had an organ transplant.

Painkillers can be used to manage severe pain, such as acetaminophen (Tylenol) or ibuprofen (Motrin).

There is a vaccine for shingles called Zostavax that can reduce the likelihood of getting shingles. It is not 100 percent effective, but if you do get shingles despite being vaccinated, it can lessen the severity and duration of the outbreak. This vaccine cannot be used to treat existing shingles.

HOMEOPATHIC RECOMMENDATIONS

Iris versicolor: This remedy is often helpful for a herpes zoster infection that is accompanied by stomach problems with burning sensations and nausea.

Mezereum: When this remedy is indicated, intense burning is followed by bright red eruptions that itch intolerably. The local pain of the eruptions worsens with heat and is relieved by cold applications.

Ranunculus bulbosus: This remedy is indicated for intensely itchy and sore shingles on the back or chest that worsen from contact with clothing or any kind of touch.

SHERRY'S NATURAL PRESCRIPTION

Dietary Recommendations

Foods to include:

• B-vitamins support nervous system function. Good food sources include whole grains, legumes, seeds, poultry, fish, and fortified soy and rice beverages.

• Citrus fruits, berries, broccoli, Brussels sprouts, red peppers, and tomatoes contain vitamin C, which supports the immune system. Orange, yellow, and red vegetables contain beta carotene, which also supports immune function and skin recovery.

• Zinc and selenium support immune function. These minerals are found primarily in whole grains and fortified cereals.

Foods to avoid:

• Sugar can hamper immune function. Minimize candy, sweets, and soft drinks.

Lifestyle Suggestions

• Acupuncture may help reduce the pain of shingles and postherpetic neuralgia.

• Do not pick or squeeze the blisters as this can lead to infection. Keep the affected area clean. Apply cool, wet compresses to relieve pain.

• Get plenty of rest. The viral infection can make you more tired, and you will need more sleep to recover.

• Moderate exercise such as walking can help relieve stress and pain and support healthy immune function.

• Reduce stress levels. Stress can trigger an outbreak and hamper recovery. Try yoga, breathing techniques, or tai chi.

• Soak in a tub of lukewarm water with bath salts or oatmeal to help relieve itching. Apply calamine lotion afterward or a product containing calendula, chamomile, or lavender.

Top Recommended Supplements

Capsaicin cream: Capsaicin is extracted from cayenne pepper. Studies have shown benefits for reducing nerve pain associated with shingles and postherpetic neuralgia. Available as Zostrix (0.025 percent) and Zostrix-HP (0.075 percent). Apply three to four times daily;

use regularly to maintain pain relief. Wash hands after application and avoid getting in the eyes, as it can burn.

Proteolytic enzymes: Include papain (from papaya), bromelain (from pineapple), and trypsin and chymotrypsin (extracted from the pancreas of various animals). They aid digestion and are thought to benefit shingles by decreasing the body's inflammatory response and regulating immune response to the virus. Dosage: Varies with the product; follow label instructions or consult your natural health care provider.

Complementary Supplements

B-complex: Helps to support the nervous system, which is under attack with the herpes zoster virus. Dosage: Take 50–100 mg of B-vitamins daily.

Vitamin C: Supports immune function and aids skin recovery. Dosage: 500 mg twice daily.

Vitamin E: May be helpful for reducing pain associated with postherpetic neuralgia. Dosage: 1,200–1,600 IU daily. Vitamin E oil (30 IU per gram) can be applied to the skin to aid recovery from blisters. Several months of taking vitamin E continuously may be needed to see an improvement.

FINAL THOUGHTS

To manage the pain of shingles and speed recovery, consider the following:

- Eat a healthy diet with lots of colourful vegetables and fruits, whole grains, legumes, seeds, poultry, fish, and fortified soy and rice beverages.
- Minimize intake of sugar.
- Reduce stress and get regular exercise and lots of rest.
- To soothe itching, soak in an oatmeal bath and apply cream containing calendula, chamomile, or lavender.
- Consider proteolytic enzymes to promote healing and capsaicin cream for treatment of pain from postherpetic neuralgia.

SECTION IV

APPENDICES

APPENDIX A

DETERMINATIONS FOR BODY FAT AND WEIGHT

Carrying extra body weight or being obese greatly increases the risks of developing health problems such as heart disease, diabetes, and certain cancers. While the words "obese" and "overweight" are used synonymously, there is a great difference between these terms in both definition and associated health risk.

"Overweight" is defined as a body weight above an acceptable weight in relation to height. This term can be misleading because it does not distinguish between body fat and lean muscle mass. For example, it is possible to be overweight without being obese, like a bodybuilder. Having a greater proportion of muscle mass would make this individual appear overweight according to standard weight/height charts, yet this person could have low body fat and be in good physical shape.

So how do you know if you are overweight or obese? There are several methods that are used to determine overweight, obesity, and the level of associated health risks. They include the body mass index (BMI), percentage of body fat, and waist circumference.

BODY MASS INDEX

The most commonly used tool to determine weight is the body mass index (BMI), which compares your height and weight to a standard. To calculate your BMI, take your weight in kilograms and divide that by your height in metres squared (kg/m^2).

- BMI less than 18.5 is *underweight*
- BMI of 18.5–24.9 is *normal weight*
- BMI of 25.0–29.9 is *overweight*
- BMI of 30.0–39.9 is *obese*
- BMI of 40.0 or higher is *severely (or morbidly) obese*

Since the BMI does not take into consideration body composition or gender differences (women have a higher amount of body fat), there are limitations with this method. However, studies have shown that the greater the BMI, the greater the risk of developing health problems, such as heart disease and diabetes.

BODY COMPOSITION

While we often look at our weight on the scale, knowing your body composition is actually more important as this reflects the level of body fat versus lean body mass (tissue, bone, and muscle), and it is excess body fat that is dangerous to health.

Body composition can be measured by the following methods:

Bioelectric impedance: A machine is used to measure an electric signal as it passes through lean body mass and fat. The higher the fat content, the greater the resistance to the current. This method is more effective than skin-fold caliper testing, but it is not 100 percent accurate.

DEXA (dual energy X-ray absorptiometry): Uses two X-ray energies to measure body fat, muscle, and bone mineral. This method is highly accurate, but also the most expensive and time consuming.

Near infrared technology: Infrared light is shone on the skin (usually the bicep area). Fat absorbs the light, while lean body mass reflects the light back. The reflected light is measured by a special sensor, transmitted into the computer, and translated into percentage of body fat. This method is highly accurate, comparable to underwater weighing, but slightly more expensive than most other methods.

Skin-fold calipers: Measures the thickness of subcutaneous fat at various locations on the body. The measurements obtained are used in special equations to obtain an estimated percent fat value. This method is not very accurate and is dependent on the skills and judgment of the person performing the test.

Underwater weighing: Involves submerging a person in a large tank of water. Lean tissue is more dense than water and fat tissue is less dense than water, so a person with more body fat will weigh less underwater and be more buoyant. Once considered the gold standard, this method is not commonly used anymore because it is complicated, requires a water tank, and is uncomfortable for the person being weighed.

Below are recommended body fat ranges for women and men along with the ranges considered to be overweight or obese:

	Women	*Men*
Normal	15–25 percent	10–20 percent
Overweight	25.1–29.9 percent	20.1–24.4 percent
Obese	Over 30 percent	Over 25 percent

WAIST CIRCUMFERENCE

Just as the degree of obesity is correlated with health risk, so is the location of the fat. Studies have shown that an apple-shaped body, which is defined by abdominal obesity or having a pot belly, greatly increases the risk of type 2 diabetes, high cholesterol and blood pressure, heart disease, stroke, and early death. In fact, waist circumference measurements have been shown to be a better predictor of health risk than the body mass index (BMI). Following are the waist measurements and their corresponding levels of risk:

For men:
• Increased risk: Waist more than 38 inches (97 cm)
• Substantially increased risk: Waist more than 40 inches (102 cm)

For women:
• Increased risk: Waist more than 32 inches (81 cm)
• Substantially increased risk: Waist more than 35 inches (89 cm)

Men often deposit weight in the waist region, whereas women tend to gain weight around the hips and buttocks, giving them the pear shape. Fat deposited primarily around the hips and buttocks does not carry the same risk as that gained around the midsection. In recent years, researchers have found that abdominal fat, which surrounds our internal organs, secretes compounds that trigger inflammation and insulin resistance, thus increasing the risk of heart disease, diabetes, and other problems.

The tendency to deposit fat around the midsection is influenced by a number of factors, including genetics and lifestyle choices. Physical activity, not smoking, and using unsaturated fat over saturated fat have been shown to decrease the risk of developing abdominal obesity.

For recommendations on weight loss, refer to the obesity section in this book.

GLYCEMIC INDEX TABLE

The glycemic index, or GI, is a ranking of carbohydrates based on how quickly they are broken down and affect blood sugar. Also called blood glucose, blood sugar is the fuel used by the cells in the body for energy. Carbohydrates that are rapidly digested and broken down quickly into blood glucose are ranked as "high GI." These include refined starches such as white bread and highly processed foods. Carbohydrates that are more slowly digested and broken down into blood glucose have a "low GI." Examples include most low-starch vegetables, non-tropical fruits, and unprocessed grains. Low-GI foods have a less dramatic impact on blood sugar and help keep levels more balanced.

A variety of other factors influence the glycemic index of a food:

- **The type of sugar:** Fructose, which is found in many fruits, some vegetables, and honey, is broken down more slowly in the body compared to sucrose (table sugar). This explains in part why fruit, which is sweet, is lower in the GI compared to other sweets (jellybeans). Fruit also contains soluble fibre, which lowers the GI.
- **The type of starch:** Amylose starch, which is found in basmati rice, contains glucose rings that are hooked together, making it harder to digest. Thus, foods containing this starch will have a lower GI. Amylopectin starch is easier to digest, so foods containing this starch (such as jasmine rice) have a higher GI value.
- **Acid content of the food:** Acid slows down the digestion of a food.
- **Fibre content:** The more soluble fibre in a carbohydrate, the lower the GI. Soluble fibre swells with water and causes the food to break down more slowly into sugar.
- **Cooking:** Heating can increase the GI ranking of a food. Cooking swells the starch molecules, making them more easily digestible. For example, raw carrots have a lower GI than cooked carrots. Cooking pasta al dente gives it a lower GI rating compared to cooking it to a soft consistency.
- **Processing of a food:** Highly processed and refined foods are usually digested more quickly and have a higher GI. For example, refining whole wheat into white flour will result in a higher GI of foods made with that flour. The same is true with rice: White rice has a higher GI than brown rice.

Continuously eating high-GI foods can lead to blood sugar imbalances, which may result in fatigue, increased appetite, and food cravings, particularly for sweets. Furthermore, numerous studies have linked diets that include large amounts of high-GI foods to obesity, increased belly fat, insulin resistance, type 2 diabetes, high cholesterol, inflammation, and increased risk of cardiovascular disease. On the other hand, research indicates that a low-glycemic diet can promote better blood sugar control, improve insulin sensitivity, reduce triglyceride levels, and assist with weight loss by reducing hunger and cravings and increasing metabolic rate. This healthy way of eating can also improve mood and energy levels and, over the long term, may cut the risk of several chronic diseases such as type 2 diabetes, heart disease, and certain cancers. For all of these reasons, it is best to minimize your intake of high-GI foods and maximize your intake of low-GI foods. Following is a table that includes low-, moderate-, and high-GI foods.

Low Glycemic (55 or less)	Moderate Glycemic (56–69)	High Glycemic (70 and over)
Apple juice	Arrowroot biscuits	Bagel (white)
Apples (fresh and dried)	Beer	Bread stuffing
Apricots (dried)	Beets (canned)	Broad beans
Bananas (ripe)	Breton crackers	Cereal (Cheerios, Crispix,
Barley	Buckwheat	Corn Flakes, Corn Pops,
Beans (haricot, lima,	Cantaloupe	Grape-Nuts, Rice
kidney, mung, navy,	Cereal (Shredded	Krispies, Total)
and pinto)	Wheat, Just Right,	Corn cakes (puffed)
Bean sprouts	Nutrigrain,	Corn chips
Broccoli	and Raisin Bran)	Dates
Carrots (raw)	Corn (sweet)	Doughnuts (cake type)
Cereals (All-Bran)	Cornmeal	English muffin
Chapati (bread)	Couscous	French baguette
Cherries	Cranberry juice	French fries
Chickpeas	cocktail	Fruit Roll-Ups
Chocolate (dark)	Croissant (white)	Glucose
Grapefruit	Digestive biscuits	Graham wafers
Grapes	Figs	Instant mashed potatoes
Kiwi fruit	Flan cake	Jellybeans
Lentils	Hamburger bun (white)	Kaiser roll
Milk	Honey	Life Savers
Oat bran bread	Jam (strawberry)	Melba toast
Oatmeal (slow-cook oats)	Mango (ripe)	Pancake syrup
Oranges	Muesli	Parsnips
Pasta (al dente/firm)	Pancakes	Pasta (corn, rice)
Peaches (fresh and dried)	Papaya	Popcorn
Pears (fresh and dried)	Pasta (white, soft)	Pop-Tarts

continued

Low Glycemic (55 or less)	Moderate Glycemic (56–69)	High Glycemic (70 and over)
Peppers	Pineapple	Potato (baked)
Plums	Pita bread	Pretzels
Pumpernickel bread	Porridge (rolled oats)	Rice (instant, jasmine, sticky)
Rice (long grain, converted, wild)	Potatoes (mashed or boiled)	Rice bread
Sourdough bread	Raisins	Rice cakes (white)
Soybeans	Rice (basmati, brown)	Rice crackers
Soy beverages	Rye bread	Rutabagas
Split peas	Split pea/green pea soup	Scone
Sushi	Sugar (sucrose)	Soda crackers
Sweet potatoes	Taco shells (corn)	Sports drinks
Syrup (pure maple)	Water crackers	Tapioca (boiled)
Taro	Wheat Thins	Watermelon
Yogurt (plain)	Whole-wheat bread	White bread

APPENDIX C

CLEANSING AND DETOXIFICATION

The purpose of doing a cleanse or detoxification (detox) program is to enhance the body's elimination of wastes and aid the reparative processes. This practice has been used for thousands of years for the treatment of a variety of health conditions. While cleansing is not widely embraced by mainstream medicine, it is highly popular and routinely recommended by natural health care practitioners.

Our bodies work hard every day eliminating toxins. Toxins are produced in the body during normal functions such as digestion, but we also get toxins from eating foods containing chemicals (preservatives, dyes, pesticides, and hormones), taking drugs, and being exposed to pollution and smoke, and from contact with household cleaners, heavy metals, and other chemicals. There is an intricate system in our bodies that transforms toxins into less harmful compounds. The liver, kidneys, colon, skin, lungs, and lymphatic system are all involved in this process. Toxins are eliminated through our sweat, stool, and urine.

WHY DO WE NEED TO CLEANSE AND DETOXIFY?

Under ideal circumstances, our bodies are capable of detoxifying chemicals that we ingest and are exposed to, but a poor diet, poor digestion or elimination, or exposure to excessive amounts of toxins can create a burden on our natural detoxification system. As well, fat-soluble chemicals that we ingest, such as pesticides and hormones from the food we eat, can be deposited and stored in our fat cells and build up over time. This can result in health problems and increased risk of disease, so by doing a cleanse we support and enhance the body's ability to eliminate toxins.

HOW DO YOU KNOW IF YOU ARE TOXIC?

Early on, the signs of toxin overload may be subtle, such as fatigue, poor digestion, and skin problems. However, there are possible serious consequences associated with some of these chemicals. Pesticides and compounds found in certain plastics contain chemicals (xenoestrogens) that are hormone disrupters. These chemicals have been linked to various cancers and other hormone-related problems such as PMS, fibroids, and thyroid disturbances. Excessive toxins are also associated with impaired immune function, nutritional deficiencies, and impaired cognitive function.

There are various lab tests that can be done to check for toxins and also to assess your body's detoxification system. These tests may involve checking urine, blood, stool, hair, and liver function. It is best to consult with a naturopathic doctor or medical doctor who practises natural and environmental medicine, as many mainstream doctors are not familiar with these tests.

HEALTH BENEFITS OF CLEANSING AND DETOXIFICATION

Most people who do a cleanse or detox program notice that they have more energy, improved concentration and memory, improved digestion and bowel function, reduced pain and inflammation, and clearer skin. It is also possible to lose some weight when doing a cleanse. Each person reacts differently.

TYPES OF CLEANSING AND DETOXIFICATION PROGRAMS

A cleanse or detox diet program may include a special diet, fasting or drinking juice only, taking herbs and supplements, colonics, exercise, chelation, and sauna therapy. There are various programs or kits available that target the organ systems involved in detoxification: the skin, liver, kidneys, colon, lungs, and lymphatic system.

A natural health care practitioner can design a program that suits your needs by targeting specific organ systems. For people trying a cleanse for the first time, a detox diet is recommended. This involves making dietary changes to avoid ingesting high-toxin foods. Fasting is another method of cleansing that is highly effective, yet more challenging to do. Below are some general guidelines for a detox diet and fasting.

Detox Diet

Eat three to four meals with the recommended foods below, which are rich in nutrients that help support detoxification. Choose organic foods as much as possible to avoid ingesting toxins. Chew your food thoroughly and eat small portions. Drink lots of purified water—at least eight to ten glasses daily between meals. Water helps to eliminate wastes from the body. The length of time that you follow this diet will depend on your existing health. You may want to do a detox diet once or twice a year to improve overall health and prevent disease. Consult with your health care provider for further recommendations.

Foods to include:
- Beans
- Condiments: celery salt, sea salt, cider vinegar, naturally fermented soy sauce
- Extra-virgin olive oil, hemp/flax/chia oil, palm fruit oil, coconut oil
- Fresh fruits and vegetables, especially artichokes, beets, broccoli, cauliflower, onions, garlic, peppers, and leafy green vegetables
- Herbal teas, including green tea
- Nuts and seeds: almonds, cashews, walnuts, flaxseed, pumpkin seeds, sesame seeds, and sunflower seeds

- Poultry and wild fish
- Whole grains: brown rice, quinoa, millet, and amaranth

Foods to avoid:
- Alcohol
- Coffee, soft drinks, and other caffeinated beverages
- Dairy products
- Fast foods, processed foods, and refined foods (white flour products)
- Food additives and preservatives
- Gluten (found in wheat, rye, barley, spelt, and kamut)
- Sugar (white or brown) and any foods with added sugar or containing artificial sweeteners
- Yeast

Fasting

Fasting is one of the oldest and most effective ways to detoxify. It gives the body a period of rest from digestion and dealing with the continual intake of toxins. It allows the body to focus on elimination of wastes and to enhance the reparative processes. Fasting has been practised for thousands of years and is commonly done in cultures around the world to improve various health conditions and to simply aid detoxification.

If this is your first fast, it is important to talk with your health care provider first. The length of a fast will depend on your health status. Many practitioners recommend one- to three-day fasts. The ideal time to do a fast is when you can get lots of rest. Do not exercise or do vigorous activities while fasting. A leisurely walk and stretching is fine.

Some people drink only water during a fast, while others drink juices, such as elderberry or vegetable juices (carrot, beet, celery, wheat grass, and barley grass). It is very important to ensure that your body gets adequate fluids because it is necessary to help flush toxins out of the body and to prevent dehydration. Drink fluids throughout the day as dictated by thirst, but be sure to have at least eight to ten glasses of water a day. Eat lightly for a few days before starting a fast; have small meals of fruits and vegetables only. The day before the fast, eat foods that are easy to digest such as soups, fruits, salads, and herbal teas. After finishing a fast, eat small, light meals, and gradually resume a healthy diet.

PRECAUTIONS

Consult with your health care provider before starting a cleanse or detox program to ensure it is appropriate for you. These programs are not recommended for pregnant or nursing women or for children. Those with serious health conditions, such as cancer, diabetes, epilepsy, heart disease, kidney disease, liver disease, hypothyroidism, low blood pressure, ulcers, and ulcerative colitis, should not try a fast or detox program unless recommended and supervised by a doctor. Fasting or restrictive detox diets are not recommended for the long term as they can result in nutrient and protein deficiencies.

Medication should never be stopped or reduced without first consulting with your health care provider.

Possible Adverse Effects

As the body is eliminating toxins, it is common to experience headache, fatigue, bad breath, dizziness, nausea, skin rash or eruptions, and mild flu-like symptoms. These symptoms often occur within the first few days and then go away. If you are currently drinking coffee or other caffeine-containing drinks, you will likely have withdrawal symptoms, such as headache and irritability when you stop consuming caffeine. This also goes away within a few days. If you are drinking a high amount of caffeinated beverages (more than three cups per day), it would help to gradually wean down before starting a detox diet or fast.

FOOD ALLERGIES AND THE ELIMINATION DIET

Allergic reactions to food, also called food hypersensitivities, are an increasingly common problem today. Hippocrates wrote about adverse food reactions and their link to various health problems back in 400 BC. However, it wasn't until the twentieth century that food allergies became understood and well documented. Today it is estimated that over 5 percent of the population suffer with some type of food allergy. Food reactions are also suspected to play a role in many health problems, such as attention-deficit/hyperactivity disorder, arthritis, asthma, eczema, fatigue, irritable bowel syndrome, migraine headache, and recurrent otitis media. As a result, a growing number of health care practitioners are using elimination diets to identify food allergies and food intolerances in their patients.

The elimination diet and food challenge test are tools that can help identify food allergies and intolerances. The elimination diet involves removing specific foods or ingredients from your diet that you and your doctor suspect may be causing your allergy symptoms. These foods are then gradually reintroduced. Some of the most common allergy-causing foods include milk, eggs, nuts, wheat, soy, and shellfish.

WHY ARE FOOD ALLERGIES ON THE RISE?

There are several reasons or theories as to why food allergies are on the rise:

Genetics: There are genetic tendencies toward food allergies and intolerances. Studies indicate that if both parents have allergies, their children have a 67 percent chance of developing food allergies. When only one parent is allergic, the child has a 33 percent chance of developing food allergies.

Hygiene hypothesis: Our overly hygienic way of living, the use of antibacterial sanitizers, and a lack of early childhood exposure to infectious agents (bacteria, viruses), beneficial bacteria (probiotics), and parasites increase the risk of allergies by suppressing the natural development of the immune system. The widespread use and abuse of antibiotics contributes to this by destroying the normal beneficial bacteria in the intestine, which leads to an overgrowth of fungi. Fungi secrete chemicals that alter normal immune function and cause allergic reactions. Antibiotic use also leads to increased intestinal permeability.

Poor digestive function: The digestive tract plays a vital role in preventing illness and disease by providing a protective barrier. When the integrity of the intestinal barrier is broken down or compromised, a condition coined *leaky gut syndrome* develops. In a person with leaky gut syndrome, partially digested dietary protein can cross the intestinal barrier and be absorbed into the bloodstream. These large molecules can cause allergic reactions in the intestines or throughout the body. There are many factors that can break down the intestinal barrier, such as stress, antibiotic use (which destroys beneficial bacteria), and parasitic infections.

Poor immune function: Stress, environmental toxins, pesticides, and other chemicals can alter immune function and cause our immune system to react inappropriately to certain foods.

Repeated consumption of certain foods: Eating the same foods over and over can be taxing to the immune system. For example, wheat, which is a common food allergen, is found in many commonly consumed food products such as breakfast cereals, bread, pasta, sauces, coatings, and fillers. Milk and eggs are other common allergens that are frequently eaten and found as ingredients in many foods, especially baked goods.

FOOD ALLERGIES VS. INTOLERANCES

Food allergies occur when your immune system mistakenly identifies a specific food or a component of food as a harmful substance. In response your immune system triggers certain cells to produce immunoglobulin E (IgE) antibodies to fight the food. The next time you eat even the smallest amount of that food, the IgE antibodies sense it and signal your immune system to release histamine and other chemicals into your bloodstream.

Food allergies are classified as either immediate or delayed. Immediate hypersensitivity reactions occur within minutes to hours after a food is eaten and cause symptoms such as a rash, hives, a runny nose, or a headache. In some cases these immediate hypersensitivity reactions can be life threatening, causing anaphylactic shock, a condition in which the throat swells and blocks the airways. These reactions are most commonly associated with milk, eggs, peanuts, tree nuts (walnuts), soy, strawberries, wheat, fish, and shellfish. People who get this type of reaction must be diligent in avoiding contact with the allergen and also carry an EpiPen with them at all times in case they have a reaction. An elimination diet is not recommended for those with immediate hypersensitivity reactions.

Delayed hypersensitivities do not appear right after consuming an allergen, making them difficult to pinpoint. These reactions may not appear for days and can cause a wide range of symptoms such as dark circles or puffiness under the eyes, fluid retention, skin rash, sinus congestion, fatigue, abdominal pain or bloating, joint inflammation, mood swings, indigestion, headaches, chronic ear infections, asthma, poor memory, anxiety, and depression. It is thought that over half of the population suffers with delayed food hypersensitivities. An elimination diet can be very helpful for determining the offending foods.

Food intolerances are food reactions that are not caused by an immune system reaction. "Food intolerance" is an umbrella term that refers to any abnormal physiological response to a food that is not caused by an immune system reaction. These reactions may be caused by enzyme deficiencies, poor function of the digestive tract, an autoimmune reaction, or sensitivity to a natural or synthetic chemical. For example, sulphites are a common food preservative added to dried fruits, wine, and processed foods that can cause severe reactions, particularly in those with asthma. Some people react to food dyes, such as tartrazine or the flavour enhancer monosodium glutamate (MSG), which is often added to Asian food.

The most common food intolerance is lactose intolerance, which occurs when the body does not produce enough of the digestive enzyme called lactase, which breaks down the milk sugar (lactose) found in dairy products. When too much undigested lactose makes its way into the large intestine, people suffer from gas and/or diarrhea. It is estimated that about 30 percent of adults are lactose intolerant. This is particularly common among Blacks and Asians.

Another common source of food intolerance is gluten, a protein found in wheat, barley, and rye. Celiac disease is one condition associated with gluten intolerance. In people with celiac disease, gluten triggers an autoimmune reaction and damages the absorptive surface of the intestine. Symptoms include diarrhea or constipation, gas, bloating, fatigue, weight loss, anemia, hair loss, and depression. It is estimated that about 1 in 100 Canadians have gluten intolerance.

There are also naturally occurring substances in foods that can cause reactions in some people, such as salicylates, which are found in many vegetables, herbs, spices, fruits, and chocolate. Salicylates have been associated with various mental health problems such as attention-deficit/hyperactivity disorder, depression, and headaches.

ELIMINATION DIET

Food allergies and food intolerances are a major source of undesirable symptoms that negatively impact the quality of life of many people. Many health care practitioners believe that the only definitive way to identify and manage adverse food reactions is through the use of an elimination diet followed by carefully organized food challenges. This can be a difficult process to follow as it requires strict dietary changes. However, it can be incredibly rewarding to identify foods that are causing unpleasant reactions.

Below are some guidelines for a standard elimination diet. It is best to work with your health care provider during this process.

Foods to include:
- All vegetables and fruits except those listed below
- Beans
- Brown rice, quinoa, amaranth, buckwheat, tapioca, and flours made of these grains
- Chicken, turkey, lamb, and cold-water fish; choose organic/free-range as much as possible
- Clarified butter (ghee)
- Nuts except soy and peanuts
- Olive, sunflower, safflower, and flaxseed oil

- Salt, pepper, garlic, and fresh herbs
- Water, herbal teas, rice milk, vegetable juice, and fruit juice (drink sparingly and avoid orange juice)

Foods to avoid:
- Alcohol, soft drinks, juice cocktails, coffee, and chocolate
- Beef, pork, veal, and deli meats
- Citrus fruit (oranges, orange juice, and grapefruit), apples, and strawberries
- Dairy products (milk, cheese, yogurt, butter, ice cream) and eggs
- Eggplant, corn, potatoes, tomatoes, and bell peppers
- Foods containing yeast (breads and baked goods unless they are yeast and gluten-free)
- MSG, food dyes, preservatives, and artificial sweeteners
- Soy products (soy nuts, soy milk, tofu) and peanuts
- Sugar (white and brown) and foods containing sugar
- Trans fatty acids (hydrogenated oils, which are found in margarines and many baked goods and processed foods)
- Wheat (found in bread, pasta, cereals, sauces, and thickeners, and as a filler in processed meats)

If salicylates or amines are a suspected allergen, then you will also need to avoid tomatoes, broccoli, olives, spinach, mushrooms, avocados, all dried fruit, smoked meats, canned fish, soy sauce, miso, and vinegars.

Follow these dietary guidelines for at least one month to cleanse the body of the offending food. Take time to plan your meals, and eat a variety of the allowed foods. Stock your cupboard and refrigerator with the allowed foods. Read food labels, and find out about food ingredients and preparation methods when dining out. Keep a food diary, noting what you are eating and any symptoms that you experience.

It is not uncommon to experience withdrawal symptoms within the first week, such as headaches, food cravings, and changes in bowel function. This occurs as the body detoxifies and adjusts to your new diet. Coffee drinkers typically experience more severe symptoms such as headache and a foggy-headed feeling when caffeine is stopped.

After following the diet for 30 days, reintroduce one food item at a time into your diet. This re-addition of foods is called the "challenge" phase of the diet. On the first day of food challenges, a food is eaten one to three times during the day. Over the next few days, return to the elimination diet, and watch for the return of any symptoms. If any symptoms develop, it is possible that you are allergic or intolerant to that reintroduced food.

It can take several months to complete an elimination and challenge diet. It is best to do this only if you can commit to following the strict guidelines. Cheating will defeat the purpose and hinder your ability to detect potential allergens or intolerances. Keep in mind that if you've had a severe (anaphylactic) reaction to certain foods, this method can't be used. It is advisable to work with a health care professional when considering an elimination diet so that you can get proper nutritional advice, recommendations on supplements, and monitoring throughout this process.

HORMONE TESTING

Throughout this book there are discussions about the importance of proper hormone balance and the impact of imbalanced hormones on health. Imbalanced hormones can affect many areas of health and cause problems such as depression, sleep disturbances, weight gain or loss, bone loss, breast swelling and tenderness, fibroids, low libido, sexual dysfunction, and many other aspects of health.

While blood tests are most commonly done to check hormone levels, testing saliva for hormones is becoming increasingly popular. In fact, if you're experiencing hormone-related symptoms, a saliva hormone test is possibly the best way to uncover hormone causes of symptoms. Generally, the best test for hormone balance involves testing the "big five" sex steroid hormones: cortisol, DHEA, estradiol, progesterone, and testosterone. The balance between these hormones is critical to good health. For example, Rocky Mountain Analytical, a Canadian saliva hormone testing lab, has data that shows that seven out of ten women with self-reported symptoms of depression and four out of five women with hot flashes or low sex drive had laboratory-confirmed hormone imbalance. This tells us that saliva hormone test results correlate very well with how patients feel. Unfortunately, blood tests do not look at symptoms, nor do they test all the same hormones.

There are basically three ways to test for hormones: in blood, in saliva, or in urine. Blood testing is the standard method most doctors use to test for hormones, but there are some drawbacks with blood tests for hormones. For example, blood or serum is less accurate for the measurement of testosterone in women because the test is calibrated for the high testosterone levels seen in men. As well, hormones in blood are often bound to proteins and may or may not be available to the tissues that require them. Consequently, blood and serum levels of hormones may not give the best picture of how hormones are behaving at the tissue level. This means that blood test results often don't match up with the symptoms you are experiencing.

Saliva, on the other hand, measures the amount of hormone that actually gets into tissue because salivary hormones have already passed through tissue (the saliva gland) to get into saliva. Saliva hormone levels tend to correlate well with symptoms. Saliva samples are also easier to collect—it can be done at home and samples can be mailed in. There are suggested ranges for women who are supplementing with hormones. In addition, there are some hormones that are not routinely measured in blood.

Saliva hormone testing has been in the scientific literature for over 50 years and is rapidly becoming the test method of choice for hormone monitoring for many practitioners. Nevertheless, saliva testing is not without controversy. Some saliva hormone-testing facilities claim that the tests can be used to determine the "right" dose of hormones for a patient, and that supplementing to achieve specific ratios of one hormone level to another is ideal. Unfortunately, there is no test—blood, saliva, or urine—that tells a doctor exactly how much hormone to give or what dose is right for you. The tests can help guide the doctor in choosing the dose (and in choosing which hormones to supplement with), but you still need to work with a doctor who understands hormone balance and hormone testing. Saliva testing is still the best choice to help uncover the cause of hormone symptoms. You are best to choose an accredited laboratory that includes symptom information in its analysis of your saliva specimen.

Hormone imbalance contributes to many common health conditions. For example, PMS is often due to estrogen dominance (or a lack of progesterone) in the last half of the menstrual cycle. Endometriosis, fibrocystic breast disease, and uterine fibroids have also been associated with estrogen dominance. And even bone loss can arise from hormone imbalance, specifically a lack of testosterone or lack of estrogen or both. In other words, keeping your hormones in balance is an important part of good health, and saliva hormone testing is a great way to find out if you're in balance.

Urine testing is less common because a 24-hour specimen is needed, which makes collection more challenging. Urine testing may be particularly helpful for determining thyroid status. Low thyroid (hypothyroidism) is common and also commonly undiagnosed. This is because it is possible to have blood results within the normal range, yet have inadequate thyroid function. Symptoms of low thyroid include weight gain, depression, dry skin, feeling cold all the time, low libido, and hair loss.

Typical blood tests for thyroid include measuring levels of the thyroid hormones T3, T4, and TSH (thyroid-stimulating hormone). Urinary thyroid assessments may be helpful for people who have normal serum TSH levels, but who still have symptoms of low thyroid function. Research from Europe has shown that the urinary thyroid test results match patient symptoms better than the serum TSH. What this means is that many people who have normal TSH results register low on a urinary thyroid assessment, which matches their symptoms.

The urinary thyroid assessment involves collecting all your urine for a full 24 hours. The sample is sent away to the laboratory and is analyzed for T3, T4, and selenium, which is an important mineral for proper thyroid function. The results are reported to your doctor along with an interpretation based on your results and the symptoms you reported.

In Canada, Rocky Mountain Analytical is an accredited laboratory that collects symptom information and provides a complete interpretation of results. Located in Calgary, Alberta, they specialize in saliva hormone testing and other prevention-focused tests, including urinary thyroid assessment, food allergy testing, omega-3 fatty acid testing,

testing for insulin resistance, and many others. Rocky Mountain Analytical is unique in that they collect symptom information prior to testing, and they use the symptoms along with the test results to provide an interpretation to your doctor. They do this because it is important to look at test results as being part of, not separate from, the person. And symptoms provide information about how a person is doing, so even if the results look fairly normal, if the symptoms are severe the interpretation gives some suggestions as to why those symptoms might be prominent.

For more information on saliva hormone testing, visit www.rmalab.com or call (403) 241–4513.

HOMEOPATHY

by Bryce Wylde, BSc, RNC, DHMHS, Homeopath

Homeopathic medicines are *micro* doses of plant, mineral, and other naturally occurring substances. Homeopathic medicines are safe and efficient with no side effects and no drug interactions, allowing people to take conventional medications, if necessary, at the same time as their homeopathic treatment.

Homeopathy has become the fastest-growing field of integrative medicine in Canada. Contemporary Canadian society's newfound understanding of health care as *prevention of disease* has led to a new perspective of natural approaches like homeopathy as mainstream. In line with this new definition of health care, homeopathy helps the body do what it should be able to do on its own to keep the body healthy and free of disease. Conventional approaches, such as drugs and surgery, are sometimes necessary, but these approaches should soon become known as the complementary approach!

HOW HOMEOPATHY WORKS

Homeopathic medicines trigger the body's natural defence mechanisms and support systems to manage ailments, as opposed to conventional medicines, which use chemicals to eradicate invading pathogens or change your body's natural chemistry. In this way, homeopathy is able to help the body regain balance by getting it to do better what it is already equipped to do on its own. If necessary, when disease has progressed too far, conventional approaches like drugs and surgery may be prudent to use adjunctively.

Homeopathic medicines work on three basic principles. The first is the law of similars, which states that the same things that cause an illness will ultimately cure it. The second is that infinitesimal doses are all that are needed to trigger the body's natural defence system. The third is that homeopathic medicines are prescribed in a very individualized way, taking into account not only physical symptoms but also the patient's behavioural and mental/emotional condition.

THE SCIENTIFIC PROOF FOR HOMEOPATHY

Research centres around the world are conducting studies of homeopathic medicines, and a growing number of these studies are being published in peer-reviewed journals. One of many such studies that has become very well known was published in the *Lancet* in 1997. K. Linde and colleagues (from Munich University) published the results of a meta-analysis of 135 clinical trials that compared homeopathic drugs with a placebo (K. Linde et al., "Are the Clinical Effects of Homeopathy Placebo Effects? A Meta-analysis of Placebo-Controlled Trials," *Lancet*, 1997, 350: 834–843). The authors concluded that "The results of this meta-analysis are not compatible with the hypothesis that the clinical effects of homeopathy are completely due to placebo."

Another meta-analysis conducted in 2000 on 24 studies relating to controlled, randomized clinical trials concluded that "There is some evidence that homeopathic treatments are more effective than placebo." (M. Cucherat et al., "Evidence of Clinical Efficacy of Homeopathy: A Meta-analysis of Clinical Trials," *European Journal of Clinical Pharmacology*, 2000, 56: 27–33)

Oddly enough, these and other trials and studies have not been given sufficient prominence, either within the scientific community or by media. But the international scientific community is quickly becoming interested in studies on homeopathy, many of which are documented in prestigious scientific journals. Scientific studies have demonstrated that highly diluted biological products (homeopathic medicines) can have a verifiable effect on humans. Homeopathy offers a simple, effective, and safe medical therapy free from known side effects. Although it is always good to consult with a qualified practitioner, there are many homeopathic remedies that are safe for self-medication.

THE HISTORY OF HOMEOPATHY IN CANADA

Homeopathy is a branch of natural medicine that has a long history of success. For over 200 years, Canadians have been using homeopathic medicines successfully to treat acute and chronic illnesses. Although homeopathy has long been thought of as "complementary" in the medical field, homeopaths were recognized under government structure before practitioners of conventional medicine. In Upper Canada in 1859, homeopathic doctors were acknowledged and regulated under the Act Respecting Homeopathy. In 1865, An Act to Regulate the Qualifications of Practitioners in Medicine and Surgery in Upper Canada was proclaimed. A clause in this act prohibited any repeal or action that would in any way affect the Homeopathic Act of 1859 and the Eclectic Act of 1861. In 1866, An Act Respecting the Medical Board and Medical Practitioners authorized the formation of a licensing board for conventional doctors, exempting homeopaths and midwives. As a consequence of these two acts, the Council of Education and Registration of Upper Canada was established in 1866, with the authority to grant licences to practise medicine in Upper Canada.

HOW HOMEOPATHY IS REGULATED IN CANADA

Health Canada regulates homeopathic medicines. They are manufactured according to the highest drug safety standards and carry a DIN-HM number (a drug identification number—homeopathic medicine). This is just like any other drug available in local pharmacies that carries a DIN. Homeopathic medicines are considered safe and effective, with no side effects and no drug interactions, allowing people to take conventional medications, if necessary, at the same time as their homeopathic treatment. It should be noted that other alternative, natural health products (NHPs) are required by the Canadian government to have an "NPN" number to identify their safety and efficacy.

Ontario is leading the way in Canada as it relates to regulations of the practice of homeopathy. For more information on finding a qualified homeopathic practitioner in Ontario and regulations around the practice of homeopathy in Ontario, contact the Transitional Council of the College of Homeopaths of Ontario: www .collegeofhomeopaths.on.ca.

INDEX